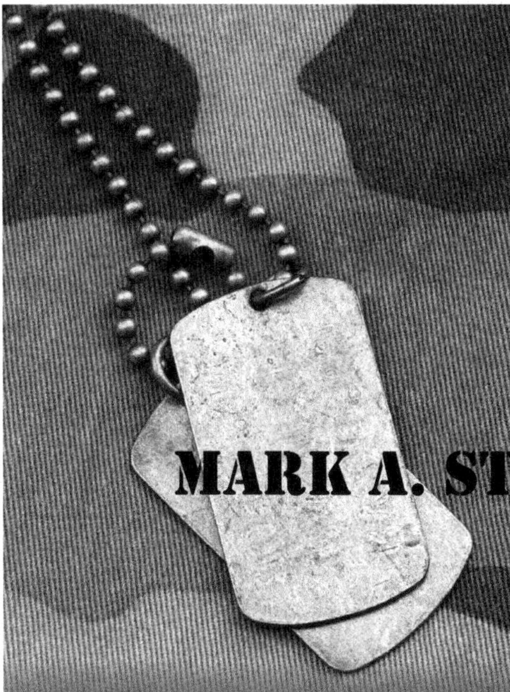

MARK A. STEBNICKI

CLINICAL MILITARY COUNSELING

GUIDELINES FOR PRACTICE

AMERICAN COUNSELING ASSOCIATION
6101 Stevenson Avenue, Suite 600
Alexandria, VA 22304
www.counseling.org

CLINICAL MILITARY COUNSELING

GUIDELINES FOR PRACTICE

AMERICAN COUNSELING ASSOCIATION
6101 Stevenson Avenue, Alexandria, VA 22304

Associate Publisher • Carolyn C. Baker

Digital and Print Development Editor • Nancy Driver

Production Manager • Bonny E. Gaston

Copy Editor • Tyler Krupa

Cover and text design by Bonny E. Gaston

LIBRARY OF CONGRESS
CATALOGING-IN-PUBLICATION DATA

Names: Stebnicki, Mark A., author.
Title: Clinical military counseling : guidelines for practice/ Mark A. Stebnicki.
Description: Alexandria, VA : American Counseling Association, [2020] | Includes bibliographical references and index.
Identifiers: LCCN 2020027778 | ISBN 9781556203992 (paperback)
Subjects: LCSH: Veterans—Mental health services. | Post-traumatic stress disorder.
Classification: LCC RC451.4.V48 S74 2020 | DDC 616.85/212—dc23
LC record available at https://lccn.loc.gov/2020027778

DEDICATION

To all my family members who have served in the U.S. Army, Navy, and Marines.

To all those serving now and who have served in the U.S. Armed Forces.

To the unseen service of those professionals who serve the military community.

To my wife Bonnie, daughter Sarah, son Mark D., and their loving spouses (Brandon and Leigh), and to my grandson Noah, who is a new light shining in this world.

★ ★ ★

TABLE OF CONTENTS

Preface vii

About the Author xi

PART I ★ The Military Culture

CHAPTER 1 The Culturally Competent Clinical Military Counselor 3

CHAPTER 2 Societal Myths, Stereotypes, and Stigma of the U.S. Military Culture 17

CHAPTER 3 Counseling Issues for Women and Other Minorities in Military Life 35

PART II ★ Medical and Psychosocial Aspects of Military Health

CHAPTER 4 Mapping the Military Brain: The Neuroscience of Military Stress and Trauma 69

CHAPTER 5 Psychosocial Aspects of Military Suicide 91

CHAPTER 6 Psychosocial Aspects of Chronic Illness and Disability in Veteran Health 111

CHAPTER 7 Psychosocial Aspects of Chronic Pain and Other Medical Conditions in Military Life 141

CHAPTER 8 Blast Injuries and Traumatic Brain Injury in the Military 163

PART III ★ Clinical Issues in Military Counseling

CHAPTER 9 Spirituality, Moral Injury, and Trauma in Military Life 185

CHAPTER 10 Military Families and the Deployment Cycle 205

CHAPTER 11 Career Transitions in Military Life: The Transition Mission 223

CHAPTER 12 Becoming a Competent Clinical Military Practitioner: Earning the Circle of Trust 239

CHAPTER 13 Complex Military PTSD and Co-Occurring Mental Health Conditions 261

CHAPTER 14 Military Resiliency and Integrative Treatment Strategies in Operation Military Counseling 297

Index 315

PREFACE

In the early morning hours of September 11, 2001, one of the deadliest attacks in the history of the United States took place, in which 2,977 Americans were killed, and more than 6,000 others were severely injured, causing permanent chronic illnesses and disabilities. Two commercial jetliners, American Airlines Flight 11 and United Airlines Flight 175, were hijacked by 19 al-Qaida terrorists and crashed into the North and South Towers of the World Trade Center in Lower Manhattan. It took only about 90 minutes for the Twin Towers to burn and collapse. A third jetliner, American Airlines Flight 77, crashed into the Pentagon, which led to a partial collapse of the building's west side. A fourth plane, United Airlines Flight 93, was heading toward Washington, DC, but crashed into a field in Stonycreek Township near Shanksville, Pennsylvania, where several heroic passengers thwarted the terrorist hijackers' efforts. Hence, the global war on terrorism ushered in the 21st century.

American citizens are now in the crosshairs of asymmetrical radicalized enemy combatants spreading hate throughout the globe perpetrated by extremist groups that go by the names of ISIS (Islamic State of Iraq and Syria), ISIL (Islamic State of Iraq and the Levant), the Taliban, Al-Shabaab, al-Qaida, and Boko Haram. The U.S. military is duty bound to bring the fight to places such as Afghanistan, Iraq, Syria, and many parts of Africa.

At the time of this writing, the Coronavirus (COVID-19) pandemic has emerged as a significant concern during its first wave of infection. The medical, physical, and mental health of military and civilians alike have been compromised. Health care workers are challenged by a lack of resources (e.g., hospital beds, N95 masks, ventilators) and readiness to fight this common viral enemy. From a military logistics, planning, and unified command and control perspective, COVID-19 requires a highly organized and collaborative effort between civilians and the military to activate a disaster response to fight a biological enemy. At times in the United States and around the globe, COVID-19 has mimicked a zombie apocalypse as seen in Hollywood-style movies. Overall, the military has an important role in filling medical gaps in service through use of materials, medical treatment facilities on land and water, medical personnel, and other resources.

I propose that we are in a paradigm shift in the counseling and psychology profession. We have trauma fatigue, which is a new type of complex acute and posttraumatic stress requiring vital healing resources. For many, the Earth does not feel like a safe place to live. Global terrorism and pandemics have fundamentally altered and behaviorally changed the way in which we live our everyday lives. This transformation is apparent in airports, shopping malls, schools, restaurants, entertainment venues, federal and state buildings, and other institutions. Homegrown terrorism is on the rise in the United States, requiring teams of first responders, disaster mental health specialists, and critical incident stress debriefers. Our own historical trauma from September 11 is reinforced and magnified by 24-hour media coverage unfolding in real time. We are consumed with graphic images of horrific scenes of terrorist attacks, wars, civil unrest, and other conflicts around the globe.

After more than 20 years of war and mission creep (i.e., the gradual expansion of a mission beyond its original scope), we have a multigenerational group of military service members and veterans who have fought in Operation Iraqi Freedom, Operation Enduring Freedom, Operation New Dawn, and Operation Inherent Resolve (which started in August 2014). There were many wars that came before these operations, and many more will follow. At this point in the war on terrorism, there are two generations of parents and their children who potentially could be enlisted together as well as training and fighting alongside one another. The long-term mental, physical, and psychological effects of warfighting are mapped into our mind, body, and spirit.

So, who are the people who represent the less than 2% of Americans in the U.S. Armed Forces? Who are the individuals who volunteer to defend the security of the United States and swear an oath to fight enemies, both foreign and domestic? The foundation for this book was inspired by family members, friends, and clients who have served in the military. My extensive experiences as a counselor educator, researcher, and practitioner working with active-duty Marines, veterans, veterans with disabilities, and military families are memorialized in this book. The designation of *clinical military counselor* throughout this book depicts professionals who work in the fields of mental health, rehabilitation, clinical addiction, and school counseling as well as psychologists, social workers, and other behaviorally licensed practitioners.

Presently, we need "all hands on deck" to train up for Operation Military Counseling. I coined this mission in 2015 when I developed the Military and Trauma Counseling certification program at East Carolina University. This mission expanded in 2016 to the Clinical Military Counseling Certificate program that I developed, which is offered through the Telehealth Certification Institute of New York.

Clinical Military Counseling takes a holistic approach to working with the military. It integrates current research and clinical practice guidelines for working with the medical, psychosocial, spiritual, psychological, vocational, career, family, and cultural aspects of the military. Guidelines for best practices are offered to assist in earning "the circle of trust" of service members and veterans to facilitate screening, prevention, treatment interventions, and other resources for the military community.

Clinical Military Counseling discusses new issues related to military medical, physical, behavioral, and psychological health. Complementary and integrative health resources are offered to practitioners for cultivating resiliency and coping skills. These approaches are critical because newer studies suggest that the use of first-line, evidence-based practices treating complex posttraumatic stress disorder (PTSD) are only 30%–50% effective. Studies suggest that 80% of service members and veterans frequently use integrative health approaches, such as mindfulness-based stress reduction, meditation, yoga, Reiki, and acupuncture.

Part I of *Clinical Military Counseling* helps differentiate military versus civilian mental health counseling practices, identifying commonly held societal myths and stereotypes of the U.S. military and discussing the military from a multicultural perspective. Historically, the military culture has reflected mostly White heterosexual men. However, today there is not just one type of military service member. Rather, the military comprises a diverse group of individuals who possess different racial, ethnic, sexual identity, and other cultural characteristics.

Part II of *Clinical Military Counseling* honors the collective wisdom of the expanding clinical military medical and mental health practices. It delivers new directions to clinicians in military policies and resources that reflect current clinical military counseling and psychological practices for the 21st century. Contemporary topics are discussed, such as the neuroscience of military stress and trauma, military suicide and co-occurring mental health conditions, psychosocial aspects of chronic illnesses and disability in veteran health, and the signature disabling conditions of blast and traumatic brain injuries.

Part III of *Clinical Military Counseling* addresses important clinical mental health issues in military life. The integration of spirituality and identification of moral injury, as it relates to military trauma, assists clinical military counselors in healing the mind, body, and spirit of service members and veterans. Military families and deployment cycle issues are discussed because of the important role that military families have in creating coping and resiliency skills for military service members and veterans. Other key aspects in Part III explore career transitions in military life and the psychosocial adjustment required to function medically, physically, and psychologically at an optimal level after a career in military service.

The essential strength woven into Part III, as well as into other chapters in *Clinical Military Counseling*, emphasizes how to provide competent and ethical clinical military counseling services. Earning the circle of trust of service members and veterans is underscored throughout this work, demonstrating the essential elements in the assessment, diagnosis, and treatment of complex PTSD and co-occurring mental health conditions.

The concluding chapter on military resiliency and integrative health approaches explores, discusses, and applies vital research on the impact that extraordinary stressful and traumatic events have on active-duty service members, veterans, and military families. There is strong evidence in the research suggesting that integrative health practices are beneficial in decreasing symptoms related to posttraumatic stress, anger, depression, anxiety, and substance misuse behaviors as well as military suicidality. Holistic health approaches—such as mindfulness-based stress reduction, breathing meditation, yoga, animal-assisted therapy, expressive art, and other integrative approaches—provide a new horizon for healing the mind, body, and spirit of service members and veterans.

Overall, the work presented in *Clinical Military Counseling* is a model for training and education in best practice for clinical military counselors. The comprehensive medical, physical, and mental health aspects of this work are driven by research and clinical practice. Clearly, both civilian and military researchers support a wellness agenda for living optimally in mind, body, and spirit throughout one's military career and beyond.

★ ★ ★

ABOUT THE AUTHOR

MARK A. STEBNICKI, PhD, LCMHC, DCMHS, CRC, CMCC, is professor emeritus and former coordinator of the Military and Trauma Counseling certificate program, which he developed in 2015 at the Department of Addictions and Rehabilitation at East Carolina University. Professor Stebnicki also developed the national Clinical Military Counseling Certificate program—a 12-hour continuing education program offered nationally through the Telehealth Certification Institute of New York. Professor Stebnicki is a counselor educator, researcher, and practitioner with more than 30 years of experience in rehabilitation and mental health. He has worked with both adolescents and adults, specializing in stress, trauma, grief, loss, and the psychosocial aspects of chronic illness and disability. His primary focus is working with military service members, veterans, veterans with disabilities, and military families. Professor Stebnicki has published nine professional textbooks as well as 40 journal articles and book chapters. In addition, he has given more than 100 national, regional, and statewide presentations. He has served on many statewide and national professional counseling boards.

★ ★ ★

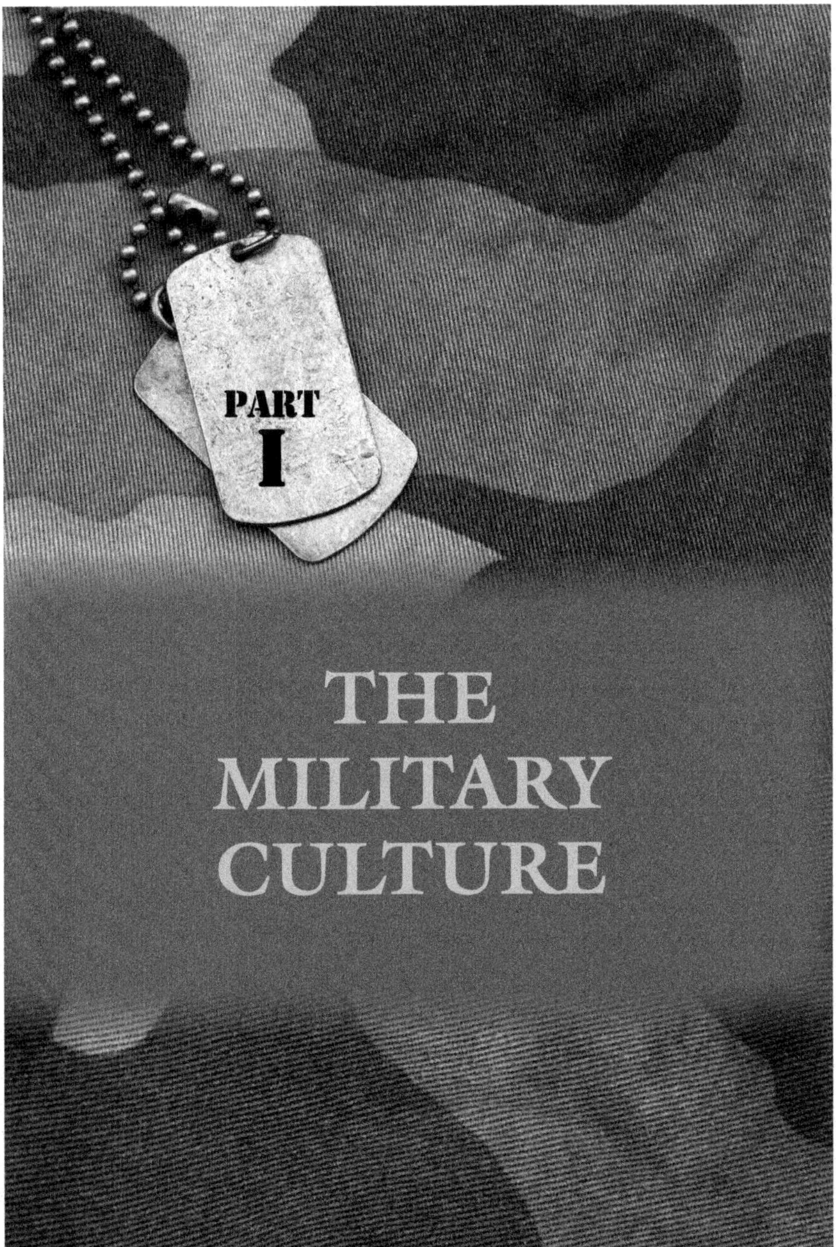

PART I

THE MILITARY CULTURE

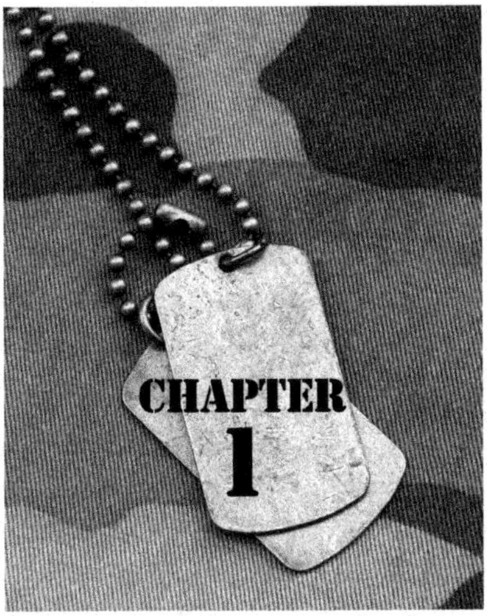

THE CULTURALLY COMPETENT CLINICAL MILITARY COUNSELOR

Three rules for a gunfight.
One, bring a gun. Two, bring all your friends with guns.
Three, never bring a knife to a gunfight.

—Anonymous

★ ★ ★

The mission I refer to as Operation Military Counseling (OMC) began in 2015 when I developed one of the first graduate certificates in military counseling within a Council for Accreditation of Counseling and Related Educational Programs (CACREP)-accredited counselor education program. The Military and Trauma Counseling certificate program, offered at East Carolina University, was designed to help bridge the gap between military and civilian or community mental health research and practice. The mission and core values of OMC are reflected in the current national certificate that I developed in 2016, the Clinical Military Counseling Certificate program, as well as the comprehensive work in this book.

Clinical Military Counseling offers extensive research and qualitative data collected from focus groups of active-duty personnel, veterans, veterans with disabilities, and military families. Guidelines for practice are also offered to the reader for consideration in the assessment, diagnosis, and mental health treatment of military clients. Thus, the present work advances the role and function of clinical military counseling as a dynamic and evolving specialty area of the counseling profession. The philosophical foundation in *Clinical Military Counseling* is for practitioners to consider the theories, knowledge, and skills that they have acquired in psychology and counseling and facilitate therapeutic strategies and approaches through the cultural lens of the military.

Historically, mental health counselors have not had the opportunities in their graduate training programs to achieve military cultural competence. This deficiency is due in part to the lack of available training in most graduate curriculums, where assessment, diagnosis, and mental health treatment for military populations is rarely discussed other than in occasional seminars, attending guest lectures, and classroom assignments for military counseling–related issues (Stebnicki et al., 2017). Recognizing that the military is a unique culture unto itself, some newer multicultural counseling texts now offer a separate chapter in military culture counseling. Some CACREP-accredited programs are now advancing their curriculum in military counselor training through departmental and college coursework that is cross-disciplinary. Indeed, graduate training in the assessment, diagnosis, and treatment of military mental health conditions (e.g., posttraumatic stress disorder, major depressive disorder, anxiety, substance use disorders, suicidality, and other co-occurring mental health disorders) has been slowly evolving in counselor education.

Historically, psychologists and clinical social workers have had a long-standing advantage of being eligible for careers as independent practitioners working within the federal government system of medical and mental health care (e.g., Veterans Health Administration) where they can obtain third-party reimbursement through private insurance (e.g., Humana Military, Medicare, TRICARE) and work on military bases and installations. Accredited programs in psychology and social work have evolved more rapidly and early on to offer academic certifications and graduate programs that prepare students to work competently and ethically with military service members and veterans. For instance, American Psychological Association–accredited programs have partnered with the U.S. Army to establish the Health Professions Scholarship Program (U.S. Army, 2019). This program provides scholarship opportunities for doctoral-level clinical and counseling psychologists to work alongside U.S. Army health care professionals. They work for 2 years and complete an active-duty training program at selected sites. Other branches of the military have similar programs.

Currently, there is movement toward parity across the various counseling disciplines. In 2018, the U.S. Department of Veterans Affairs (VA) issued new qualifications and standards allowing licensed mental health counselors to be eligible for jobs and careers within the VA system. The revised standards clarify the scope of practice that enables licensed mental health professionals to fully participate as independent practitioners. At the time of this writing, interpretive guidelines by the federal government's Office of Human Resources Management are slow in being issued to the VA hospitals and clinics across the United States (American Counseling Association, 2018). Regardless of educational and professional background, clinical military counselors have the competence to understand the unique cultural and within-group differences by earning the "circle of trust" while engaging in therapeutic interactions with military clients.

TRAINING UP FOR OMC

Becoming a culturally competent clinical military counselor requires an understanding that there is not one homogeneous group labeled "the military culture." Rather, the military comprises individuals who identify with various racial and ethnic groups (e.g., Hispanic Latino/a, African American, Native American, Asian American); the lesbian, gay, bisexual, and transgender community; as well as many other cultural groups. The U.S. Armed Forces of the 21st century, unlike previous generations, have multiple identities that demographically represent the U.S. population.

The military culture also reflects within-group differences, which are illustrated by the distinct military occupational specialty (MOS) types (e.g., infantry, special forces/operations, mechanic, cook, communications officer, counterintelligence). There are personnel who are assigned to combat and noncombat units. Service members are deployed and mobilized on humanitarian missions. Some service members are deployed to hostile geographic locations outside the continental United States (referred to as OCONUS), whereas others are mobilized to bases within the continental United States (CONUS), such as Hawaii or Alaska. Other service personnel are deployed to ally nations across Europe (e.g., Italy, Spain) and Asia (e.g., Japan, South Korea). There are also cultural differences in officer versus enlisted and non-commissioned officer ranks.

One of the most notable differences in the military culture relates to the specific branch of service defined under the general title of the U.S. Armed Forces, which include the Army, Navy, Marine Corps, Air Force, and Coast Guard (U.S. Department of Defense [DoD], 2020). In December 2019, the U.S. Congress created a sixth and independent branch of the Armed Services: the Space Force (Gould & Insinna, 2019). The command structure for the Space Force is organized under the Air Force. A Chief of Space Operations command position has been created; this person will report directly to the Secretary of the Air Force and will become a member of the Joint Chiefs of Staff. At the time of this reporting, Congress prohibited any new billets given the already enormous costs of adding another branch of service to the DoD budget. Therefore, the newly formed Space Force staff will be composed of existing staff, with about 151 Air Force, 24 Army, as well as 14 Navy and Marine Corps personnel. There will be an additional nine members from the Joint Chiefs of Staff, the Office of the Secretary of Defense, and the intelligence community. Given this newly created branch of service, the organizational structure will be dynamic and fluid at various points in its early history. Overall, each branch of service reflects different mission objectives, weapon systems utilized, ranks, organizational structures, values, as well as many more characteristics.

There is a shortage of qualified mental health practitioners to work competently with military service members, veterans, veterans with disabilities, and their families. Although most mental health professionals are not veterans themselves, they can still serve as allies in forming therapeutic alliances with their military clients by earning the circle of trust. The literature in military psychology and counseling recognizes the unique cultural differences between military and civilian mental health (Adler & Castro, 2013; Carrola & Corbin-Burdick, 2015; France, 2018; Hobbs, 2008; Redmond et al., 2015; Stebnicki, 2016; Stebnicki et al., 2017; Westwood et al., 2014).

Training in clinical military counseling practices becomes problematic when guidelines for the assessment, diagnosis, and mental health treatment of service members and veterans do not translate well from nonmilitary or civilian populations. The assumption appears to be that generally the principles, theories, and strategies in psychology and counseling can apply to all clients regardless of cultural identity. However, the military clients whom I have had in my psychotherapy practice discussed past negative experiences with mental health treatment from providers who reportedly were not familiar with military culture. Anecdotally, common concerns of military clients have been that their therapist (a) did not understand the military culture, which was not related to the mental health provider being of veteran status; (b) appeared to feel uncomfortable when they discussed their combat experiences, and in many cases the therapist shifted the conversation to another topic; (c) was not a TRICARE provider, so it was difficult to find a therapist or continue in therapy as a private-pay client; or (d) worked for the VA, which had long waiting lists and would frequently have a different therapist for each visit, resulting in their therapist always wanting them to retell stories of their combat experiences.

UNDERSTANDING THE MILITARY AS A CULTURE

Clearly, the military meets the definition of a culture. For instance, the military has its own operational language, rituals, customs, traditions, values, beliefs, mission, as well as organizational and sociopolitical structures. Within-group differences exist regarding mission, values, language, and other cultural characteristics that exist across the different branches of the U.S. Armed Forces (i.e., Army, Navy, Marine Corps, Air Force, Coast Guard, Space Force). The indoctrination process into the military culture is exemplified in boot camp or basic training, where the ethos, or cultural identity, is formed as it relates to the occupation itself. The culture is contextualized especially by the jargon of written, spoken, and nonverbal language.

As an example of military culture, the Marine Corps has the core values of honor, courage, and commitment. These values translate into mission objectives and determine how each Marine thinks, acts, and fights. The Marines were founded in 1775 and have a proud and long-standing legacy of being a forward-deployed fighting force on land, at sea, and in the air. As many Marines will state with pride, "We are the first in and last out," or "We are the tip of the spear." Another cultural aspect that I have learned through my family members and clients who served in the military is that many Marines tend to state in the present tense "I am a Marine" even long after they have separated from service, whereas those who have served in the other branches of service typically state, "I am retired from [or used to be in] the Navy/Army/Air Force/Coast Guard." The motto "Once a Marine, always a Marine" is a strong cultural trait of this branch of service. Another example within the military culture is that the term "soldier" is specifically designated for those attached to the Army. You should never call a Marine a "soldier" because this designation will hinder credibility and make it difficult to earn the circle of trust with your military clients.

As in many cultures, if the active-duty service member does not comply with the military code of conduct—or accept or acculturate into its branch of service, mission, values, beliefs, customs, traditions, and so forth—then military life can be harsh in some circumstances. In other situations, the service member may be rejected by their culture because they did not accept prominent aspects of military life. Other unique characteristics that prevail in military culture are the strict laws, ethics, and policies that govern military behavior and conduct. If these policies are not followed correctly, it can lead to punitive actions and consequences enforced by the Judge Advocate General's Corps guided by the military's code of conduct (DoD, 1993).

It may appear to some outside the clinical military counseling profession that there is only one culture that represents "the military." This view is easily understood because military life has a unique indoctrination, ethos, and cultural shaping that require all those in service to accept the same identity, traditions, rules, and laws that govern behaviors and other operational and mission-related values and beliefs. However, there are within-group differences in its language and jargon. For instance, as a cultural greeting or expression of enthusiasm, Marines say "Oohrah" and "Booyah," Army soldiers say "Hooah," Navy sailors say "Hooyah," and Air Force airmen say "HUA" (loosely described as an acronym for "heard, understood, acknowledged"). There is also jargon you may have heard and other common military expressions, such as "Whiskey Tango Foxtrot," "roger that," "zero dark thirty," "outside the wire," or "got your six." To gain some level of acceptance, service members must know how to speak the language of their culture. This ability helps service personnel both personally and professionally.

The military culture is defined from the core values and skills earned during specialized training, such as acquired for one's MOS. Most individuals in the military will tell you that their military achievements were "earned"; there are no "participation trophies" awarded after boot camp; and promotion, rank, and other achievements such as patches and medals are based on stringent productivity requirements. Military service members, regardless of gender, must function optimally by passing regular mental and physical fitness evaluations. There is unit pride because the service member understands that they have achieved much more in the military than they could on their own in civilian life. This is due in part to the high levels of motivation, drive, and leadership skills acquired while in service to their country.

In civilian life, there are many employees who have contributed high levels of energy and effort to their job, company, or organization where they work. They are proud of what they do, and some give 100% productivity. In military life, high levels of productivity are required by all, not just a few. Unlike civilian occupations, the military contract asks individuals for a long-term commitment—24 hours a day, 7 days a week, 365 days a year. Particularly during mobilizations or deployments, there are no days off. The life and safety of others in the kinetic environment of the battlefield and military culture depend on the quick and decisive actions of others in the unit. Thus, during deployment, your "head is always on a swivel," there may not be regular mealtimes, and sleep deprivation is common. Any pain experienced by the service member is known as "weakness leaving the body."

Operation tempo is critical to the mission. The DoD describes and measures this component by the service members' speed, intensity, pace, and response time based on critical events that unfold in whatever environment they are placed. The U.S. military does a good job of preparing, planning, organizing, and executing mission objectives for multiple situations and environments. As a result, job performance and productivity are constantly being assessed. Overall, there are multiple challenges for individuals in the military to do their job well. Ultimately, failure is not an option because it risks the health, safety, and lives of others in their unit.

The point is that military culture itself is founded on individuals adopting, accepting, and acculturating into this same identity regardless of gender, race, and ethnicity. There is little flexibility and, in many situations, zero tolerance for those actions and behaviors that differentiate self from others in the unit and command structure. The service member must wear the uniform with pride and honor. Individuals who enlist in the military are contractually (legally) and culturally bound to accept military life for an average of 4 years, depending on the branch of service and MOS. Overall, there is no other occupation like the military in the U.S. labor market. Those who do not adjust well to military life often experience a psychological, emotional, physical, and occupational or career cost. Competent clinical military counselors understand these unique aspects of the military culture. Otherwise, clinicians may misrepresent, stereotype, and even reinforce negative myths about the military culture. However, having awareness, knowledge, and skills will assist you to gain credibility, earn the circle of trust, and form a therapeutic relationship with your military clients.

Becoming a competent and ethical clinical military counselor will take some time and experience. The reader should consult the Military Resources to Explore (MRE) section at the end of this chapter. As a side note, the acronym MRE is also used to describe "meals, ready-to-eat," which is an operational field ration introduced in 1975 and typically used during times of combat deployments. C-rations, the older version, were considered inedible by many service members because of the texture and taste. Current MREs average 1,250 calories, 13% protein, 36% fat, and 51% carbohydrates; contain many food sources; are prepared in approximately 24 different entrees; and taste better when heated (U.S. Army, 2018). Just as in many cultures, food is an important aspect of the culture itself.

MILITARY VERSUS CIVILIAN TRAUMA: REACTIONS AND CONSEQUENCES

One important area to highlight in military culture is how exposure to trauma is expressed. As suggested by Adler and Castro (2013), one of the unmistakable cultural differences between military and civilian life is that the demands of killing, avoiding being killed, caring for the wounded, and witnessing death and injury are all part of military service training. In addition, there are frequent geographic relocations; separations from family, friends, and loved ones; and the demands of 24 hours, 7 days per week availability where one is always on call. The occupation requires that the service member be optimally mentally and physically fit for duty.

As Adler and Castro (2013) have suggested, one of the fundamental aspects of exposure to trauma in the military is that service members are not passive victims of a critical incident. Rather, military personnel train for the physical and psychological demands of combat on an ongoing basis, whereas civilians do not. Thus, for military service members, the physiological and psychological reaction to combat is to "aggress—not stress." In civilian life, most individuals naturally react as victims because they are not prepared mentally and physically to be confronted or aggress against such unpredictable traumatic experiences such as combat.

Therefore, civilians typically experience an acute onset of the full range of posttraumatic stress symptoms (PTSSs), such as intrusive, intense, and prolonged traumatic memories; persistent avoidance of the trauma triggers; hypervigilance; detachment; isolation; and withdrawal. When military personnel experience catastrophic injury or death on the battlefield, it is "mission forward" because the life and safety of their fellow comrades depend on their quick and decisive actions to neutralize any enemy combatants or targets. Thus, the service member must perform at a high level, physically and mentally, to adapt and cope during combat operations.

A critical point in military versus civilian exposure to extraordinary stressful and traumatic incidents is that it is not possible to begin the grieving process while one is fighting for survival. Hence, military personnel typically do not experience the full range of PTSSs or symptoms related to loss and grief during a state of high alert or sympathetic arousal. Consequently, PTSSs may be delayed, and the full range of negative medical and mental health conditions may not be experienced until after deployment. These important issues are dealt with in greater detail in the chapters that follow.

Veterans' reactions to PTSSs and their consequences may be transient as they go through periods of exacerbation and remission, whereas others experience chronic and persistent symptoms with varying degrees of intensity throughout their lifetime. Although both civilians and military service members may experience extraordinary stressful and traumatic events, many civilians have much earlier access to mental health services than military personnel.

One reason for the delayed onset of both symptoms and treatment is that there are no rewards for active-duty service members to seek mental health counseling or to be diagnosed with a mental health condition (e.g., posttraumatic stress disorder, major depressive disorder, anxiety, substance use disorder). The stigma of seeking mental health services can compromise the service member's security clearance, rank, and promotions as well as produce a negative perception of their ability or fitness to serve (DoD, 2013). Indeed, there are multiple lost opportunities for mental health treatment throughout the deployment cycle, which has long-term medical, physical, and mental health consequences, particularly after the service member transitions to civilian life.

WAR STORIES IN THE MILITARY CULTURE

One common characteristic in the military community is the untold stories of warfighting. I have been told by many veterans that the "real warfighters" (e.g., Army Special Forces; Delta Force; Marine Corps Special Operations Command; Navy Sea, Air, and Land [SEAL] teams) never talk to anyone about their missions. There are multiple war biographies, historical books, and personal accounts of warfighting as seen in videos, movies, and documentaries by individuals who were at the epicenter of conflict. However, outside of these storytelling platforms, many veterans do not want to discuss their experiences with civilian friends, families, intimate partners, or anyone else who was not present with them during combat operations. There is a certain level of trust between military service members who can communicate their combat experiences to one another.

Vietnam War veterans were particularly closed to discussing their wartime experiences with anyone other than unit members or members of some military service–related organizations, such as the Veterans of Foreign Wars. For Vietnam veterans, the awareness, knowledge, and acceptance of medical and mental health treatment for complex posttraumatic stress disorder (e.g., traumatic brain injury, blast injury) had minimal support. VA disability treatment and benefits were offered only to those who exhibited severe medical and mental health symptoms. Some of these attitudes and perceptions toward the silence of warfighting prevail today among military service members deployed to hostile regions OCONUS. I have heard some of the most horrific stories imaginable from my active-duty and veteran clients. I felt that it was both a privilege and therapeutic opportunity after they disclosed the deepest, darkest level of their humanity. This point in therapy is always where posttraumatic growth and combat resiliency can be achieved.

There is a common jargon of warfighting, as many military counselors can attest to. Many of my active-duty and veteran clients have expressed phrases to me such as "I only got 2 hours of sleep while on deployment," "I've seen some of my unit buddies blown up and burned alive," and "One of my worst fears was not that I would be killed in action but the thoughts of being captured and tortured." There are countless other stories that depict the mental, emotional, psychological, and physical exhaustion related to being at the epicenter of combat operations. The upcoming chapters address these issues that clients bring to the therapeutic environment. Guidelines and best practices for the reader are offered because it is critical that we offer our full attention to a military client who may want to discuss issues related to reconciliation and forgiveness of their sins or explore the "ghosts of past enemy combatants or civilians" whom they have killed. There is indeed a moral injury, existential anxiety, and a psychological cost to killing another person—particularly if the enemy combatant was a military-age adolescent.

Regardless of the issues, therapists should not anticipate or expect that service members and veterans will discuss war stories, which may be the deepest and darkest moments of their lives, for several reasons. One reason is because of the operational security nature of the mission and the inability to disclose sensitive information, as found in an *after-action report* (i.e., a summary of the multiple details related to a combat mission, such as its analysis, the nature of the operation, the unit personnel involved, and successes and challenges of the mission). Circling back to the foundation of the culturally centered therapeutic environment is the critical lesson of earning the circle of trust with your military clients.

Regarding war stories, it is critical to be present with the individual military client who may want to discuss their combat-related experiences. Competent clinical military counselors use a high level of attending, listening, and empathy skills to earn the circle of trust. They allow their military clients to (a) disclose at the level they feel most comfortable, (b) facilitate approaches and strategies that give permission in a confidential and safe environment to discuss their warfighting experiences, and (c) be open to the idea that therapy is difficult but has rewards. Facilitating a safe environment for military clients to communicate thoughts, feelings, and experiences is essential for optimal therapeutic value and moving forward in the therapeutic process. Restoring the mind, body, and spirit after warfighting or military life can be exhausting work for the client and therapist.

GUIDELINES FOR PRACTICE

The following guidelines for practice are offered to military counselors for cultivating optimal therapeutic engagements. These principles will assist military counselors during their assessment, diagnosis, and treatment of mental health conditions and related issues:

- Apply the theories, knowledge, skills, and therapeutic strategies in psychology and counseling by facilitating therapeutic approaches through the cultural lens of active-duty service members, veterans, veterans with disabilities, and family members.
- Know that being a service member or veteran mental health practitioner may not assist you in earning the circle of trust because there is not just "one military" service member or veteran. Rather, there are many within-group differences among the different branches of service, MOS types, and enlisted versus officer ranks; in addition, individuals also have different gender, racial, ethnic, and cultural traits. Becoming a competent clinical military counselor extends beyond knowledge of the military culture. It involves an understanding of the medical, psychosocial, vocational, transition, mental health treatment, and family dynamics within the military.
- Demonstrate the core and foundational skills of person-centered counseling through attending, listening, and using the skills of empathy to earn the circle of trust. There may be language used in session that you do not understand (e.g., "I was on a FOB"; "I did reconnaissance"; "I am an E-4 11 Bravo"; "My gunny told me we had CAS"; "A 60-cal round hit near me";

"I ran exfil-ops in a CH-47"). However, asking unnecessary or irrelevant questions (e.g., "What is 11 Bravo?" "Who is gunny?" "What is a CH-47?") will only hinder the flow of the therapeutic relationship and will demonstrate your lack of knowledge of the military culture itself.

CONCLUDING REMARKS

The demands of being trained to kill enemy combatants, avoiding being killed, caring for the wounded, and witnessing death and injury indeed have a medical, physical, psychological, emotional, social, spiritual, and occupational cost. Military service members must be in a constant state of mental and physical readiness with a total focus on the mission. Thus, it is difficult to turn off sympathetic arousal as the service member transitions to veteran status in society. The shift from active duty to civilian life is a major cultural shift in which the veteran is challenged with integrating a new identity and life sometimes after years of military service that has been indoctrinated into their mind, body, and spirit. Competent and ethical clinical military counselors understand some of the unique cultural differences in the assessment, diagnosis, and treatment of active-duty personnel, veterans, veterans with disabilities, and military family members.

REFERENCES

Adler, A. B., & Castro, C. A. (2013). An occupational mental health model for the military. *Military Behavioral Health, 1*(1), 41–51. https://doi.org/10.1080/21635781.2012.721063

American Counseling Association. (2018, July 20). VA issues new qualification standards for professional counselors. *ACA Government Affairs Blog*. https://www.counseling.org/news/aca-blogs/aca-government-affairs-blog/aca-government-affairs-blog/2018/07/20/va-issues-new-qualification-standards-for-professional-counselors

Carrola, P., & Corbin-Burdick, M. F. (2015). Counseling veterans: Advocating for culturally competent and holistic interventions. *Journal of Mental Health Counseling, 37*(1), 1–14. https://doi.org/10.17744/mehc.37.1.v74514163rv73274

France, D. (2018). *Combat vet don't mean crazy: Veteran mental health in post-military life*. NCO Historical Society.

Gould, J., & Insinna, V. (2019, December 10). Congress creating Space Force with limited headroom. *Defense News*. https://www.defensenews.com/congress/2019/12/10/congress-creating-space-force-with-limited-head-room/

Hobbs, K. (2008). Reflections on the culture of veterans. *Workplace Health & Safety, 56*(8), 337–341. https://doi.org/10.1177/216507990805600803

Redmond, S. A., Wilcox, S. L., Campbell, S., Kim, A., Finney, K., Barr, K., & Hassan, A. M. (2015). A brief introduction to the military workplace culture. *Work, 50*(1), 9–20. https://doi.org/10.3233/WOR-141987

Stebnicki, M. A. (2016). Military counseling. In I. Marini & M.A. Stebnicki (Eds.), *The professional counselor's desk reference* (2nd ed., pp. 499–506). Springer.

Stebnicki, M. A., Clemmons-James, D., & Leierer, S. (2017). A survey of military counseling content and curriculum among Council on Rehabilitation Education- and Council for Accreditation of Counseling and Related Educational Programs-accredited programs. *Rehabilitation Research, Policy, and Education, 31*(1), 40–49.

U.S. Army. (2018, March 8). *Lifestyles: Meals, ready-to-eat.* https://www.goarmy.com/soldier-life/fitness-and-nutrition/components-of-nutrition/meals-ready-to-eat.html

U.S. Army. (2019, April 25). *Army medicine: Health Professions Scholarship Program (HPSP).* https://www.goarmy.com/amedd/education/hpsp.html

U.S. Department of Defense. (1993, August). *Joint Ethics Regulation (JER)* (DoD 5500.7-R). https://www.esd.whs.mil/Portals/54/Documents/DD/issuances/dodm/550007r.pdf

U.S. Department of Defense. (2013, February). *2011 Department of Defense Health Related Behaviors Survey of Active Duty Military Personnel.* https://www.murray.senate.gov/public/_cache/files/889efd07-2475-40ee-b3b0-508947957a0f/final-2011-hrb-active-duty-survey-report.pdf

U.S. Department of Defense. (2020, January). *DOD dictionary of military and associated terms.* https://www.jcs.mil/Portals/36/Documents/Doctrine/pubs/dictionary.pdf

U.S. Department of Veterans Affairs. (2018). *VA handbook 5005/106: Licensed Professional Mental Health Counselor qualification standards.* Office of Human Resources Management. https://www.va.gov/ohrm/

Westwood, M., Kuhl, D., & Shields, D. (2014). Counseling military clients: Multicultural competence, challenges, and opportunities. In C. C. Lee (Ed.), *Multicultural issues in counseling: New approaches to diversity* (4th ed., pp. 275–293). American Counseling Association.

MILITARY RESOURCES TO EXPLORE (MRE)

Books and Reference Works

Mullaney, C. M. (2009). *The unforgiving minute: A soldier's education.* Penguin Books.

Tick, E. (2014). *Warrior's return: Restoring the soul after war.* Sounds True.

Tzu, S. (2013). *The art of war: Classics of Eastern thought* (L. Giles, Trans.). Barnes & Noble. (Original work published ca. 500 B.C.E.)

U.S. Department of Defense. (2020, January). *DOD dictionary of military and associated terms.* https://www.jcs.mil/Portals/36/Documents/Doctrine/pubs/dictionary.pdf

Other Resources

Center for Deployment Psychology—
Common military acronyms and terminology
http://deploymentpsych.org/system/files/member_resource/Common%20Military%20Acronyms%20and%20Terminology_CDP_8May13.pdf

Center for Deployment Psychology—
Military culture course modules
http://deploymentpsych.org/military-culture-course-modules

Enlisted and officer rank and insignia
https://www.defense.gov/Resources/Insignia/#enlisted-insignia

Military alphabet
http://www.militaryspot.com/military-alphabet/

Military code of conduct
https://www.esd.whs.mil/Portals/54/Documents/DD/issuances/dodm/550007r.pdf

Military time chart
http://military.onlineclock.net/chart/

Military Times
http://www.militarytimes.com/

Military unit size/structure
http://www.cfr.org/world/modern-military-force-structures/p11819

National Guard
http://www.nationalguard.mil/

Security clearances
https://www.clearancejobs.com/security_clearance_faq.pdf

U.S. Air Force
https://www.af.mil/

U.S. Army
https://www.army.mil/

U.S. Coast Guard
https://www.uscg.mil/

U.S. Marines
https://www.marines.mil/

U.S. Navy
https://www.navy.mil/

U.S. Space Force
https://www.spaceforce.mil/

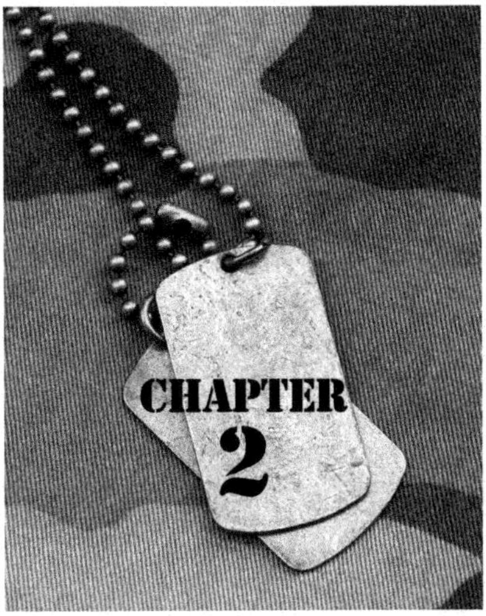

SOCIETAL MYTHS, STEREOTYPES, AND STIGMA OF THE U.S. MILITARY CULTURE

Me: Thank you for your service!
Him: Well I didn't do much except drink a lot . . .
but the Navy did help me refine my drinking skills.

—Conversation with one
of my military clients

★ ★ ★

Myths, stereotypes, and stigma have existed throughout the centuries concerning military service members. Approximately 2,500 years ago, Sun Tzu (ca. 500 B.C.E./2013) wrote *The Art of War*, a text on warfighting and the classical philosophies of Eastern thought. It addressed such issues as preparing for battle during wartime and taking tactical advantages on enemy armies; it also contained reflections on the writings of Confucius and philosophies of Taoism that, in part, have formed the foundation of today's military culture. In this extensive work, Tzu also discussed expected behaviors, morals, and ethics of conscripted military personnel and high-ranking officers as well as many more military-related issues that reflected the culture at the time. The influence of this and other historical references (e.g., writings of Carl von Clausewitz and Napoleon, memoirs of great generals of past wars) may have been responsible in part for Western societies' perceptions and attitudes regarding the military culture within the United States.

Numerous studies address the myths, stereotypes, and stigma associated with the military culture's impact on various racial and ethnic groups; gender-related issues; the lesbian, gay, bisexual, and transgender community; persons with HIV/AIDS; as well as persons with disabilities. However, few studies have explored the myths, stereotypes, and stigma relating to the military culture (Ashley & Constantine Brown, 2015; Griffin & Stein, 2015; Kim et al., 2016; Pietrzak et al., 2009; Quartana et al., 2014; Stebnicki et al., 2016; Vogt et al., 2014). The purpose of this chapter is to highlight some of the more prevalent societal and clinician myths, perceptions, and attitudes regarding the military culture and how these factors hinder, challenge, and affect service members' and veterans' motivation for seeking medical and mental health treatment.

THE IMPACT ON MILITARY CULTURE

Cultural myths and stereotypes regarding the military community can be both negative and positive. Some individuals in American society as well as clinical providers see military service members as possessing a high level of courage, honor, loyalty, confidence, toughness, and resiliency. Others in society may portray this group as possessing the potential to act in violence, having low impulse control, or having poor mental and physical health (Ahern et al., 2015; Currier et al., 2017; Quartana et al., 2014; Vogt et al., 2014). Theoretically, stigmas regarding the military culture are based on public perceptions of individuals not associated with the military. Service members and veterans can also internalize public stigma and adopt these negative perceptions of themselves, which may hinder good mental health and wellness.

Skopp et al. (2012) developed the Military Stigma Scale, a 26-item scale designed to measure public and self-stigma within two dimensions (public and self-stigma). Interested readers should consult the references section for details of this scale development study. However, public and self-stigma have been shown to produce lasting negative effects on the mental health and well-being of service members and veterans. The most harmful effects are that stigma is directly associated with mental health treatment seeking and may even counteract or nullify positive treatment outcomes.

As a direct result of negative military cultural myths, stereotypes, and stigma, medical and mental health professionals may directly/indirectly or consciously/unconsciously be facilitating treatment approaches based on cultural myths. The psychosocial impact on the service member or veteran may include the following:

- The client may feel "broken," possess low self-esteem, and have difficulties assimilating or transitioning into the civilian culture.

- Clinicians and society may project negative attitudes and perceptions that can create a reluctance and resistance on the part of the service member or veteran seeking medical and mental health treatment. This behavior reinforces the military identity that no one understands the culture except those who have served. Consequently, they may reject nonmilitary medical and mental health providers altogether.
- Many indigenous cultural groups or foreign nationals distrust the American military, particularly while they are on deployment in hostile countries. Many indigenous groups were taught to fear Americans. They are viewed and portrayed as violent people, which is reinforced by American movies, electronic media, and political propaganda. Thus, if the service member overpersonalizes this stereotype, they may endorse this belief about themselves or not feel committed to a combat mission.
- Stigma associated with the "suck it up" mentality, warrior ethos, indoctrination rituals, and other cultural attributes in the military hinders service members' and veterans' ability to seek mental health treatment. Submitting to the values of seeking psychotherapy disavows military cultural philosophy and ideology.

Many factors influence clinical providers' and society's attitudes and perceptions toward social and interpersonal interactions with the military culture. Some of these factors relate to the unique characteristics of each war and generation. For instance, rarely did Vietnam War veterans hear the phrase "thank you for your service," whereas this phrase is commonly heard today by those who have served in the war on terrorism after 2001. Additionally, many Vietnam veterans rarely sought mental health treatment, primarily because conditions such as posttraumatic stress disorder (PTSD), major depressive disorder, anxiety, and substance use disorders—as well as military suicidality—were not readily recognized by the U.S. Department of Veterans Affairs (VA) system of health care.

The level of screening, assessment, diagnosis, and treatment did not exist then like it does now in veteran health care. The numbers of Vietnam War veterans with a VA disability rating of PTSD pale in comparison with Operation Iraqi Freedom, Operation Enduring Freedom, and Operation Inherent Resolve veterans. The veteran psychiatric treatment facilities for Vietnam veterans were reserved only for those with the most severe, chronic, and persistent symptoms of PTSD.

Other influences that mediate attitudes and perceptions toward the military community are related to political rhetoric, governmental policies (i.e., VA, U.S. Department of Defense [DoD]), and various veteran organizations. These influences help to shape both negative and positive attitudes and perceptions toward active-duty service members, veterans, veterans with disabilities, and military families.

Unfortunately, many clinical providers who are not culturally competent in providing medical and mental health services to the military may unintentionally accept "Hollywood's" version and portrayal of the military culture.

As a consequence of military cultural myths, stereotypes, and stigma, clinicians may create barriers that harm the service member's or veteran's (a) reintegration and transition into employment and educational opportunities within the labor market (Currier et al., 2017; Farley, 2013; Griffin & Stein, 2015); (b) perceptions of seeking mental health treatment (Quartana et al., 2014; Vogt et al., 2014); (c) security clearance, rank, promotions, and perception of their mental or psychological fitness to serve (DoD, 2013; Stebnicki, 2016); (d) willingness to utilize professional mental health and substance abuse counseling services (Rae Olmsted et al., 2011); (e) utilization of alternative mental health treatment (Kim et al., 2016); (f) psychosocial transition from active duty to civilian life (Derefinko et al., 2019; Gibbons et al., 2014); (g) reconnection and readjustment with family members and intimate relationships (Ahern et al., 2015); and (h) ability to overcome the mental and physical health disparities that exist within the veteran culture (Hobbs, 2008; Stebnicki et al., 2016).

MILITARY MYTHS COMMON TO THE CULTURE

In this section, I present an extensive list of myths attributable to the military culture that potentially may affect the clinician's perception and attitude toward serving their military clients. Clinical military counselors who are culturally competent understand these cultural myths and the value of earning the circle of trust within the therapeutic relationship with active-duty personnel, veterans, veterans with disabilities, and family members. In addition, they understand the importance of the working alliance and how unintentional actions could adversely affect the therapeutic relationship. The cultural dynamics in session are of paramount importance, and unintended consequences could occur any number of ways, such as verbal and nonverbal communication as well as language that portrays a cultural bias, negative attitude, or perceptions toward a group of individuals. Clinical military counselors should understand that 75% of what we communicate to one another is done by metacommunication.

All military troops serve in combat operations: This myth assumes that all military service members and veterans are warfighters and have served in combat operations. The Pew Research Center's analysis of information gathered from the DoD's Defense Manpower Data Center (https://www.dmdc.osd.mil/appj/dwp/dwp_reports.jsp) indicates that in June 2018, there were approximately 1.3 million active-duty military personnel across the U.S. Armed Forces. Approximately 15% of all active-duty service members were deployed overseas—the lowest numbers of troops deployed since 1957. Most troops (70%) were deployed to Asian and European military installations. Only 15% of troops were deployed to Middle Eastern countries (e.g., Iraq, Afghanistan, Syria) and North African nations, whereas 3% were deployed to sub-Saharan Africa or the Americas (e.g., El Salvador). The remainder (14%) were located at sea or in other undisclosed locations around the globe. There was a surge in U.S. troops sent to Iraq in 2007 and 2019. However, these numbers pale in comparison with the Vietnam War, in which 45% of all troops were deployed to combat operations overseas.

Although the United States has one of the most highly trained and well-funded military forces in the world, most active-duty service members are not involved in combat operations. For every "trigger puller" in the military, there are at least five others deployed to assist with food, ammunition, and intelligence. Thus, most military service members' military occupational specialty (MOS) is to support combat operations (although there may be times when units within a battalion may be called up to the front lines to engage enemy combatants). There are hundreds of MOSs across all branches of the military, such as cooks, mechanics, embarkation and logistics specialists (i.e., shipping and receiving clerks), truck drivers, and vehicle mechanics, just to name a few. The smallest number of military service members are part of an elite, highly trained, specialized group of warfighters who are members of the Army Special Forces (i.e., Green Berets, Night Stalkers, Rangers), Navy (i.e., Sea, Air, and Land [SEAL] teams; Navy Special Warfare Combatant Craft Crew), Marine Corps (i.e., Marine Corps Special Operations Command, Marine Corps Force Reconnaissance), Air Force (i.e., Air Force Special Tactics), and the 1st Special Forces Operational Detachment–Delta (an elite special operations force of the Army tasked with specialized missions primarily involving counterterrorism and special reconnaissance).

Psychosocial implications of this myth: There are indeed distinct within-group cultural differences between combat versus noncombat service members and veterans. Although each branch of service has a different mission (e.g., boots on the ground, fighting in the air, commanding the seas), there is a misperception that all military troops have engaged in combat operations. As a result, one common issue related to some service members and veterans is that they may have low self-worth or self-esteem because they have trained up for combat operations, yet they were never called to duty or never served in a combat unit deployed to a hostile region. Even those who deployed to hostile areas may have spent their entire deployment on a Forward Operations Base and did not go out on patrols, go on reconnaissance missions, or engage in enemy firefight. Those not involved in the fight may have lost a unit buddy and may feel survivor's guilt for not being there for their fellow comrades. It becomes ambiguous and complicated for some service members who may have screened positive for a mental health disorder (i.e., PTSD or anxiety) who were not directly involved with enemy combatants.

Additionally, because most service members serve outside the continental United States on military installations in allied Asian and European countries, the phrase "thank you for your service" implies that the service member is worthy of society's view of the warfighter. Alternatively, there may be the negative public perception by some that because the service member was not exposed to combat operations, they should be seen in a lesser status primarily because they, for example, served as "just a cook" in the Navy, a truck mechanic, or an embarkation and logistics specialist. Overall, there are unintentional psychological consequences to reinforcing negative stereotypes, attitudes, and perceptions toward the military culture. Clinical providers may project communication that devalues the service member because of their status (combat vs. noncombat operator, enlisted vs. officer rank, MOS of infantry vs. counterintelligence).

It is respectful to say "thank you for your service": Saying "thank you for your service" is indeed respectful. However, there is a mixture of anecdotal evidence and testimonials to support the notion that this saying should not always be expressed to active-duty personnel or veterans (Brennan, 2017; Kelly, 2018; Richtel, 2015). Alternative accolades include phrases such as "thank you for your sacrifice," "thank you for defending our country," "thank you for your willingness to serve," or "welcome home." Yet, these expressions have much of the same meaning. Civilians who really want to express gratitude for the military can volunteer at multiple service organizations (e.g., Wounded Warrior Project, Veterans of Foreign Wars, United Service Organizations, military base activities). At times, actions speak louder than words. Given the ratio of combat versus noncombat operators, if you express "thank you for your service," statistically, 30% have served in a combat-related role, whereas 70% have not. Thus, you may have to deal with the awkwardness of this situation that may not be consistent with the warfighter stereotype.

Most active-duty service members and veterans I have had in my psychotherapy practice, and most veterans who attend my clinical military counseling workshops, have indicated that they do not like the expression "thank you for your service." Many indicate that (a) civilians do not understand what they have seen or experienced so it is disingenuous to say "thank you" because they have never been in the military; (b) most politicians say "thank you for your service," which also sounds disingenuous and does not reflect authenticity; (c) they are jaded by their experiences in the military, so this expression triggers an anger reaction because they were not honored by their own branch of service; and (d) it is a superficial comment, particularly if they served in a noncombat role. Many service members and veterans view their enlistment in the military as an occupational choice; therefore, if this logic is applied, people should also say "thank you for your service" to mental health counselors, firefighters, law enforcement officials, farmers, or coal miners—all of whom can also have dangerous jobs at times. Interestingly, when I selectively expressed "thank you for your service" in past interactions with friends and colleagues who have served, they in turn expressed "thank you for your service Mark" because of the active-duty Marines and veterans across all branches whom I serve in my psychotherapy practice and the clinical military counselor training that I do.

Psychosocial implications of this myth: First and foremost, it is important that each expression of "thank you" be taken individually rather than used impulsively with every service member whom you encounter. Many are jaded or cynical about their military service because they are struggling with medical, physical, and mental health conditions that created their present situation. Some have a moral injury based on their horrific experiences in combat. Others find this expression disingenuous because it is repeated by multiple civilians they meet who will never understand their military experiences. A major point is that clinical practitioners should avoid "sounding like everyone else," such as individuals seen in the media, politicians, and uninformed civilians.

Second, there are other ways to express your gratitude that are more proactive, such as volunteer service–related activities. Lastly, as helping professionals, it is critical to understand the psychosocial implications of stereotypes and stigmas placed on service members or veterans living in the civilian world. Also, it is essential to understand that many family members and spouses are left out of the conversation and acknowledgment of "thank you for your service" even though they too have sacrificed their life alongside their loved one's deployments. These issues are discussed at length in the chapter on military families.

Most veterans have PTSD and other mental health conditions: The prolonged war on terrorism that began in 2001 reflects more than 20 years of warfighting, with frequent and longer deployments and increased mental health and co-occurring disorders. The epidemiological significance of military suicide completions is unlike any other war. However, the incidence and prevalence of suicide completions do not differ significantly in combat versus noncombat participants. At least half of all suicide completions involve active-duty service members who were never deployed to a combat theater (Kessler et al., 2015; Kline et al., 2016; Reger et al., 2015). Adjustment disorders are some of the most frequently diagnosed conditions among both active-duty service members and civilians, whereas PTSD is not (Fielden, 2012; Morgan & Kelber, 2018). Some studies have shown that among active-duty service members, 23%–49% met the diagnostic screening criteria for PTSD (Institute of Medicine, 2013; Kim et al., 2016), 7% met the criteria for major depressive disorder, and 7.5% met the criteria for anxiety disorders (Witkiewitz & Estrada, 2011).

As far as substance use disorders, approximately 23%–50% of active-duty service members reported binge drinking at least once during a 30-day period, whereas 17% were considered moderate drinkers, and 8% were considered heavy drinkers (DoD, 2013). Interestingly, the literature suggests that the rates of substance use disorders and co-occurring mental health conditions are only slightly higher in incidence and prevalence in military versus civilian populations (Witkiewitz & Estrada, 2011). So how do we account for the approximately 50%–70% of service members and veterans who do not meet the criteria for PTSD or a co-occurring mental health disorder? Increasing awareness and access to military mental health treatment has never been more apparent than in the print and electronic media's coverage of veteran suicides. The media's coverage reinforces the public perception that most service members have severe psychiatric disorders. They tend to deemphasize success stories of those who have bounced back from adversity (Edwards-Stewart et al., 2011).

Overall, statistically, the research does not support the myth that most service members and veterans have PTSD and other co-occurring mental health conditions. The myth concerning severe mental health issues in the military sets up the stereotype that civilians have better mental health and wellness than the military culture. Military researchers are now examining the coping and resiliency skills possessed by service members and veterans. Generally, finding solutions to increase military mental health access and to destigmatize treatment requires a more sophisticated and complex analysis.

Psychosocial implications of this myth: Truly, there are negative societal attitudes and perceptions toward psychiatric disabilities in the military. This harmful myth hinders service members and veterans from seeking medical and mental health treatment. Some researchers have suggested that the electronic and print media's coverage of veteran suicides tends to overemphasize the lack of mood regulation and behavioral health. Consequently, if the focus is on military service members' "pathology" and their mental health disorders, then this stigma becomes pervasive (Edwards-Stewart et al., 2011).

The essential point is that if people focus solely on military mental health disorders, then service members and veterans can be denied job and career opportunities because employers may not want to hire a veteran for fear of mental and behavioral health concerns or that the veteran may be prone to violence. The focus on poor veteran mental health also creates conflicts in social-emotional relationships with family members and intimate partners. Overall, the media's portrayal of veteran mental health problems creates stigma to the extent that the individual may want to socially detach, isolate, and not identify themselves as a member of the military community. Society's image of the warfighter who is "broken" or "damaged goods" intensifies service members' and veterans' negative emotion, mood, and affect. Consequently, if one cultural attribute or trait is overemphasized and becomes generalized to all aspects of the military culture (i.e., all veterans have mental health disorders), this generalization leads to negative attitudes and stereotypes regarding the culture itself.

All veterans are seeking or receive disability benefits: Active-duty service members and veterans are eligible to receive disability benefits for a comprehensive list of medical, physical, and mental health conditions as well as many different chronic illnesses and diseases (VA, 2020). All conditions that are service connected must be evaluated and diagnosed by medical and mental health professionals connected with the U.S. Armed Forces and VA clinics. The VA oversees the disability program. A medically determinable and objective disability rating system is used and expressed in terms of the percentage of impairment (0%–100%). A medical board examines the alleged medical, physical, and mental health conditions in terms of etiology, functional limitations, and other evidence that contributes to the condition(s). Other extensive documentation is required, such as the personnel record associated with the person's MOS, after-action reports of combat deployments and other critical incidents involving the service member, as well as other reports.

Complex formulas and guidelines are associated with receiving benefits. In some cases, the service member or veteran may have temporary or partial disability benefits before a total and permanent rating is established; it can sometimes take up to 5 years to receive a favorable determination. Disability benefits in the military are different than the Social Security Administration's program of Social Security Disability Income. The principles of receiving disability benefits are to offset the average earnings lost due to the person's disabling condition(s) preventing them from performing their military duties. Also considered is the future anticipated and expected treatment that will likely occur over the lifetime of the service member or veteran. In 2013, about 3.5 million of the nation's 22 million veterans received some form of service-connected disability benefits (Congressional Budget Office, 2014).

Approximately 1.1 million veterans have a disability rating of 70% or more and are medically retired. There are some 60,000 veterans who receive income from three different sources for which they are eligible: retirement income from the branch of service where they served, the VA, and Social Security Disability Income benefits. Some active-duty service members may have a disability rating and are assigned to light duty work until maximum medical improvement is determined. Most who have a severe disability (e.g., moderate-severe traumatic brain injury, spinal cord injury, amputation, severe muscular skeletal conditions) cannot serve and are forced to medically retire. Statistically, not everyone in the military qualifies for disability benefits. However, most service members when asked whether they would rather be working and not disabled indicate that they would like to return to their jobs but cannot because of their medical, physical, and mental health conditions. Overall, eligibility for disability benefits is not automatic, and not all service members receive the same exact benefits because of variances in rank, length of time in service, MOS, types of disabling conditions sustained while in service, as well as other factors.

Psychosocial implications of this myth: The U.S. military has a long history of caring for the wounded and injured during wartime. Currently, 45% of veterans who served in Iraq and Afghanistan report having some type of service-connected disability, whereas less than 21% of Gulf War veterans receive disability benefits (National Veterans Foundation, 2015). Although there are many theories as to why disability claims have risen after 2001, the one viable explanation is that the service-connected disability eligibility standards have been expanded. Additionally, many service members are encouraged by unit commanders, veteran service organizations, and other government entities to apply for disability benefits to document their medical, physical, and mental health conditions. The intention of receiving disability benefits and compensation due to injury, whether you are a veteran or civilian, is to avoid the excessive out-of-pocket expenses over your lifetime for medical, physical, or mental health treatment as well as to obtain financial stability for you and your family. There has also been a change in the military culture's attitude and perceptions toward mental and physical disability. Many veterans communicate that there is "no shame" in receiving disability benefits that were earned while in service to their country.

Today, being a veteran with a disability has a much different meaning because of the documented serious mental and physical health conditions (i.e., PTSD, suicidal ideation, opioid addiction, traumatic brain injury, amputation). However, there continues to be a reoccurring myth or stereotype in society that "all veterans are on disability benefits." Unfortunately, this negative attitude only serves to stigmatize the veteran as being a member of a disenfranchised group possessing medical, physical, or mental health "deficits," further separating the veteran from society, which tends to see mental and physical disability as an aberration. The psychosocial impact of such attitudes is pervasive and harms veterans' mental health and well-being. One reason is because of the ambiguity of physical (visible) disabling conditions versus mental health (invisible) disabilities. According to the attitude and perception of some in society, those with a mental health (invisible) disability may not deserve the same financial benefits as those who have suffered medical and physical disabilities.

Women in the military have less dangerous jobs and have it easier: An in-depth discussion of women in the military is covered in the chapters that follow. It is recognized in the literature that women have had a long history of serving in various capacities and were particularly utilized in medical units during World War II. Yet, women in the military are rarely recognized for their valor, strength, resiliency, and high level of job performance, primarily because of the hypermasculine nature of the military culture. Part of the issue is that there have been fewer job opportunities and billets available to women that could advance their military careers. Currently, women compose more than 16% of all active-duty service members (Reynolds & Shendruk, 2018). Women are now assigned to combat operations and are also casualties of war. The number of women varies across the branches of service. Of the 200,000 women in the military, approximately 8.4% are Marines, whereas 20% are in the Air Force (Katzenberg, 2019). Women have a mandatory boot camp but are separated from their male counterparts during their basic training. However, women are integrated into many of the same units and missions as men. In 2016, Secretary of Defense Ash Carter mandated that all MOSs be open to women across all branches of the military.

However, despite this action, most military branches have been extremely slow to accept these changes. Although women are offered the same billet opportunities as men, most definitely do not receive the same rate as their male counterparts (Snow, 2018). In the Marines, only 11 enlisted women served in the traditional "03 Infantry" career field. The Army, for example, has only 78% of their MOSs open and available to women. In 2017, the Navy's elite special warfare operating billet (Navy SEALs) accepted women into SEAL training school. Overall, more than 75% of SEAL candidates drop out of this highly intense training. The Army Rangers special operations group also graduated one female soldier in 2019. Although women in the military have many more career opportunities than ever before, there are still discrepancies in the number of employment opportunities, and many are perceived as not equivalent in status to their male counterparts.

Psychosocial implications of this myth: Military research at the Pew Research Center and demographic data gathered by the DoD have provided more statistics than in the past regarding women in the military. For example, survey research suggests that gender integration within the various branches across the military has no effect on unit cohesion. However, the myths persist because of the attitude and perception of what characteristics should compose the image of the warfighter. Most women in the military show much resiliency for mental and physical toughness, and they have earned the right to become highly skilled at their MOS and wear the uniform within their branch of service. One of the more critical issues challenging women in the military today is the troubling statistics on the prevalence and incidence of military sexual trauma. The psychological and emotional cost of unwanted sexual advances, harassment, assault, and rape is a dark reality that women face in military life. Consequently, many women present with the clinical symptoms associated with complex PTSD and co-occurring mental health conditions.

All veterans are gun owners: There are relativity few contemporary studies describing firearm ownership among U.S. veterans. Firearm ownership for some in mental health treatment can be a risk factor for harm. Although most veteran suicide completions are a result of self-inflicted fatal gunshot wounds, a national survey conducted in 2015 indicated that only 45% of all veterans possess one or more firearms (Cleveland et al., 2017), whereas 20%–30% of nonveterans own firearms (Gramlich & Schaeffer, 2019). Reducing access to firearms is increasingly supported by clinical military counselors because 66% of male veteran suicides involve guns (VA Suicide Prevention Program, 2016). However, suicide by firearm is not unique to the military, and most suicides by civilian men (56%) are the result of self-inflicted gunshot wounds. Firearms are deeply entrenched in the American lifestyle, and guns are a major part of the entertainment experience of Americans while watching movies and TV as well as playing video games. Guns are deeply rooted within the history of the United States, beginning as early as the Revolutionary War, in which the Regulators wanted political asylum from Great Britain. The myth and stereotype that "all service members and veterans are gun-toting, right-wing, National Rifle Association conservatives" should come as no surprise, even though many veterans do not own firearms. This unfounded myth serves to reinforce stereotypes and stigmas that are attributed to the military culture, thus making it easier to form negative attitudes and perceptions regarding this culture.

Most veterans whom I have had the privilege to serve in my psychotherapy practice have indicated that guns are an insignificant part of their civilian lives. Those who have good mental health and well-being also have meaningful family and intimate partner relationships, careers, and recreational activities that do not involve weekends at the gun range. Most veterans understand the lethality of assault weapons. Many gladly relinquish the role of having to carry a firearm as required by their occupation. Some of my more high-risk veteran clients refuse to keep firearms in their home as a self-initiated suicide prevention method they learned when they transitioned from active duty to civilian life. Overall, many healthy functioning combat veterans have separated themselves from their experience with the use of weapons of war, because a gun itself does not define who the person is socially, emotionally, and psychologically.

Psychosocial implications of this myth: All myths and negative stereotypes harm the psychological and emotional well-being of service members and veterans. The perception that "all veterans own guns" is intricately tied to veterans' mental health, particularly when it comes to issues related to veteran suicide. Although men are at least 4 times more likely than women to end their life violently, it further reinforces the stigma that all male veterans are at risk for suicidal ideation, attempts, or completions. This stigma alone takes the focus off important issues in female veteran mental health because female veterans are 2.4 times more likely than civilian women to die from suicide (VA Suicide Prevention Program, 2016).

BEST PRACTICES FOR CLINICIANS

Competent and ethical counselors are aware of the attitudes, perceptions, beliefs, values, and behaviors that are imposed on their clients as guided by the *ACA Code of Ethics* (American Counseling Association, 2014). Competent and ethical clinical military counselors are aware of the myths, stereotypes, and stigma surrounding the military culture. Regardless of whether you are a civilian or a veteran mental health clinician, it is essential that cultural awareness, knowledge, and skills guide your practice. The following guidelines are offered to assist in informing a culturally competent practice that is mindful of myths, stereotypes, and stigma that could hinder personal growth and optimal well-being with military clients:

- Remember that the service member or veteran, not the practitioner, defines their own unique identity within the branch of service where they served, their MOS, the unit they were attached to, their rank, and any exposure they had to combat operational stress.
- Avoid harmful attitudes and stereotypes by listening for the service member's or veteran's experience of their military life and how others in society or family members may attribute negative characteristics toward them, ultimately affecting their self-worth, self-esteem, and identity.
- Recognize how service members or veterans choose to assimilate, acculturate, or transition to civilian culture and understand how the environment itself affects optimal mental and physical functioning.
- Explore how psychosocial adjustment and adaptation to service-connected mental and physical disabilities can hinder the service member's or veteran's coping and resiliency.
- Be aware that psychosocial adjustment and adaptation to service-connected mental and physical disabilities can hinder the service member's or veteran's coping and resiliency because of stigma and negative attitudes associated with persons with disabilities.
- Interpret how negative perceptions and attitudes can follow the service member or veteran in civilian jobs, intimate partner and family relationships, and social-recreational activities as well as how they may affect their overall quality of life.

- Recognize that exposure to combat does not imply that the service member or veteran will have a life of PTSD and co-occurring mental and physical health conditions.
- Differentiate between PTSD and moral injury. Not all combat veterans have a moral injury. Competent practitioners recognize the meaning, purpose, and experience of each military client's deployment and mission.
- Identify trauma exposure acquired during combat versus non-combat situations and how stress and trauma are experienced and assigned by the individual. Appraise one's perception and attitude toward critical events, how they turn on their stress mechanisms, as well as the individual's coping and resiliency skills.

CONCLUDING REMARKS

This chapter highlights some of the more prevalent myths and negative stereotypes about the military culture. Few studies exist that explore military myths, stereotypes, and stigma and how they ultimately affect the mental health and well-being of persons who have served their country. Many scholars in the multicultural counseling literature underscore the relevance of how negative myths and stereotypes create harmful psychological effects when they are generalized to all members of a culture. Accordingly, culturally competent clinical military counselors work intentionally in meaningful ways to reduce negative stigma in therapy.

REFERENCES

Ahern, J., Worthen, M., Masters, J., Lippman, S. A., Ozer, E. J., & Moos, R. (2015). The challenges of Afghanistan and Iraq veterans' transition from military to civilian life and approaches to reconnection. *PLoS One, 10*(7), Article e0128599. https://doi.org/10.1371/journal.pone.0128599

American Counseling Association. (2014). *ACA code of ethics.*

Ashley, W., & Constantine Brown, J. (2015). The impact of combat status on veterans' attitudes toward help seeking: The hierarchy of combat elitism. *Journal of Evidence-Informed Social Work, 12*(5), 534–542. https://doi.org/10.1080/15433714.2014.992695

Brennan, M. B. (2017, November 9). Should you say "thank you for your service"? *Psychology Today.* https://www.psychologytoday.com/us/blog/the-war-within/201711/should-you-say-thank-you-your-service

Cleveland, E. C., Azrael, D., Simonetti, J. A., & Miller, M. (2017). Firearm ownership among American veterans: Findings from the 2015 National Firearm Survey. *Injury Epidemiology, 4*(1), Article 33. https://doi.org/10.1186/s40621-017-0130-y

Congressional Budget Office. (2014, August 7). *Veterans' disability compensation: Trends and policy options.* https://www.cbo.gov/publication/45615

Currier, J. M., McDermott, R. C., & McCormick, W. H. (2017). Mental health treatment–related stigma and professional help seeking among student veterans. *Psychological Services, 14*(4), 531–542. https://doi.org/10.1037/ser0000129

Derefinko, K. J., Hallsell, T. A., Isaacs, M. B., Colvin, L. W., Salgado Garcia, F. I., & Bursa, Z. (2019). Perceived needs of veterans transitioning from the military to civilian life. *Journal of Behavioral Health Services & Research, 46,* 384–398. https://doi.org/10.1007/s11414-018-9633-8

Edwards-Stewart, A., Kinn, J. T., June, J. D., & Fullerton, N. R. (2011). Military and civilian media coverage of suicide. *Archives of Suicide Research, 15*(4), 304–312. https://doi.org/10.1080/13811118.2011.615692

Farley, J. I. (2013). *Quick military transition guide: Seven steps to landing a civilian job.* JIST Works.

Fielden, J. S. (2012). Review: Management of adjustment disorders in the deployed setting. *Military Medicine, 177*(9), 1022–1027. https://doi.org/10.7205/milmed-d-12-00057

Gibbons, S. W., Migliore, L., Convoy, S. P., Greiner, S., & DeLeon, P. H. (2014). Military mental health stigma challenges: Policy and practice considerations. *The Journal for Nurse Practitioners, 10*(6), 365–372. https://doi.org/10.1016/j.nurpra.2014.03.021

Gramlich, J., & Schaeffer, K. (2019, October 22). *7 facts about gun ownership in the U.S.* Pew Research Center. https://www.pewresearch.org/fact-tank/2018/12/27/facts-about-guns-in-united-states/

Griffin, C. L., Jr., & Stein, M. A. (2015). Self-perception of disability and prospects for employment among U.S. veterans. *Work, 50*(1), 49–58. https://doi.org/10.3233/WOR-141929

Hobbs, K. (2008). Reflections on the culture of veterans. *Workplace Health & Safety, 56*(8), 337–341. https://doi.org/10.1177/216507990805600803

Institute of Medicine. (2013). *Returning home from Iraq and Afghanistan: Assessment of readjustment needs of veterans, service members, and their families.* https://www.nap.edu/catalog/13499/returning-home-from-iraq-and-afghanistan-assessment-of-readjustment-needs

Katzenberg, L. (2019, March 8). 40 stories from women about life in the military. *The New York Times Magazine.* https://www.nytimes.com/2019/03/08/magazine/women-military-stories.html

Kelly, J. (2018, November 9). *Why saying thank you for your service offends some veterans.* InMilitary.com. https://inmilitary.com/why-saying-thank-you-for-your-service-offends-some-veterans/

Kessler, R. C., Stein, M. B., Bliese, P. D., Bromet, E. J., Chiu, W. T., Cox, K. L., Colpe, L. J., Fullerton, C. S., Gilma, S. E., Gruber, M. J., Heeringa, S. G., Lewandowski-Romps, L., Millikan-Bell, A., Naifeh, J. A., Nock, M. K., Petukhova, M. V., Rosellini, A. J., Sampson, N. A., Schoenbaum, M., . . . Ursano, R. J. (2015). Occupational differences in US Army suicide rates. *Psychological Medicine, 45*(15), 3293–3304. https://doi.org/10.1017/S0033291715001294

Kim, P. Y., Toblin, R. L., Riviere, L. A., Kok, B. C., Grossman, S. H., & Wilk, J. E. (2016). Provider and nonprovider sources of mental health help in the military and the effects of stigma, negative attitudes, and organizational barriers to care. *Psychiatric Services, 67*(2), 221–226. https://doi.org/10.1176/appi.ps.201400519

Kline, A., Weiner, M. D., Interian, A., Shcherbakov, A., & St. Hill, L. (2016). Morbid thoughts and suicidal ideation in Iraq war veterans: The role of direct and indirect killing in combat. *Depression and Anxiety, 33*(6), 473–482. https://doi.org/10.1002/da.22496

Morgan, M., & Kelber, M. (2018, October 29). *Adjustment disorders: How are they relevant to military mental health?* Psychological Health Center of Excellence. https://www.pdhealth.mil/news/blog/adjustment-disorders-how-are-they-relevant-military-mental-health

National Veterans Foundation. (2015, October 23). *What do we do with the staggering number of veterans?* https://nvf.org/staggering-number-of-disabled-veterans/

Pietrzak, R. H., Johnson, D. C., Goldstein, M. B., Malley, J. C., & Southwick, S. M. (2009). Perceived stigma and barriers to mental health care utilization among OEF-OIF veterans. *Psychiatric Services, 60*(8), 1118–1122. https://doi.org/10.1176/appi.ps.60.8.1118

Quartana, P. J., Wilk, J. E., Thomas, J. L., Bray, R. M., Rae Olmsted, K. L., Brown, J. M., Williams, J., Kim, P. Y., Clarke-Walper, K., & Hoge, C. W. (2014). Trends in mental health services utilization and stigma in US soldiers from 2002 to 2011. *American Journal of Public Health, 104*(9), 1671–1679. https://doi.org/10.2105/AJPH.2014.301971

Rae Olmsted, K. L., Brown, J. M., Vandermaas-Peeler, J. R., Tueller, S. J., Johnson, R. E., & Gibbs, D. A. (2011). Mental health and substance abuse treatment stigma among soldiers. *Military Psychology, 23*(1), 52–64. https://doi.org/10.1080/08995605.2011.534414

Reger, M. A., Smolenski, D. J., Skopp, N. A., Mezger-Abamukang, M. J., Kang, H. K., Bullman, T. A., Perdue, S., & Gahm, G. A. (2015). Risk of suicide among US military service members following Operation Enduring Freedom or Operation Iraqi Freedom deployment and separation from the US military. *JAMA Psychiatry, 72*(6), 561–569. https://doi.org/10.1001/jamapsychiatry.2014.3195

Reynolds, G. M., & Shendruk, A. (2018, April 24). *Demographics of the U.S. military.* Council on Foreign Relations. https://www.cfr.org/article/demographics-us-military

Richtel, M. (2015, February 21). Please don't thank me for my service. *The New York Times*. https://www.nytimes.com/2015/02/22/sunday-review/please-dont-thank-me-for-my-service.html

Skopp, N. A., Bush, N. E., Vogel, D. L., Wade, N. G., Sirotin, A. P., McCann, R. A., & Metzger-Abamukong, M. J. (2012). Development and initial testing of a measure of public and self-stigma in the military. *Journal of Clinical Psychology, 68*(9), 1036–1047. https://doi.org/10.1002/jclp.21889

Snow, S. (2018, March 5). Where are the female Marines? *Marine Corps Times*. https://www.marinecorpstimes.com/news/2018/03/05/where-are-the-female-marines/

Stebnicki, M. A. (2016). Military counseling. In I. Marini & M.A. Stebnicki (Eds.), *The professional counselor's desk reference* (2nd ed., pp. 499–506). Springer.

Stebnicki, M. A., Grier, P. J., & Thomas, J. F. (2016). Best practices in the healthcare of LGB military service members, partners, and families. *Journal of Military and Government Counseling, 3*(3), 150–171.

Tzu, S. (2013). *The art of war: Classics of Eastern thought* (L. Giles, Trans.). Barnes & Noble. (Original work published ca. 500 B.C.E.)

U.S. Department of Defense. (2013, February). *2011 Department of Defense Health Related Behaviors Survey of Active Duty Military Personnel*. https://www.murray.senate.gov/public/_cache/files/889efd07-2475-40ee-b3b0-508947957a0f/final-2011-hrb-active-duty-survey-report.pdf

U.S. Department of Veterans Affairs. (2020, April 1). *Compensation*. https://www.benefits.va.gov/compensation/dbq_ListBySymptom.asp

VA Suicide Prevention Program. (2016, July). *Facts about veteran suicide*. https://www.va.gov/opa/publications/factsheets/Suicide_Prevention_FactSheet_New_VA_Stats_070616_1400.pdf

Vogt, D., Brooke, A. L., Leone, D., Wang, J. M., Sayer, N. A., Pineles, S. L., & Litz, B. T. (2014). Endorsed and Anticipated Stigma Inventory (EASI): A tool for assessing beliefs about mental illness and mental health treatment among military personnel and veterans. *Psychological Services, 11*(1), 105–113. https://doi.org/10.1037/a0032780

Witkiewitz, K., & Estrada, A. X. (2011). Substance abuse and mental health treatment in the military: Lessons learned and a way forward. *Military Psychology, 23*(1), 112–123. https://doi.org/10.1080/08995605.2011.548651

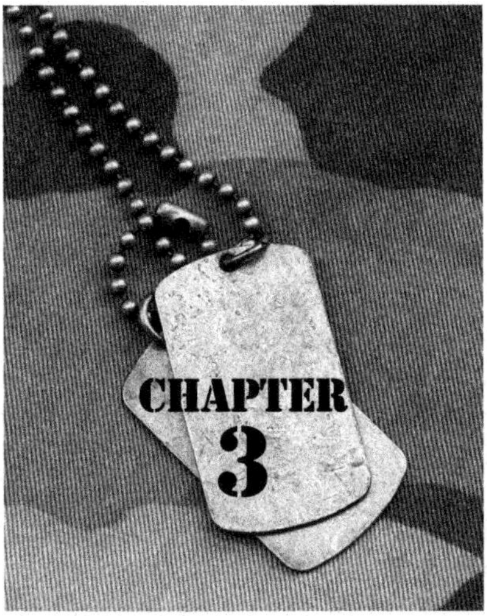

COUNSELING ISSUES FOR WOMEN AND OTHER MINORITIES IN MILITARY LIFE

Suck it up Buttercup!
DID YOU HEAR WHAT I SAID RECRUIT?

—Common military expression

★ ★ ★

Historically, the military has primarily been composed of White men. The U.S. Armed Forces currently reflect, although not proportionally, the different racial, ethnic, and cultural groups that exist in the U.S. population. However, the military also reflects the prevailing political ideology, sociocultural views, attitudes, and perceptions regarding race, gender, and ethnicity. For example, in a 2019 survey of active-duty military personnel (*N* = 1,630), 36% of the troops surveyed directly witnessed White nationalism or ideologically driven racism (Shane, 2020). This behavior has created serious concerns among the House Armed Services Committee, which has held hearings regarding issues of racism in the military. Extremist activities in the military have been a major concern in the Pentagon and the U.S. Department of Defense (DoD), particularly considering a 2015 study reporting that racial and ethnic minorities make up 40% of all active-duty service members (Parker et al., 2017).

Few empirical studies exist in military counseling and psychology that define the unique mental health characteristics of racial and ethnic minorities within the U.S. Armed Forces. Clearly, military life is a much different experience for men and women as well as those individuals who identify culturally and racially as African American; Hispanic and Latino/Latina; lesbian, gay, bisexual, and transgender (LGBT); American Indian; Asian American; or members of other minority groups. In this chapter, I explore the changing demographics in the military and the dynamic issues associated with providing therapeutic services to women and other minority groups in military service.

It is of paramount importance that medical and mental health practitioners know how to facilitate therapeutic services with a diverse group of individuals. Military multicultural researchers, much like in the civilian literature, have emphasized the importance of building a strong rapport with clients who are culturally different because the rates of retention with minorities in psychotherapy treatment are typically lower. In a large study of veteran patients (N = 506,471) being treated for posttraumatic stress disorder (PTSD) in the U.S. Department of Veterans Affairs (VA) system, it was found that Hispanics and Latinos/Latinas, African Americans, and Native Americans had significantly lower rates of retention (defined as psychotherapy treatment for eight sessions or 3 months) compared with White veterans (Shiner et al., 2017). Higher rates of retention were found when same-gender therapists were matched with same-gender patients—particularly when female therapists were matched with female patients. Further research is needed to explore culturally matching therapists and patients who come from diverse cultural backgrounds.

The burgeoning literature in the general area of multicultural counseling consistently reflects two similar points. First, building a strong rapport and earning the circle of trust with clients who are culturally different is critical in establishing a strong therapeutic working alliance. Second, receiving training in multicultural awareness, knowledge, and skills offers therapeutic advantages for sustaining clients for longer periods of time in therapy. Thus, high-functioning clinical military counselors have the competence to work optimally in today's military, which reflects a significantly more diverse group of individuals from different racial and ethnic backgrounds.

Some of the most notable differences among minority individuals in the military are the discrepancies in rank, promotions, branch of service, and other human resource issues. For example, of the 37 current highest ranking military personnel (i.e., generals in the U.S. Army, U.S. Air Force, and U.S. Marine Corps [USMC] and admirals in the U.S. Navy), 32 are White men. The other high-ranking officials are White women (n = 2), African American men (n = 2), and one Asian American man (Bernal, 2018). Additionally, active-duty women and other minorities in lower enlisted non-commissioned officer ranks (e.g., sergeant major, master chief petty officer) and officer ranks (e.g., lieutenant, captain, major) have not been promoted at the same pace. This same lack of diversity is also seen among civilian employees within the Pentagon. The obvious benefits of rank or earned promotions in the military are recognition, pay, benefits, and other privileges afforded to higher ranking officers.

Demographic reporting of gender, race, and ethnicity in the U.S. military will vary somewhat depending on the reporting source. For instance, the U.S. Census Bureau (2019b) categorizes race into five groups: White, Black or African American, American Indian or Alaska Native, Asian and Native Hawaiian, or other Pacific Islander. Ethnicity is divided into two categories: Hispanic and non-Hispanic. Thus, statistical analyses can be somewhat sophisticated and seem to conflict at times because the U.S. Census Bureau reports total resident population estimates that include persons in the military and those living in institutions (e.g., correctional facilities, nursing homes). Therefore, some proportional statistics can have several interpretations. Overall, this chapter cites governmental and nongovernmental sources to statistically describe and depict various racial and ethnic groups.

WOMEN IN THE MILITARY

Women have had a long history in the U.S. military of serving on active duty beginning first in the Army (1901) and then the Navy (1909). The number of women in the military increased during World War I and World War II, when the majority served as nurses, clerks, and communications specialists. After 2001, more than 300,000 women were deployed in support of Operation Iraqi Freedom (OIF) and Operation Enduring Freedom (OEF). By 2013, former Defense Secretary Leon Panetta, who served in President Obama's administration, lifted the ban on women participating in combat operations (Psychological Health Center of Excellence, n.d.), which has paved the way for expanding military occupational specialties (MOSs) and the careers of military women.

Today, the military culture has a distinctive profile. Women compose approximately 16% of the U.S. Armed Forces. Compared with military men, a greater proportion of military women are Black, are not married, and are commissioned officers (Patten & Parker, 2011). Female veterans are just as likely as male veterans to experience the same mental health concerns after separation from military service. Furthermore, studies examining gender differences in PTSD have reported that women are at higher risk than men for postdeployment PTSD (Crum-Cianflone & Jacobson, 2014; Jacobson et al., 2015). This occurrence is due in part to the high incidence and prevalence of unwanted sexual advances, sexual assault, and military sexual trauma (MST) among military women versus men. Additionally, there are other preenlistment mental health conditions (i.e., depression, anxiety, trauma exposure) that have adverse effects on the well-being of military women that may not show up on clinical screenings at the time of separation from service into civilian life. Consequently, in comparison with female veterans from wars prior to 2001, women who serve are more vulnerable to homelessness, unemployment, impaired mental and physical functioning, and other critical issues (Mankowski & Everett, 2016).

MST

Sexual violence, unwanted sexual contact, and harassment among individuals in the U.S. military are pervasive. Data on the range of these critical incidents are difficult for researchers to obtain because there are restricted and unrestricted reporting sources in the military. These acts begin early on in one's career at military academies and during initial military training among enlisted service members, where it has been reported that the number of unwanted sexual encounters jumped more than 30% between 2018 and 2019 (Meyers, 2020). Previously, it was reported in 2018 that MST reached an all-time high with individuals in the military. An estimated 17% of military women and 2.4% of men reported a sexual assault in 2018, showing a dramatic increase over the last several years (Office of People Analytics, 2019).

In survey research, it was estimated that 13,000 women and 7,500 men experienced sexual assault by penetration. Yet, only 6,053 or 1 in 3 service members self-reported their incidents of sexual assault to their unit command (S. G. Smith et al., 2018). Sexual assault in the military most often occurs between junior enlisted ranks (E3 and E4) and against those 17–24 years old, and it is perpetrated by peers who they work, train, and live with. The use of alcohol was involved in 62% of sexual assault cases reported and investigated. Of military women who were sexually assaulted, 85% knew their offender. Of military men, 30% reported that their sexual assault was perpetrated by a woman, whereas 50% were perpetrated by other men. Additionally, 13% of those reporting sexual assault indicated that their offenders were a mix of men and women acting together.

Military women who reported sexual harassment were 3 times more likely to encounter a sexual assault. Additionally, it was reported during the DoD's investigation of assault charges that military women were able to take disciplinary action in only 65% of cases brought to the military courts (S. G. Smith et al., 2018). Overall, there is a positive correlation between unhealthy working environments and sexual assault (Office of People Analytics, 2019). Unhealthy working environments on military bases and installations are marked by sexual harassment (reported by 24.2% of active-duty women and 6.3% of active-duty men), sexual assault, gender discrimination, and workplace hostility. Researchers on MST have indicated that there are multiple barriers to seeking mental health treatment, including (a) stigma, (b) practical barriers to reporting the incident, (c) negative perceptions among some medical and mental health providers, and (d) the belief of the sexual assault survivor that they can handle the mental health symptoms associated with this particular stressful and traumatic event (Zinzow et al., 2015).

In 2018, the DoD launched the Catch a Serial Offender Program, which improved reporting incidents of sexual assault through the use of confidential, anonymous, and nonretaliatory measures as well as hotlines. Beginning in 2018, system-wide DoD sexual assault prevention training and treatment programs have been implemented across all branches of the military for individuals in both the enlisted and officer ranks (DoD, 2019a). At the time of this writing, it is too early in the process to report on data from the strategic plan implemented across the military branches. However, funding is available for several more years to try and make a difference in deterring and reducing sexual assaults among active-duty personnel.

Sexual assault prevention programs, such as the Catch a Serial Offender Program, have been slow in developing over the many years women have enlisted in the military. The program's public relations slogan of "Protecting Our People Protects Our Mission" recognizes that (a) sexual assault is real for all individuals in military life, (b) sexual assault is a crime punishable by military laws, and (c) reporting unwanted sexual advances and sexual assault is encouraged.

Most active-duty and veteran women whom I have seen in my psychotherapy practice reported that they had been sexually harassed, had received unwanted sexual advances, or had been sexually assaulted during their time in military service. Most of these women did not report incidents of MST for fear of repercussions that would harm their career. Many had been told by their drill sergeants during basic training, "Don't report every incidence of sexual harassment because it will hurt your career." In fact, more than half (59%) of sexual assaults were reported to military legal officials. Most women (70%) were discouraged from following through on their sexual assault charges (Campbell & Raja, 2005).

MST is associated with significant mental health problems and other risk factors for women in the military. Most sexual assault survivors are at a significantly higher risk for being diagnosed and treated for PTSD (Kimerling et al., 2007), particularly if they have served in combat operations. Thus, veteran women have a higher incidence of experiencing more frequent and severe clinical symptoms related to depression, PTSD, anxiety, and substance use disorders. Overall, women have poorer mental and physical health outcomes after separation from military service (Frayne et al., 2006).

Most women (62%) who report MST have a history of intimate partner violence (IPV) and other related sexual trauma (Campbell

& Raja, 2005). Active-duty and veteran women who report sexual trauma are sometimes subjected to secondary victimization. This act occurs when medical and mental health providers, regardless of gender, believe that the reported sexual assault did not occur or that somehow the person was responsible for their own sexual assault. In most cases, secondary victimization is primarily projected onto female, rather than male, veterans. Secondary victimization can occur directly and indirectly, as well as consciously and unconsciously, whereby the provider may "blame the victim" for being sexually assaulted. Campbell and Raja (2005) suggested there are few, if any, studies that have examined secondary victimization of active-duty female personnel because of the lack of reporting that occurs during incidents of sexual assault.

It is critical that practitioners evaluate any incidents of unwanted sexual advances or assault during the intake interview and comprehensive clinical assessment. Competent practitioners understand that earning the circle of trust is paramount to self-disclosure. Thus, it is essential that professional providers maintain objectivity before implementation of any therapeutic approaches and when addressing MST. It is also critical that clinicians provide appropriate screening and assessments for high-risk clients who may have sustained MST and IPV, with the intention of integrating these issues into the therapeutic relationship (Tinney & Gerlock, 2017).

It has been reported that the VA system's universal screening of MST has been problematic because policies on administering or approaching such issues are dealt with somewhat sporadically. This omission occurs, in part, because MST itself is not a syndrome or diagnosable mental health condition; thus, many forms of sexual assault tend to be overlooked during initial assessments (Kimerling et al., 2007). During the initial assessment of active-duty and veteran women, practitioners should explore questions about the elements of coercive control or IPV that have occurred before enlistment as well as during and after their military service. IPV is experienced by many couples in the military. Researchers have suggested that IPV is co-occurring with a pattern of chronic mental health problems that are critical to address in session. The intention is to educate your clients about disrupting the cycle of violence, to decrease the risk of harm and lethality, and to maintain a plan of safety (Tinney & Gerlock, 2017).

The Health Insurance Portability and Accountability Act of 1996 (HIPAA), as it applies to the DoD and disclosure of medical and mental health information, allows practitioners to *not disclose* information to base commanders related to mental health and substance abuse education. Disclosure aspects of MST are particularly relevant for service members. HIPAA standards as they relate to those in the U.S. Armed Services are addressed in Title 45 of the Code of

Federal Regulations, Section 164.512(k), and DoD 6025.18-R of the Health Information Privacy Regulation (DoD, 2011). Although it could be implied that education (or psychoeducation) is part of mental health treatment, Title 45 does not provide this level of detail. Thus, the intent of the HIPAA standards allows medical and mental health providers to disclose only a minimum amount of information to military base commanders to satisfy the purpose of the request for any information pertaining to mental health treatment (Psychological Health Center of Excellence, n.d.).

The disclosure aspects of HIPAA are particularly relevant to service members who have experienced MST or IPV and, as a result, may have a mental health condition (i.e., PTSD) requiring treatment or psychoeducation. This component may be viewed by some military mental health advocates as perhaps a move forward with the intention to reduce the stigma of seeking mental health and substance abuse treatment. Under these regulations, the DoD lists nine circumstances in which disclosure is required. The reader is encouraged to review treatment protocols for both MST and IPV as well as the section of the HIPAA standards pertaining to active-duty personnel because this discussion goes beyond the scope and intent of this chapter.

The essential point is that if mental health and substance abuse issues arise as a direct result of MST or IPV, the client can be treated and protected in confidence except under the nine circumstances outlined by the DoD regarding the HIPAA standards. For example, under the category of "Harm to Mission," medical and mental health practitioners in their expert opinion may conclude that the service member's mental health conditions may hinder their ability to stay focused on the mission or exhibit good insight and judgment to fulfill their responsibilities. Thus, mental health professionals may have to disclose such information to the appropriate unit or organization commanders because such an individual may be a harm to themselves and others. Another example is whether the service member is "fit for duty" after inpatient psychiatric or substance abuse hospitalization. Professional practitioners are always encouraged to review the VA's and DoD's practice guidelines and other clinical issues that can provide the best form of treatment in a confidential environment driven by the client's needs.

AFRICAN AMERICANS IN THE MILITARY

Brown (2020) documented African American military achievements dating back to the American Revolutionary War. On March 5, 1770, Crispus Attucks became the first African American to die during a skirmish with British soldiers. On September 21, 1866, the 10th Cavalry Regiment of the U.S. Army was formed during the Indian wars, and African Americans fought in a unit known as the "Buffalo Soldiers," a name created by the Comanche tribe and other Natives they fought against. One of the most decorated African American military units was the 369th Infantry, an all African American unit, under the command of all White officers, who fought in World War I, known as the "Harlem Hellfighters." This brave group of warriors fought back against German offenses and spent 191 days on the front lines, longer than any other American unit at the time. By World War II, African Americans were recognized through military medals and other awards for their heroism. In 1941, during Pearl Harbor, Doris "Dorrie" Miller was awarded the Navy Cross for bravery, placing himself in harm's way while rendering aid to his other unit members while fighting the Japanese. It was not until October 25, 1940, that the first African American, Benjamin O. Davis Sr., held a senior officer rank in the U.S. Army and was later promoted near the end of his career to brigadier general. General Davis, an original member of the famed Buffalo Soldiers, had a son, Benjamin O. Davis Jr., who was the first African American West Point graduate. Davis Jr. followed in his father's footsteps, and at the end of his career, he was awarded the rank of four-star general on December 9, 1998. General Davis Jr. founded and commanded an elite unit of fighters known as the "Tuskegee Airmen," who were attached to the Tuskegee Army Airfield base in Alabama.

The list of achievements and military accomplishments of heroism are recorded in the African American civilian and military literature and can be seen in military museums. Some of the African American military historical events that may not be reported include the testimonials of African American service members who were ignored and passed over for multiple military medals of achievement. Historically, White service members earned promotions to more skilled MOSs, received better military benefits, and had other opportunities that were not afforded to African American service members. There are other countless stories of racial discrimination, isolationism, as well as brutal physical and mental abuse that African American service members had to endure just to achieve the same status as White service members.

It was not until June 1941 that President Truman signed an Executive Order establishing the Fair Employment Practices Commission. Executive Order 9981 on July 26, 1948, abolished racial discrimination in the U.S. Armed Forces. Despite the federal government's well-intentioned efforts, the U.S. Armed Forces were a much different experience for African American service members and veterans. One example is the segregated USMC Camp Montford Point in Jacksonville, North Carolina. This USMC base recruited and trained the largest group of African American Marines, many of whom were deployed during World War II to capture Okinawa (National Montford Point Marine Association, n.d.). Camp Montford Point was commissioned on August 26, 1942, and decommissioned on September 9, 1949. It is attached to the largest USMC amphibious base in the world

(Camp Lejeune) and remains as a historical example of how African Americans began their military careers in segregated military units. Despite the DoD's desegregation movement of U.S. military bases, some Vietnam War veterans have described fighting in all African American units segregated from White troops.

The military barracks of the 21st century reflect significant racial and ethnic diversity (Mershon & Schlossman, 2002). Moskos and Butler (1996) have pointed to the historical fact that social justice, educational opportunities, and other civil and human rights were actually instituted in the U.S. Armed Forces well before the civil rights movement of the 1960s. Leal and Teigen (2018) have suggested that a small but growing group of scholars investigating African Americans, Latinos, and other minorities in the military have largely concluded that military service has had a positive impact on the individual and minority communities, which has afforded career development opportunities that would not otherwise be available in civilian life. For many African Americans, enlistment in military service is viewed as a form of career development, potential for increased socioeconomic benefits, challenge and adventure, a way to increase one's self-esteem and dignity, and opportunities for financial security for their family members (Eighmey, 2006; Gifford, 2005).

African Americans currently in the military continue to experience struggles. I have heard anecdotally from multiple clients in my psychotherapy practice stories of verbal and physical abuse; additional requirements to achieve the same rank, recognition, and career advancement; and many other opportunities that have only been available to White service members. In an independent study on racial disparities and military justice, it was reported that African American service members were substantially more likely than their White counterparts to be punished for infractions and incidents as codified in the Uniform Code of Military Justice (Christensen & Tsilker, 2017). Data obtained independently through the Freedom of Information Act, not furnished by the DoD, show a much different military experience for African Americans and other minority groups in terms of fair and equal treatment as it relates to behaviors punishable by the military code of justice (e.g., substance use, physical altercations, job performance requirement). Military justice may reflect judicial bias, much like civilian courts, in terms of criminal convictions of African Americans and other minorities who are incarcerated at significantly higher rates than their White counterparts.

HISPANICS AND LATINOS/LATINAS IN THE MILITARY

The U.S. Census Bureau (2018) reported that there are more than 58.9 million Americans who identify as Hispanic or Latino/Latina, which represents the largest ethnic minority group in the United

States today. The U.S. federal government considers only two ethnic groups and divides ethnicity into two categories: Hispanic or Latino/Latina and non-Hispanic or non-Latino/Latina (U.S. Census Bureau, 2019b). Many Hispanics or Latinos/Latinas identify with a certain race (White, African American, Asian, Pacific Islander, or Native American). Accordingly, Hispanics encompass a highly diverse group in terms of country of origin, geographic region, immigrant generation from which they came, sociopolitical ideology, religious and spiritual beliefs, as well as many other variables.

The Office of Management and Budget (2020) requires federal agencies to collect and report statistical data on the two categories of ethnicity and then describe Hispanics or Latinos/Latinas as descendants of Mexico, Puerto Rico, Cuba, South or Central America, or another Latin American country. The federal government classification of "Hispanic" does not have full acceptance among the culture, and many prefer a national or panethnic identity based on their country of origin or ancestral birthplace (Delgado-Romero et al., 2008; Sue et al., 2019). For instance, some prefer the term "Mexican American," "Latino/Latina," or "Spanish American," whereas others identify and state their cultural identity as "I am an American." Salinas and Lozano (2017) have examined the literature that advocates the term *Latinx* to describe persons of Hispanic and Latino/Latina culture. Latinx is typically used in higher education and is a gender-neutral term that advocates for individuals living along the gender continuum. The DoD does not use the term Latinx when describing Hispanics or Latinos/Latinas in the military. Thus, for consistency with DoD policies, terms, and definitions, I use the terms Hispanic or Latino/Latina.

The number of Hispanics enlisting in military service each year has risen significantly from 11.5% in 2003 to almost 17% in 2010 (Patten & Parker, 2011). In 2019, recruiters across all branches of the military had difficulty recruiting military personnel, except for Hispanic individuals. In fact, each year more than 20,000 Hispanics have enlisted in the U.S. military. Hispanic women (ages 18–44) represent about 16% of the U.S. civilian population and 13% of the total military population. In North Carolina alone, Hispanic Army recruits grew by 66% between 2014 and 2017 (Linford & Raynor, 2018).

Aside from demographic and statistical representation of Hispanics, a better understanding of some unique attributes within the Hispanic military culture is important to improve the quality of medical and mental health care as well as when considering career counseling approaches. For example, researchers have reported a positive correlation between military service and Hispanic veterans obtaining good careers, particularly in more technical fields (Cancio, 2018). As shown in the career development literature, industries that employ persons with good technical skills (i.e., internet technology support, telecommunications, computer software support engineering) have higher salaries with an excellent occupational outlook. Military service provides advance schools of training and college tuition support to acquire such skills—most of which are transferable to civilian occupations.

Accordingly, higher levels of education and job skills are critical when considering that Hispanics graduate from high school at substantially lower rates than non-Hispanic Whites or African Americans. In fact, only 51% of male Hispanics and 65% of female Hispanics, ages 17–21, earn a high school diploma (Asch et al., 2009). Although military service is a significant predictor of educational achievement beyond high school for Hispanic service members and veterans, multiple variables can affect positive career growth, transition from active duty to civilian life, and optimal mental and physical health. Many factors—including the number and length of deployments, negative critical events that occurred during military service, and other critical incidents—have affected Hispanic veterans' mental and physical health. In addition, service-connected disabilities and multiple other factors can hinder successful transition to education, occupations, and careers for Hispanic veterans.

Hispanic military veteran health is an important topic to discuss because they are a population of interest among epidemiologists and other behavioral health researchers. The critical health issue of tobacco use among Hispanic veterans appears in the literature because of the long-term health effects involving multiple body systems and diseases. Few studies have analyzed and reported on tobacco use and nicotine addiction in the Hispanic military population. In a secondary analysis of the 2014–2015 Tobacco Use Supplement of the Current Population Survey administered by the U.S. Census Bureau, Hammett et al. (2019) compared a nationally representative cohort of Hispanic veterans' and nonveterans' smoking cessation behaviors. Currently, Hispanics are the third largest smoking demographic in the United States and receive less access to good medical and mental health care. Additionally, they receive significantly fewer interventions than White military service members in terms of smoking cessation treatment resources.

Tobacco use and nicotine addiction among all service members and veterans, regardless of race and ethnicity, have long-term health implications because tobacco is one of the most addictive substances in the U.S. military. Tobacco use among service members is part of acculturating to military life. It is a health concern particularly for Hispanics and Latinos/Latinas because of the frequency of use, abuse, and long-term health implications. The Hispanic and Latino/Latina population is projected to almost double within the next 20 years (National Center for Veterans Analysis and Statistics, 2019). Thus, looking ahead, it is critical for military medical and mental health providers to encourage smoking prevention and cessation programs within the overall military behavioral and mental health system.

Few studies have untangled the statistical inconsistencies of the incidence and prevalence of the multiple medical, physical, and mental health experiences of Hispanics. One challenging aspect about delving into the medical and mental health military literature is the conflicting conclusions in the research. For example, the literature in epidemiology supports that Hispanics tend to experience better health outcomes than non-Hispanic Whites, despite having a lower socioeconomic status and less access to health care in the United States (Franzini et al., 2001). Some researchers have reported that Hispanics, as a group, have a higher life expectancy and lower death rate than non-Hispanic Whites. Extensive research in epidemiology and other health-related fields has examined this phenomenon, which was first noted by Markides and Coreil (1986) as the "Hispanic paradox." Part of the paradox may begin with the ambiguity of the term *Hispanic* itself and how individuals within the culture identify with other racial and ethnic groups in North America. D. P. Smith and Bradshaw (2006) have suggested that the Hispanic paradox does not exist. They reached this conclusion primarily because of inconsistencies in the way in which Hispanic data have been previously collected by vital statistics and the U.S. Census Bureau.

In one study, Andersen and Newman (2005) used the behavioral model for health service utilization and compared the mental health treatment–seeking behaviors of Latino and non-Latino White veterans of the Iraq and Afghanistan wars. The findings suggest that, when adjusting for various demographic and mental health variables, there were no significant differences between the Latino and non-Latino White groups seeking mental health treatment at the VA's system of health care (Pittman et al., 2019). Interestingly, Latino and non-Latino White veterans appear more similar than different in regard to clinical symptoms, characteristics, and utilization of mental health referral and treatment resources in the post-9/11 era. These findings suggest that perhaps the common factor is that OEF and OIF veterans are similarly affected medically, physically, cognitively, psychologically, emotionally, and socially as a result of fighting in one of the longest wars in U.S. history.

Some researchers have noted that Hispanics' level of acculturation to the military culture is different than Whites'. Complicating the multicultural mental health researcher's conundrum is the person's attitude and perception toward achieving good medical and mental health. For example, it has been reported that many of the psychological and emotional needs of Hispanic and Latino/Latina military service members relate more to issues of ethnic identity, immigration, acculturation, discrimination, and negative cultural stereotypes (Manoleas & Garcia, 2003). The level of acculturation may be a causal effect in Hispanic and Latino/Latina health outcomes. For example, the U.S. population as a whole has poorer health outcomes than other countries because of poor nutrition; sedentary activities; lack of movement throughout one's day; and the resultant conditions of obesity, heart disease, and cancers that all relate to the "American lifestyle" habits. Consequently, multiple deficits exist in the mind, body, and spiritual wellness of American society (Gordon, 1996; Schlitz et al., 2005; Shannonhouse et al., 2016; Stebnicki, 2016; Weil, 1995).

As for Hispanics who have maintained certain family values, alternative health care practices, and other beliefs, there may be a resiliency factor in their overall health—hence, the Hispanic paradox. For example, some authors have pointed to several factors, including the strength of Hispanic family values and extended social networks. The Hispanic folk healing traditions of *curanderismo* may also heal the mind, body, and spirit and have a positive effect on health outcomes (Gonnering & Riley, 2017; Gonzalez-Chevez, 2005; Romero-Ramirez, 2016).

I bring these issues forward because of the significant increase in the Hispanic military population and the need for developing medical and mental health treatment approaches consistent with the culture's values and belief system. Heavy reliance on traditional Western models of health and healing, which are solely evidence-based practices and approaches, may hinder earning the circle of trust with the Hispanic military culture. The emerging field of multicultural military health deserves increased attention to advance optimal medical and mental health treatment approaches that are culturally sensitive.

ASIAN AMERICANS AND PACIFIC ISLANDERS IN THE MILITARY

Few studies exist that describe mental health counseling issues as they relate to Asian Americans and Pacific Islanders serving in the U.S. military. This group is primarily identified by the DoD as Asian Americans and Pacific Islanders. Thus, little is known about the specific medical and mental health issues concerning this group of veterans (Colpe et al., 2015; Tsai, Whealin, & Pietzak, 2014). Asian American culture has been studied extensively in the nonmilitary population and multicultural counseling literature. This strong base of research may be helpful in elucidating some of the more important issues for military mental health practice.

Asian Americans and Pacific Islanders have had a relatively short history in U.S. military service given that this population began immigrating to North America in the mid-1800s. Although it is recognized that persons of Asian descent served in the War of 1812 and fought in the Civil War on both sides in the Union and Confederate Armies, it was not until the desegregation of the U.S. military in 1948 and late into the 20th century that Asian Americans and Pacific Islanders were allowed into military school and academies and were awarded with military rank, promotions, medals, and other honors afforded to White military service members.

It is difficult to generalize and culturally contextualize persons of Asian and Pacific Island ancestry because they compose a diverse racial and ethnic group of 60 different subgroups typically depicted by the various sociocultural backgrounds and geographic regions of the world (Tsai, Whealin, & Pietzak, 2014). The major groups, in order of size, include Filipinos, Chinese, Koreans, Vietnamese, Asian Indians, and Japanese. These groups are unique in that they differ in terms of language, religious and spiritual beliefs, family composition and values, level of education, and income (Sue et al., 2019). Asian Americans experience varying degrees of assimilation or acculturation both in the United States and in military life. Thus, it is difficult to generalize and attribute the same cultural characteristics with this group identified by the U.S. Census Bureau and DoD as Asian American and Pacific Islander.

Collectively, Asian Americans and Pacific Islanders compose about 5% of the U.S. population and approximately 1.5% of U.S. military veterans (Tsai, Whealin, & Pietzak, 2014). They are projected to be one of the fastest growing minority groups and will almost double in size by 2060. It is projected that Asian Americans and Pacific Islanders will climb from 15.6 million to 34.4 million or compose 8%–9% of the total U.S. population (U.S. Census Bureau, 2012b). Historically in the United States, Asian Americans and Pacific Islanders have been excluded from society and incarcerated in camps; they have also sustained similar racial stereotypes, discrimination, and loss of human rights as other minority groups. For instance, the Chinese Exclusion Act of 1882—as well as the Exclusion Acts of 1875, 1917, and 1924—resulted in historical trauma and the "perpetual foreigner" stereotype of Americans who were of Asian descent. After the bombing of Pearl Harbor, this practice of racism led to the eventual incarceration of 110,000–120,000 Americans of Japanese descent in "relocation centers," authorized and signed into law by President Franklin D. Roosevelt on February 19, 1942 (Pollard, 2017).

Given the historical adversity faced by Asian Americans and Pacific Islanders, it is difficult for one to reconcile how this cultural group could "swear an oath" to protect America from all enemies foreign and domestic when at one point in history, persons of Asian descent were perceived as the enemy. Also, given the backdrop of the Asian culture being forced into relocation camps, much like the history of other minority groups in America, it is important to recognize that many Asian Americans and Pacific Islanders retain many of their cultural values and beliefs. Asian Americans and Pacific Islanders assimilate and acculturate at differing levels in the United States and live by the individual norms, standards, and family traditions that are based on their overall value system (Sue et al., 2019). From an outsider perspective, one can observe conflicts with Asian family values and the U.S. military, which is composed of predominantly White men.

In attempts to overcome Asian stereotypes, the U.S. military celebrates the heritage of Asian Americans and Pacific Islanders each year during the month of May. This is another indication that today's military is motivated to understand the unique cultural differences reflected in the changing demographics. May is distinct because it marks the anniversary month of the first Japanese immigrants to North America (May 7, 1843). This celebration also recognizes Chinese immigrant laborers for their contributions toward American society and the work they performed in the completion of the transcontinental rail system in the United States (Defense Equal Opportunity Management Institute, 2016).

There are several major differences observed between Asian Americans and other minorities in the U.S. military. From a career perspective, Asian Americans and Pacific Islanders rise through their promotion and rank at a more rapid pace than any other minority group in the military. Asian Americans and Pacific Islanders have enlisted in the military in growing numbers since the war on terrorism began in 2001. Since this time, this group is 28% more likely to achieve officer ranks than other minorities in the military. For example, Asian American and Pacific Islander officers in the U.S. Army have seen a 41% increase between 2004 and 2016. This rate compares with a growth of just 4% for other ethnic minority groups in the U.S. military and an overall decline of 3.1% for African Americans (Heubl, 2018).

There are mental health differences in Asian American and non–Asian American military service members worth noting. The Army Study to Assess Risk and Resilience in Service members, also known as Army STARRS (Colpe et al., 2015), sampled a representative group of nondeployed soldiers (N = 5,428) and collected data on the prevalence of mental health treatment, history of deployments, and other sociodemographic characteristics. This study revealed that Asian Americans and Pacific Islanders had a higher rate of suicide than all other racial and ethnic groups during deployment and those who never deployed. Comparatively, civilian Asian Americans and Pacific Islanders have been found to have much lower suicide rates than other racial and ethnic groups (Leong et al., 2007).

Findings of other studies (e.g., Tsai, Whealin, & Pietzak, 2014) related to the approximately 1.5 million U.S. veterans identifying as Asian American and Pacific Islander also deserve closer attention when it comes to utilization of medical and mental health services. For instance, Asian American and Pacific Islander troops who served during OEF and OIF, who were mostly female, were less likely to be deployed than other minority groups. Asian Americans and Pacific Islanders have also reported better general health, fewer service-connected disabilities or VA ratings, a lower smoking rate, and higher income levels than other veteran minorities. However, one study that used a national sample of Asian American and Pacific Islander veterans, when adjusting for differences in sociodemographic and health characteristics, indicated that this group utilized the VA system of health care at about the same rates as other racial and ethnic groups in terms of outpatient, inpatient, and emergency services (Tsai, Desai, et al., 2014). Asian American and Pacific Islander veterans were also more likely to be permanently homebound than all other racial and ethnic groups, even though most Asian Americans live in urban and not rural areas of the country. In terms of differences, the research suggests that Asian American veterans reported fewer symptoms of PTSD and had better overall physical health compared with Pacific Islander veterans. Further analysis in all studies would be required.

Overall, the research and clinical practice in mental health and multicultural counseling support the notion that Asian Americans and Pacific Islanders seek mental health services less frequently than other racial and ethnic minority groups. However, the analysis and discussion in this area are not clearly elucidated in the literature. Thus, within-group differences and level of acculturation in the military culture may need to be considered. One aspect that is clear is the negative stigma and stereotypes that exist among Asian Americans and Pacific Islanders regarding mental health issues, which complicates treatment-seeking behaviors.

AMERICAN INDIANS AND ALASKA NATIVES IN THE MILITARY

Historically, the relationship between the U.S. government and American Indians in the military is quite complicated. The DoD and the VA continue to publish data gathered from various research projects with the intention of educating military health care providers on the unique cultural attributes of the American Indian population, with a special emphasis on the health disparities of this at-risk group of service members and veterans (VA, 2012). Another intention of such DoD and VA research projects is to educate practitioners on the accomplishments, achievements, and honors earned by Native American military service members and veterans. To honor the American Indian and Alaska tribes who have served in the U.S. military, the DoD has proclaimed National Native American Heritage Month, which is celebrated each November. This recognition was only recently instituted and was inaugurated in November 2011.

Native American warriors have a rich history of service in the U.S. Armed Forces. They understand the sacrifice of protecting their homeland. In World Wars I and II, the Navajo, Comanche, Choctaw, Hopi, Cherokee, and other American Indian tribes provided essential communications and intelligence-gathering information to troops using their native languages. After the Navajo code was developed, the USMC developed a code-talking school where more than 400 Navajos were recruited (National Museum of the American Indian, n.d.). The U.S. Army also deployed code talkers who used tribal languages to communicate sensitive material. These sophisticated methods of communication were critical in many missions where American troops required top secret and sensitive information to be shared within special units.

Native American Indian is a term that reflects the various indigenous peoples of North America, including Alaska Natives. Just as with the other cultures highlighted in this chapter, additional resources and skills would be beneficial to work competently with this diverse group of individuals. The intention of this section is to feature important considerations for medical and mental health care of American Indians and Alaska Natives. Many interrelated variables intersect with civilian and military life, which challenges even the most experienced providers. It is of paramount importance to consider that Native people, just like other minorities, may be reluctant to seek Western medical and mental health treatment because of the historical trauma inflicted by White ethnic cultures.

Before 1900, few Indian tribes were included in the decennial federal census. None were recognized in the 1790–1840 censuses. It was not until 1860 that the general population of American Indians was included for the first time in a federal census (U.S. Census Bureau, 2019a). This exclusion speaks volumes about the lack of early recognition by the federal government to acknowledge the 567 Native American nations (Bureau of Indian Affairs, 2018), who speak approximately 252 different languages. The National Congress of American Indians (2020) recognizes 573 Indian nations, tribes, bands, pueblos, communities, and villages. The 10 largest American Indian tribes in order of population include the Cherokee, Navajo, Choctaw, Blackfeet, Muscogee, Iroquois, Chippewa, Apache, Pueblo, and Chickasaw (Centers for Disease Control and Prevention, 2018). The largest Alaska Native tribes in order of population include Alaskan Athabascan, Aleut, Inupiat, Tlingit-Haida, and other various smaller tribes (U.S. Census Bureau, 2012a). By the end of the 18th century in North America, the American Indian population was annihilated by wars, disease, extermination, and seizure of Indian lands (Sue et al., 2019), resulting in the majority of American Indian nations decreasing to about 10% of their original population (Richardson, 1981).

Eventually, the U.S. government forced isolation and segregation of American Indians by requiring them to live on reservations—land originally owned by their Native ancestors. Around this period, the U.S. government instituted American Indian boarding schools, where frequent mental and physical abuse and cruel punishments were perpetrated by White ethnic teachers and staff. The primary task was to sequester Native children, contain and control their environment, and then provide a White education, teaching the children to speak English only. Essentially, these boarding schools basically forced Native peoples to give up their languages, beliefs, values, spirituality, and most other cultural aspects of their identity. Various court rulings provided U.S. citizenship to all native-born Indians in the United States around 1924 (Simms, 2016). Despite citizenship, acts of racism, discrimination, and isolation persisted on reservations, which continued to perpetrate the historical trauma experienced.

Just like other groups, American Indians' ancestry can vary racially and ethnically because of consenting and nonconsenting sexual contact and the rape perpetrated by Europeans and Africans. For at least the last 500 years, American Indians also have had a heritage that is mixed intertribally. It is estimated that at least 98% of the Native population is tribally mixed and approximately 75% is racially mixed (Russell, 1997). The term "full blood" refers to Native Americans who consider themselves to be 100% descended from one Indian tribe, which would be about 2% of the Native population. The term Native American Indian is legally defined and is based on "blood quantum" (one fourth or more Native American blood) and ancestry (Bureau of Indian Affairs, 1988). Native nations across the United States set different standards and criteria for membership in a tribe. For instance, the Cherokee Nation of Oklahoma enrolls members with a blood quantum as little as 1/512. Most tribes or nations require one-fourth blood quantum (Russell, 1997). The issue of blood quantum is quite controversial among Native tribes and is a sensitive topic related to ethnic and racial identity. The culture itself decides who can participate in the various tribal traditions and rituals, be involved with social and political affairs, as well as benefit from any tribal revenues earned (Garrett, 2008).

Indeed, there are the extraordinary social stressors placed on Indian tribes by the non-Native culture's ignorance and discrimination of the American Indians' legal and political structure; system of religious and spiritual beliefs; and health care practices integrating the mind, body, and spirit (Mehl-Madrona, 1997; Rainbow Eagle, 2003; Solomon & Wane, 2005). Additionally, there are significantly high levels of poverty, socioeconomic distress (with the lowest median income of any racial or ethnic group), unemployment, illiteracy, and low education (Mehl-Madrona, 1997; Office of the Surgeon General, 2001; Simms, 2016; VA, 2012). The medical and mental health disparities with the American Indian population have the highest prevalence and incidence among any minority group. Epidemiological data in this area are difficult to obtain because Native American Indians are not frequent users of medical and mental health care because of a distrust of Western or European medicine.

Prominent in the mental health literature are the high incidence and prevalence of depression, substance use disorders, PTSD, and suicide (Harley, 2018; Simms, 2016; Yurkovich & Hopkins-Lattergrass, 2004).

In a 2012 VA report, there were approximately 31,500 American Indian and Alaska Native active-duty service members, of whom 84% were male and 16% female. The total population of Native veterans is 154,305, with approximately 89% male and 11% female. Harley's (2018) extensive research on American Indian and Alaska Native civilians has indicated that this group experiences a higher rate of disability than any other minority group in the United States. Today, Native nations are extremely high risk and have higher mortality rates because of stroke, tuberculosis, chronic liver disease (linked to alcoholism), substance use disorders, motor vehicle accidents, diabetes, heart disease, and obesity.

The epidemiological characteristics of American Indians should be of interest to medical and mental health providers and researchers given that, before enlistment, the Native culture is predisposed to multiple high-risk medical, physical, and behavioral lifestyle risk factors. After American Indian service members transition to civilian life, they may be returning to the same high-risk environment. This designation would be defined by a lack of adequate resources for medical and mental health care given the backdrop of the culture's status as socioeconomically disadvantaged, societal stigma and discrimination of the culture itself, and other behavioral lifestyle risk factors that place individuals in harm's way, such as substance use and co-occurring disorders as well as suicidality.

Overall, it should be noted that access to statistical data regarding American Indian health disparities is challenging for researchers because (a) Indian reservations are sovereign nations and can determine what aspects of the culture can be disclosed publicly; (b) there is a general distrust of non-Natives given the historical trauma inflicted by Western cultures; and (c) tribal communities are often located geographically in rural areas of the United States, which makes access difficult. Accordingly, data collected by the DoD and VA may only offer partial discovery of health risk factors because of the Native nonveteran health of the culture, which has many challenges.

LGBT MILITARY SERVICE MEMBERS, PARTNERS, AND FAMILIES

The stress of military life has multiple mental and physical health challenges for all service members, veterans, and military families. It becomes significantly more challenging for the estimated 50,000–150,000 active-duty and ready-reserve service members who are LGBT (Gates, 2010; Gates & Herman, 2014; Meadows et al., 2018). These challenges relate with the negative cultural stereotypes directed at and stigma associated with the LGBT community. It becomes confounding for some military service providers because the LGBT military culture comprises other racial, ethnic, and cultural identities.

LGBT military service members have a long history of serving honorably in the U.S. Armed Services despite some exclusionary policies that have created stigma and institutionalized heterosexism (W. B. Johnson et al., 2015). In September 2011, with the repeal of the "Don't Ask, Don't Tell" (DADT) federal law (DADT Repeal Act, 2010), LGB individuals were afforded civil protections to serve in the military. Basically, the repeal of DADT allowed LGB persons to openly discuss their sexual orientation with medical and mental health providers without fear of retribution, denial of promotions, discrimination, and other aspects of military life that might compromise their physical safety, mental health, and overall well-being (W. B. Johnson & Buhrke, 2006).

In April 2019, in accordance with the Trump administration's policies, the Pentagon initiated a ban on service members who openly identify as transgender, transsexual, or queer (C. Johnson, 2019b). The current DoD (2019b) policies under the Trump administration view different categories of eligibility by current service members versus individuals who self-identify as LGB and want to enlist in the U.S. Armed Services. Policies on enlistment and active-duty service members further segregate service members who identify as transgender and those with and without a diagnosis of gender dysphoria. At the time of this writing, there are no civil protections afforded to military service members who come out, who are diagnosed with gender dysphoria, or who are in gender transition-related medical care such as cross-sex hormone therapy or sexual reassignment surgery. The Trump administration's policy exempts transgender individuals who came out during the Obama administration from a military discharge. Thus, in some situations, depending on the branch of service and which direction the "political winds" are blowing, LGBT service members are able to serve under a "grandfathering" policy.

The DoD (2019b) has stated that their policies are meant to ensure that the U.S. military maintains the highest standards necessary to achieve maximum readiness, deployability, and lethality. Historically, many conflicts have arisen between the DoD and the Trump administration's policies. For example, a spokesperson from the Pentagon indicated that transgender persons will be grandfathered in and that they do not anticipate enforcing any military discharges (C. Johnson, 2019b). Although the DoD (2019b) policy indicates that transgender service members may continue serving in their current MOS, eligibility determination is typically handled on a case-by-case basis.

The consequences of governmental policies are confusing and frustrating, and they anger many LGBT service members and veterans. The policies oftentimes result in transgender concealment, which ultimately amplifies the service member's feelings of vulnerability and sense of belongingness, which subsequently affects mental and physical well-being (W. B. Johnson et al., 2015; Stebnicki et al., 2015; Witten, 2007). Basically, there are no career benefits to openly coming out in a typical hypermasculine, heterosexual, and primarily White male work environment. Because of the negative attitudes, perceptions, and stigma associated with LGBT service members, this group requires advocates for justice. Most importantly, LGBT service members and veterans require a confidential and secure environment for medical, physical, and mental health treatment.

Without protections for active-duty LGBT personnel, these individuals will likely face continued sexual stigma and discrimination, and they will not be afforded equal job opportunities, much like what occurred historically with women and people of color in the military (Burkes, 2011; Fassinger, 2008). As a result of the Trump administration's ban on transgender service members, two important military LGBT advocacy organizations merged in 2019. The American Military Partner Association and OutServe-SLDN (Servicemembers Legal Defense Network) formed one organization: the Modern Military Association of America (C. Johnson, 2019a).

LGBT service members who have enlisted in military service must be evaluated on the basis of individual merit, productivity, job performance, as well as mental and physical fitness for duty, just like all other qualified service members. Fitness for duty has rarely been an issue for LGBT military service members. Despite the Trump administration's policies on LGBT service members, research has clearly shown that LGBT service members do not compromise military readiness, unit cohesion, security, or mission success (Bateman & Dalvi, 2004; Frank, 2010; W. B. Johnson & Buhrke, 2006).

In a meta-analysis, Stebnicki et al. (2015) found that LGBT active-duty service members and veterans had significantly poorer physical and mental health outcomes compared with their heterosexual counterparts in the military. There are multiple causes of health disparities among LGBT military service members, partners, and families. Despite the repeal of DADT, the act of coming out to medical or mental health providers continues to have real career consequences for many active-duty personnel (Goldbach & Castro, 2016; Valentine et al., 2019). These repercussions are especially prevalent on military installations because treatment notes are recorded in the electronic medical record, making patient confidentiality vulnerable because the system is open to a larger group of individuals who have access to patient records. Consequently, LGBT service members may delay or avoid going to medical or mental health appointments because of the fear of stigma and discrimination regarding their sexual orientation that may be recorded in the clinical records (Gay and Lesbian Medical Association, 2006; L. Johnson & Federman, 2013).

There are also concerns related to medical and mental health practitioners' deficits in screening, assessment, treatment, and professional training in regard to the unique cultural differences in LGBT service members (McNair & Hegarty, 2010). For instance, if the professional provider is not attuned to the individual's guilt, self-blame, anxiety, anger, or depression that may have resulted from workplace harassment, assault, and stigmatization of the person's sexual preference, then the provider may attribute the etiology of these behaviors and symptoms to a mental health disorder (Dworkin, 2000; Fassinger, 2008). The LGBT service member may be naturally responding to the stereotypes and stigma within the unhealthy military workplace environment.

BEST PRACTICES FOR CLINICIANS

The following guidelines are offered for military counselors to consider when cultivating therapeutic multicultural relationships with women and other minority groups in the military. Exploration and application of these principles will assist in rapport building and the working alliance:

- Facilitate comprehensive clinical assessments, diagnosis, and treatment by demonstrating multicultural competence. Competent clinical military counselors examine their cultural assumptions, myths, stereotypes, and other aspects that could hinder the therapeutic relationship.
- Explore written materials and attend continuing education seminars and workshops on multicultural counseling with intention to increase your awareness, knowledge, and skills on earning the circle of trust to work optimally with persons who are culturally different.
- Identify service members and veterans who are at higher risk for MST and IPV and who may be targets of workplace or unit discrimination. Consider the environmental, sociocultural, and psychosocial aspects and their interactional effects on your client's mental health and well-being.
- Recognize elements of coercive control, IPV, and MST that occurred before, during, and after clients' military service. Identify this pattern of behavior with service members and veterans and facilitate psychoeducation, harm-reduction approaches, and assessment of client lethality for a possible plan of safety.
- Acknowledge that military sexual assault is a crime under the Uniform Code of Military Justice. As a clinician, consider the ethical implications and weigh potential risks and benefits, or any foreseeable harm, that may come to your military client who reports sexual assaults or MST. Support and advocate for your military client's decisions regarding confidentiality.
- Recognize the risk factors, consequences, and psychosocial impact of LGBT service members and veterans coming out to others in their unit. Assist LGBT service members to identify potential risks for workplace discrimination, harassment, and assaults.

- Maintain objectivity with LGBT military clients during therapeutic interactions to ensure that they are free to express their preferred gender and cultural identity. Although the LGBT literature suggests that coming out is generally associated with positive personal growth and optimal well-being, concealment—at times—is a personal preference and a coping mechanism for one's military career.
- Recognize and facilitate therapeutic strategies to assist military service women and other minorities choose how they want to assimilate or acculturate into the larger military culture.
- Acknowledge that all service members and veterans belong to many different racial, ethnic, and cultural groups besides the military culture. Recognize the within-group differences in the military culture itself (e.g., officer, non-commissioned officer, or enlisted service member), MOS types (e.g., infantry, Osprey pilot, reconnaissance), and gender identity (e.g., male, female, LGBT).
- Facilitate therapeutic strategies that assist service members to choose the degree and level of affiliation and acculturation they desire within the military culture or community. Competent and ethical clinical military counselors understand, support, and recognize their choices.
- Explore the importance of your military client's family's cultural values; the influences acculturation and assimilation have; and any cultural practices that serve as a natural resource and support for optimal mental, physical, and spiritual well-being.
- Understand how to assess the high-risk behavioral health and lifestyle factors that could potentially lead to long-term medical, physical, and mental health consequences. Recognize health disparities in veterans' medical and mental health while balancing this vulnerability with acceptance into the military culture.

CONCLUDING REMARKS

This chapter emphasizes that military life can be a much different experience for women, African Americans, Hispanics or Latinos/as, Asian Americans and Pacific Islanders, American Indians and Alaska Natives, LGBT individuals, and other cultural minorities. Historically, the U.S. Armed Services have been predominantly composed of heterosexual White men. However, with the considerable increases in women and minority military service members, it is essential that competent clinical military counselors understand and recognize some of the unique cultural and within-group differences among active-duty personnel and veterans. Thus, it is essential that medical and mental health clinicians integrate multicultural practices into their comprehensive clinical assessment. These cultural differences affect how clinicians assess, diagnose, and treat mental health conditions.

REFERENCES

Andersen, R. N., & Newman, J. F. (2005). Societal and individual determinants of medical care utilization in the United States. *The Milbank Memorial Fund Quarterly, 83*(4), 1–32. https://doi.org/10.1111/j.1468-0009.2005.00428.x

Asch, B. J., Buck, C., Klerman, J. A., Kleykamp, M., & Loughran, D. S. (2009). *Military enlistment of Hispanic youth: Obstacles and opportunities.* RAND.

Bateman, G., & Dalvi, S. (2004, February). *Multinational military units and homosexual personnel.* University of California, Santa Barbara. https://escholarship.org/uc/item/0tj9033f

Bernal, R. (2018, July 22). Latinos aren't reaching top military positions, study shows. *The Hill.* https://thehill.com/latino/398139-latinos-arent-reaching-top-military-positions-study-shows

Brown, S. M. (2020). *African-American heroism in the military.* Military.com. https://www.military.com/history/african-american-heroism-in-the-military

Bureau of Indian Affairs. (1988). *American Indians today.*

Bureau of Indian Affairs. (2018, January 30). *Indian entities recognized and eligible to receive services from the United States Bureau of Indian Affairs.* https://www.federalregister.gov/documents/2018/01/30/2018-01907/indian-entities-recognized-and-eligible-to-receive-services-from-the-united-states-bureau-of-indian

Burkes, D. J. (2011). Lesbian, gay, and bisexual victimization in the military: An unintended consequence of "Don't Ask, Don't Tell"? *American Psychologist, 66*(7), 604–613. https://doi.org/10.1037/a0024609

Campbell, R., & Raja, S. (2005). The sexual assault and secondary victimization of female veterans: Helping-seeking experiences with military and civilian social systems. *Psychology of Women Quarterly, 29*(1), 97–106. https://doi.org/10.1111/j.1471-6402.2005.00171.x

Cancio, R. (2018). Examining the effect of military service on education: The unique case of Hispanic veterans. *Hispanic Journal of Behavioral Sciences, 40*(2), 150–175. https://doi.org/10.1177/0739986318761849

Centers for Disease Control and Prevention. (2018, December 21). *Tribal population.* https://www.cdc.gov/tribal/tribes-organizations-health/tribes/state-population.html

Christensen, D., & Tsilker, Y. (2017, May 5). *Racial disparities in military justice: Findings of substantial and persistent racial disparities within the United States Military Justice System.* Protect Our Defenders. https://www.protectourdefenders.com/wp-content/uploads/2017/05/Report_20.pdf

Colpe, L. J., Naifeh, J. A., Aliaga, P. A., Sampson, N. A., Heeringa, S. G., Stein, M. B., Ursano, R. J., Fullerton, C. S., Nock, M. K., Schoenbaum, M. L., Zaslavsky, A. M., & Kessler, R. C. (2015). Mental health treatment among soldiers with current mental health disorders in the Army Study to Assess Risk and Resilience in Service Members (Army STARRS). *Military Medicine, 180*(10), 1041–1051. https://doi.org/10.7205/MILMED-D-14-00686

Crum-Cianflone, N. F., & Jacobson, I. (2014). Gender differences in postdeployment post-traumatic stress disorder among service members and veterans of the Iraq and Afghanistan conflicts. *Epidemiologic Reviews, 36*(1), 5–18. https://doi.org/10.1093/epirev/mxt005

Defense Equal Opportunity Management Institute. (2016, May). *Asian American Pacific Islander Heritage Month: Walk together, embrace differences, build legacies.* https://dod.defense.gov/Portals/1/features/2016/0516_aapi/Asian_American_Pacific_Islander_Heritage_Month_2016_slide_3.pdf

Delgado-Romero, E. A., Galvan, N., Hunter, M. R., & Torres, V. (2008). Latino/Latina Americans. In G. McAuliffe (Ed.), *Culturally alert counseling: A comprehensive introduction* (pp. 323–352). Sage.

Don't Ask, Don't Tell Repeal Act of 2010, Pub. L. 111-321, 124 Stat. 3515.

Dworkin, S. H. (2000). Individual therapy with lesbian, gay, and bisexual clients. In R. P. Perez, K. A. DeBore, & K. J. Bieschke (Eds.), *Handbook of counseling and psychotherapy with lesbian, gay, and bisexual clients* (pp. 157–181). American Psychological Association.

Eighmey, J. (2006). Why do youth enlist? Identification of underlying themes. *Armed Forces & Society, 32*(2), 307–328. https://doi.org/10.1177/0095327X05281017

Fassinger, R. E. (2008). Workplace diversity and public policy: Challenges and opportunities for psychology. *American Psychologist, 63*(4), 252–268. https://doi.org/10.1037/0003-066X.63.4.252

Frank, N. (2010, March 3). *What does the empirical research say about the impact of openly gay service on the military? A research memo.* Palm Center. https://www.palmcenter.org/wp-content/uploads/2017/12/WhatDoesEmpiricalResearchSayAboutOpenlyGayService.pdf

Franzini, L., Ribble, J. C., & Keddie, A. M. (2001). Understanding the Hispanic paradox. *Ethnicity & Disease, 11*(3), 496–518.

Frayne, S. M., Parker, V. A., Christiansen, C. L., Loveland, S., Seaver, M. R., Kazis, L. E., & Skinner, K. M. (2006). Health status among 28,000 women veterans: The VA Women's Health Program Evaluation Project. *Journal of General Internal Medicine, 21*(3), 540–546. https://doi.org/10.1111/j.1525-1497.2006.00373.x

Garrett, M. T. (2008). Native Americans. In G. McAuliffe (Ed.), *Culturally alert counseling: A comprehensive guide* (pp. 220–254). Sage.

Gates, J. (2010, May). *Lesbian, gay, and bisexual men and women in the US military: Updated estimates.* The Williams Institute. https://escholarship.org/uc/item/0gn4t6t3

Gates, J., & Herman, J. L. (2014, May). *Transgender military service members in the United States.* The Williams Institute. https://escholarship.org/uc/item/1t24j53h

Gay and Lesbian Medical Association. (2006). *Guidelines for care of lesbian, gay, bisexual, and transgender patients.* http://www.glma.org/_data/n_0001/resources/live/GLMA%20guidelines%202006%20FINAL.pdf

Gifford, B. (2005). Combat casualties and race: What we can learn from the 2003–2004 Iraq conflict. *Armed Forces & Society, 31*(2), 201–225. https://doi.org/10.1177/0095327X0503100203

Goldbach, J. T., & Castro, C. A. (2016). Lesbian, gay, bisexual, and transgender (LGBT) service members: Life after "Don't Ask, Don't Tell." *Current Psychiatric Reports, 18*(6), Article 56. https://doi.org/10.1007/s11920-016-0695-0

Gonnering, R., & Riley, W. (2017). The paradoxical "Hispanic paradox": The dark side of acculturation. *Emergence: Complexity and Organization, 19*(3–4), 1–10.

Gonzalez-Chevez, L. (2005). Latin American healers and healing. In R. Moodley & W. West (Eds.), *Integrating traditional healing practices into counseling and psychotherapy* (pp. 85–99). Sage.

Gordon, J. S. (1996). *Manifesto for a new medicine: A guide to healing partnerships and the wise use of alternative therapies.* Perseus Books.

Hammett, P. J., Nelson, D., Burgess, D. J., Fu, S. S., & Pinsker, E. A. (2019). Population smoking characteristics and smoking cessation behaviors in a nationally representative cohort of Hispanic veterans and Hispanic non-veterans. *Military Medicine, 184*(11–12), e594–e600. https://doi.org/10.1093/milmed/usz102

Harley, D. A. (2018). American Indians and Alaska Natives with disabilities in rural, tribal lands, frontier regions, and plain states. In D. A. Harley, N. A. Ysasi, M. L. Bishop, & A.R. Fleming (Eds.), *Disability and vocational rehabilitation in rural settings: Challenges to service delivery* (pp. 239–268). Springer.

Health Insurance Portability and Accountability Act of 1996 (HIPAA), Pub. L. 104-191, 42 U.S.C. § 300gg, 29 U.S.C. §§ 1181–1183, and 42 U.S.C. §§ 1320d–1320d9.

Heubl, B. (2018, July 29). Asian-Americans' rise through the U.S. military ranks—In charts. *Nikkei Asian Review.* https://asia.nikkei.com/Spotlight/Datawatch/Asian-Americans-rise-through-the-US-military-ranks-in-charts

Jacobson, I. G., Donoho, C. J., Crum-Cianflone, N. F., & Maguen, S. (2015). Longitudinal assessment of gender differences in the development of PTSD among U.S. military personnel deployed in support of the operations in Iraq and Afghanistan. *Journal of Psychiatric Research, 68,* 30–36. https://doi.org/10.1016/j.jpsychires.2015.05.015

Johnson, C. (2019a, May 12). LGBT groups merge to form Modern Military Association of America. *Washington Blade*. https://www.washingtonblade.com/2019/05/12/lgbt-groups-merge-to-american-military-association-of-america/

Johnson, C. (2019b, April 12). Trump's transgender military ban now in effect. *Washington Blade*. https://www.washingtonblade.com/2019/04/12/trumps-transgender-military-ban-now-in-effect/

Johnson, L., & Federman, E. J. (2013). Pathways and barriers to care for LGBT veterans in the U.S. Department of Veterans Affairs (VA). *Journal of LGBT Issues in Counseling, 7*(3), 218–235. https://doi.org/10.1080/15538605.2013.812928

Johnson, W. B., & Buhrke, R. A. (2006). Service delivery in a "Don't Ask, Don't Tell" world: Ethical care of gay, lesbian, and bisexual military personnel. *Professional Psychology: Research and Practice, 37*(1), 91–98. https://doi.org/10.1037/0735-7028.37.1.91

Johnson, W. B., Rosenstein, J. E., Buhrke, R. A., & Haldeman, D. C. (2015). After "Don't Ask Don't Tell': Competent care of lesbian, gay, and bisexual military personnel during the DoD policy transition. *Professional Psychology: Research and Practice, 46*(2), 107–115. https://doi.org/10.1037/a0033051

Kimerling, R., Gima, K., Smith, M. W., Street, A., & Frayne, S. (2007). The Veterans Health Administration and military sexual trauma. *American Journal of Public Health, 97*(12), 2160–2166. https://doi.org/10.2105/AJPH.2006.092999

Leal, D. L., & Teigen, J. M. (2018). Military service and political participation in the United States: Institutional experience and the vote. *Electoral Studies, 53*, 99–110. https://doi.org/10.1016/j.electstud.2017.09.004

Leong, F. T., Leach, M. N., Yeh, C., & Chou, E. (2007). Suicide among Asian Americans: What do we know? What do we need to know? *Death Studies, 31*(5), 417–434. https://doi.org/10.1080/07481180701244561

Linford, A., & Raynor, D. (2018, June 14). NC leads the nation in Army recruits. And much of the growth is from Hispanics. *The News & Observer.* https://www.newsobserver.com/news/local/article213010354.html

Mankowski, M., & Everett, J. E. (2016). Women service members, veterans, and their families: What we know now. *Nurse Education Today, 47*, 23–28. https://doi.org/10.1016/j.nedt.2015.12.017

Manoleas, P., & Garcia, B. (2003). Clinical algorithms as a toll for psychotherapy with Latino clients. *American Journal of Orthopsychiatry, 73*(2), 154–166. https://doi.org/10.1037/0002-9432.73.2.154

Markides, K. S., & Coreil, J. (1986). The health of Hispanics in the southwestern United States: An epidemiologic paradox. *Public Health Reports, 101*(3), 253–265. https://www.jstor.org/stable/4627869

McNair, R. P., & Hegarty, K. (2010). Guidelines for the primary care of lesbian, gay, and bisexual people: A systematic review. *Annals of Family Medicine, 8*(6), 533–541. https://doi.org/10.1370/afm.1173

Meadows, S. O., Engel, C. C., Collins, R. L., Beckman, R. L., Cefalu, M., Hawes-Dawson, J., Waymouth, M., Kress, A. M., Sontag-Padilla, L., Ramchnand, R., & Williams, K. M. (2018). *2015 Department of Defense Health Related Behaviors Survey (HRBS)*. RAND. https://www.rand.org/pubs/research_reports/RR1695.html

Mehl-Madrona, L. (1997). *Coyote medicine: Lessons from Native American healing*. Fireside.

Mershon, S., & Schlossman, S. (2002). *Foxholes and color lines: Desegregation in the U.S. Armed Forces.* John Hopkins University Press.

Meyers, M. (2020, January 30). Sexual assault reports are up a third this year at military service academies. *Military Times.* https://www.militarytimes.com/news/your-military/2020/01/30/sexual-assault-reports-are-up-a-third-this-year-at-the-military-service-academies/?utm_source=Sailthru&utm_medium=email&utm_campaign=EBB%2001.31.20&utm_term=Editorial%20-%20Military%20-%20Early%20Bird%20Brief

Moskos, C. C., & Butler, J. S. (1996). *All that we can be: Black leadership and racial integration the Army way.* Basic Books.

National Center for Veterans Analysis and Statistics. (2019, May 3). *Veteran population projection model 2016.* https://www.va.gov/vetdata/docs/Demographics/VetPop_Infographic_2019.pdf

National Congress of American Indians. (2020, February). *Tribes, nations, and the United States: An introduction.* http://www.ncai.org/about-tribes

National Montford Point Marine Association. (n.d.). *Who is a Montford Point Marine?* https://montfordpointmarines.org/

National Museum of the American Indian. (n.d.). *Code talking: Intelligence and bravery.* https://americanindian.si.edu/education/codetalkers/html/chapter4.html

Office of Management and Budget. (2020, April 21). *About Hispanic origin.* https://www.census.gov/topics/population/hispanic-origin/about.html

Office of People Analytics. (2019, May). *2018 Workplace and Gender Relations Survey of Active Duty Members: Overview report.* https://www.sapr.mil/sites/default/files/Annex_1_2018_WGRA_Overview_Report.pdf

Office of the Surgeon General. (2001). *Mental health: Culture, race, and ethnicity: A supplement to Mental health: A report of the Surgeon General.* Substance Abuse and Mental Health Services Administration. https://www.ncbi.nlm.nih.gov/pubmed/20669516

Parker, K., Cilluffo, A., & Stepler, R. (2017, April 13). *6 facts about the U.S. military and its changing demographics.* Pew Research Center. https://www.pewresearch.org/fact-tank/2017/04/13/6-facts-about-the-u-s-military-and-its-changing-demographics/

Patten, E., & Parker, K. (2011). *Women in the U.S. military: Growing share, distinctive profile.* Pew Research Center. https://www.pewresearch.org/wp-content/uploads/sites/3/2011/12/women-in-the-military.pdf

Pittman, J. O. E., Baer, J., Everett, J., Dozier, M. E., Almklov, E., & Afari, N. (2019). Post-9/11 Latino veteran mental health service utilization. *Military Behavioral Health, 7*(4), 414–425. https://doi.org/10.1080/21635781.2019.1595228

Pollard, T. (2017). Hollywood's Asian-Pacific pivot: Stereotypes, xenophobia, and racism. *Perspectives on Global Development and Technology, 16*(1–3), 131–144. https://doi.org/10.1163/15691497-12341424

Psychological Health Center of Excellence. (n.d.). *Women's mental health: Women in the U.S. military.* https://www.pdhealth.mil/clinical-guidance/women-s-mental-health

Rainbow Eagle. (2003). *Native American spirituality: A walk in the woods.* Rainbow Light and Company.

Richardson, E. H. (1981). Cultural and historical perspectives in counseling American Indians. In D. W. Sue (Ed.), *Counseling the culturally different: Theory and practice* (pp. 216–255). Wiley.

Romero-Ramirez, M. G. (2016). Mental health counseling with Hispanic/Latinos: The role of culture in practice. In I. Marini & M.A. Stebnicki (Eds.), *The professional counselor's desk reference* (2nd ed., pp. 145–150). Springer.

Russell, G. (1997). *American Indian facts of life: A profile of today's tribes and reservations.* Russell Publications.

Salinas, C., Jr., & Lozano, A. (2017). Mapping and recontextualizing the evolution of the term *Latinx*: An environmental scanning in higher education. *Journal of Latinos and Education, 18*(4), 302–315. https://doi.org/10.1080/15348431.2017.1390464

Schlitz, M., Amorok, T., & Micozzi, M. S. (2005). *Consciousness and healing: Integral approaches to mind-body medicine.* Elsevier.

Shane, L., III. (2020, February 6). Signs of White supremacy, extremism up again in poll of active-duty troops. *Military Times.* https://www.militarytimes.com/news/pentagon-congress/2020/02/06/signs-of-white-supremacy-extremism-up-again-in-poll-of-active-duty-troops/?utm_source=Sailthru&utm_medium=email&utm_campaign=EBB%2002.06.20&utm_term=Editorial%20-%20Military%20-%20Early%20Bird%20Brief

Shannonhouse, L. R., Myers, J. E., & Sweeney, T. J. (2016). Counseling for wellness. In I. Marini & M. A. Stebnicki (Eds.), *The professional counselor's desk reference* (pp. 617–623). Springer.

Shiner, B., Westgate, C. L., Harik, J. M., Watts, B. V., & Schnurr, P. P. (2017). Effect of patient-therapist gender match on psychotherapy retention among United States veterans with posttraumatic stress disorder. *Administrative Policy Mental Health, 44*(5), 642–650. https://doi.org/10.1007/s10488-016-0761-2

Simms, W. F. (2016). The Native American Indian client. In I. Marini & M. A. Stebnicki (Eds.), *The professional counselor's desk reference* (pp. 127–131). Springer.

Smith, D. P., & Bradshaw, B. S. (2006). Rethinking the Hispanic paradox: Death rates and life expectancy for US non-Hispanic White and Hispanic populations. *American Journal of Public Health, 96*(9), 1686–1692. https://doi.org/10.2105/AJPH.2003.035378

Smith, S. G., Zhang, X., Basile, K. C., Merrick, M. T., Wang, J., Kresnow, M., & Chen, J. (2018). *The National Intimate Partner and Sexual Violence Survey (NISVS): 2015 data brief update release.* National Center for Injury Prevention and Control, Centers for Disease Control and Prevention.

Solomon, A., & Wane, N. N. (2005). Indigenous healer and healing in a modern world. In R. Moodley & W. West (Eds.), *Integrating traditional healing practices into counseling and psychotherapy* (pp. 52–60). Sage.

Stebnicki, M. A. (2016). Integrative approaches in counseling and psychotherapy: Foundations of mind, body, and spirit. In I. Marini & M. A. Stebnicki (Eds.), *The professional counselor's desk reference* (2nd ed., pp. 593–604). Springer.

Stebnicki, M. A., Grier, P. J., & Thomas, J. F. (2015). Best practices in the healthcare of LGBT military service members, partners, and families. *Journal of Military and Government Counseling, 3*(3), 150–171.

Sue, D. W., Sue, D., Neville, H. A., & Smith, L. (2019). *Counseling the culturally diverse: Theory and practice.* Wiley.

Tinney, G., & Gerlock, A. (2017, December). *Screening, assessment, and intervention model for intimate partner violence perpetration and co-occurring combat-related conditions.* Battered Women's Justice Project. https://www.bwjp.org/assets/screening-assessment-intervention-model-for-intimate.pdf

Tsai, J., Desai, M. U., Cheng, A. W., & Chang, J. (2014). The effects of race and other socioeconomic factors on health service use among a nationally representative sample of U.S. veterans. *Psychiatry Quarterly, 85*(1), 35–47. https://doi.org/10.1007/s11126-013-9268-0

Tsai, J., Whealin, J. M., & Pietzak, R. H. (2014). Asian American and Pacific Islander military veterans in the United States: Health service use and perceived barriers to mental health services. *American Journal of Public Health, 104*(Suppl. 4), S538–S547. https://doi.org/10.2105/AJPH.2014.302124

U.S. Census Bureau. (2012a, January). *The American Indian and Alaska Native population: 2010.* https://www.census.gov/library/publications/2012/dec/c2010br-10.html

U.S. Census Bureau. (2012b, December 12). *U.S. Census Bureau projections show a slower growing, older, more diverse nation a half century from now.* https://www.census.gov/newsroom/releases/archives/population/cb12-243.html

U.S. Census Bureau. (2018, September 13). *Hispanic Heritage Month 2018.* https://www.census.gov/newsroom/facts-for-features/2018/hispanic-heritage-month.html

U.S. Census Bureau. (2019a, December 17). *Census of American Indians.* https://www.census.gov/history/www/genealogy/decennial_census_records/censuses_of_american_indians.html

U.S. Census Bureau. (2019b, May 2). *Combining data—A general overview.* https://www.census.gov/about/what/admin-data.html

U.S. Department of Defense. (2011, August 17). *Command notification requirements to dispel stigma in providing mental health care to service members.* https://www.esd.whs.mil/Portals/54/Documents/DD/issuances/dodi/649008p.pdf

U.S. Department of Defense. (2019a, April 9). *Department of Defense annual report on sexual assault in the military: Fiscal year 2018.* https://www.sapr.mil/sites/default/files/DoD_Annual_Report_on_Sexual_Assault_in_the_Military.pdf

U.S. Department of Defense. (2019b, March 13). *5 things to know about DoD's new policy on military service by transgender persons and persons with gender dysphoria.* https://www.defense.gov/explore/story/Article/1783822/5-things-to-know-about-dods-new-policy-on-military-service-by-transgender-perso/

U.S. Department of Veterans Affairs. (2012, September). *American Indian and Alaska Native servicemembers and veterans.* https://www.va.gov/tribalgovernment/docs/aian_report_final_v2_7.pdf

Valentine, S. E., Shipherd, J. C., Smith, A. M., & Kauth, M. R. (2019). Approving affirming care for sexual and gender minority veterans. *Psychological Services.* Advance online publication. https://doi.org/10.1037/ser0000378

Weil, A. (1995). *Spontaneous healing: How to discover and enhance your body's natural ability to maintain and heal itself.* Fawcett Columbine.

Witten, T. M. (2007). Transgender bodies, identities, and healthcare: Effects of perceived and actual violence and abuse. In J. J. Kronenfeld (Ed.), *Inequalities and disparities in health care and health: Concerns of patients, providers and insurers* (pp. 225–249). Emerald Group.

Yurkovich, E., & Hopkins-Lattergrass, I. (2004). *A needs assessment focused on defining health and health seeking behaviors of Native American Indians experiencing severe and persistent mental illness. Phase II: Preliminary findings.* University of North Dakota, College of Nursing.

Zinzow, H. M., Britt, T. W., Pury, C. L. S., Jennings, K., Cheung, J. H., & Raymond, M. A. (2015). Barriers and facilitators of mental health treatment-seeking in U.S. active duty soldiers with sexual assault histories. *Journal of Traumatic Stress, 28*(4), 289–297. https://doi.org/10.1002/jts.22026

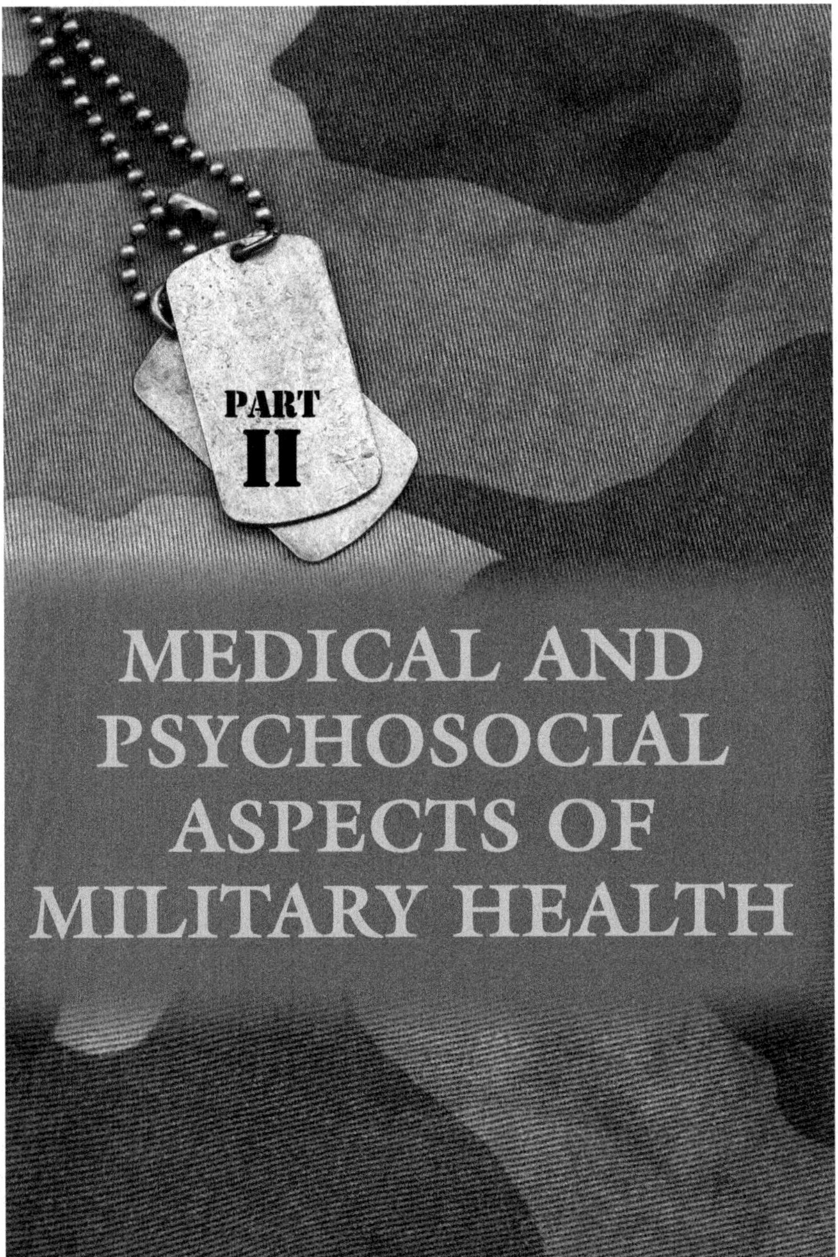

PART II

MEDICAL AND PSYCHOSOCIAL ASPECTS OF MILITARY HEALTH

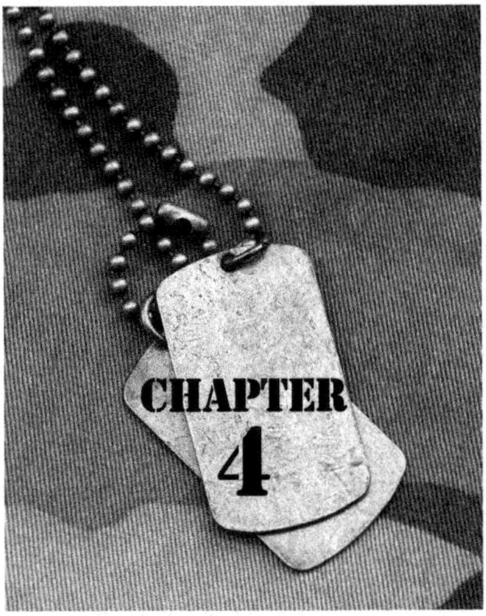

MAPPING THE MILITARY BRAIN: THE NEUROSCIENCE OF MILITARY STRESS AND TRAUMA

If "the body keeps the score,"
it's always going to be a tie between the mind and body.
However, the spirit will always send things into overtime.

—Mark A. Stebnicki, 2019
(based on the book
The Body Keeps the Score
by B. Van Der Kolk, 2014)

★ ★ ★

Service members exposed to combat operational stress are at high risk for a wide range of psychiatric, neurobehavioral, and neurocognitive conditions. Compelling new research in neuroscience is at the forefront of understanding the physiological, psychological, emotional, and neurocognitive significance of trauma survivors in military and civilian life. Indeed, the brains of service members are mapped differently than those of civilians, given the nature of the military as a high-risk occupation. This chapter focuses on the multiple complex mediating variables within the brain's complex neuropathways that record, transpose, replicate, and reproduce a wide range of psychological responses that underlie optimal brain health, neurocognitive functioning, and performance. The neuroscience of mapping the military brain has practical applications for coping and resiliency after trauma that extend beyond the clinical laboratory.

THE MILITARY NEUROSCIENCE RESEARCH AGENDA

The dynamic neural structure and function of the brain, as they relate to human emotions and acquired trauma, are quite complex and go well beyond the scope and intention of this chapter. However, a discussion of this subject matter is paramount because the literature in neuroscience has risen dramatically over the last 10 years and has multiple applications to the military culture. Kosal and Huang (2015) reported that multiple government agencies and collaboratives have applied for grant funding through the National Institutes of Health, which operates a budget to fund approximately $1.9 billion in neuroscience research. There is a 12-year initiative to fund multiple government agencies and private partners working on everything from the impact of stress to solving life-threatening neuromuscular diseases (i.e., Alzheimer's disease, amyotrophic lateral sclerosis, dementia).

Kaku (2014) remarked that perhaps one of the most ambitious neuroscience projects to date is taking place in Switzerland with Dr. Henry Markham, who is the driving force behind the Human Brain Project. Markham has received more than $1 billion in support thus far to reverse engineer the human brain in terms of its DNA using the Blue Gene computer system. The research agenda is somewhat akin to the Human Genome Project, which uses scientists around the world to unravel the mysteries located within people's DNA. One motivation for the Human Brain Project is to aid in the research of serious mental health conditions that have reached epidemic proportions around the globe. Such endeavors are closely tied to the military's research agenda.

Besides the civilian side of grant-funded initiatives in neuroscience research, the military has demonstrated a need by underscoring the link between peak human performance on the battlefield and maintaining operational tempo that would enhance troop readiness. Currently, it appears that the U.S. Department of Defense (DoD) and private military research contractors are at the forefront of cutting-edge research illuminating the potential of human performance as it relates to neuroscience and warfighting. It is difficult to estimate brain research and development activities within the U.S. military primarily because of "black budget" items. However, the DoD has spent more than $3 billion in the last decade on innovative research projects (Kosal & Huang, 2015) that depict Hollywood-style, science-fiction action movies complete with all the computer-generated imagery effects and scenarios that approximate everyday life in the distant future. For example, one project uses invisible energy beams that can produce severe burns on enemy combatants at a remote distance of approximately 600 yards. Other projects are not reported publicly because of operational security issues.

Besides defense weapon systems research, the Defense Advanced Research Projects Agency is funding neuroscience research regarding brain implants to decrease the symptoms of combat-related posttraumatic stress. The U.S. Army has requested more than $55 million for a research program involving human engineering, neuroergonomics, robotics, human behavior, and other related projects intended to predict and enhance the warfighter's cognitive performance on the battlefield and to lessen the symptoms of posttraumatic stress (Howell, 2017; Kosal & Huang, 2015). There is also an increased interest in developing pharmaceuticals that work on neurotransmitters, such as dextroamphetamine (i.e., "speed"), which is used by the U.S. Air Force to enhance alertness. Other neuropharmaceuticals have been authorized for use to assist in improving cognition and fatigue (i.e., Ritalin) and lessen the need for sleep (i.e., Provigil).

Given the current pathway of grant funding to the DoD and larger government contractors, the use of neuroscience research by defense and intelligence agencies has raised concerns by neuroscientists and bioethicists who have concluded there is a strong need for institutional review and oversight (Howell, 2017; Kosal & Huang, 2015). For example, the new technology could be utilized by defense and intelligence agencies as a type of lie-detector examination or to control one's emotions and thoughts (Rippon & Senior, 2010; Rosenberg & Gehrie, 2007). Lower ranking service members and recruits could be vulnerable to experimentation within highly classified projects by command, peer pressure, and the manipulation and promise of promotional and career opportunities.

The use of neuropharmaceuticals in eliminating or suppressing traumatic memories in combat operators has also been called into question because of ethical concerns (Henry et al., 2007). For example, in a mission-forward environment where the life and safety of others in the unit depend on each operator's quick and decisive action, any distraction can hinder operational tempo and safety. Accordingly, one of the primary functions of field medics and military medical practitioners is to return the warfighter to combat. Thus, the use of a beta-blocker to reduce posttraumatic stress symptoms (PTSSs) could be of value to infantry or elite fighting units. All these matters, and many more, are ethically complex and take on the important issues related to human rights and consent for treatment, which are commonly monitored and reviewed in civilian health care and clinical settings. There are indeed realities of utilizing human participants in experiential designs.

EARLY BEGINNINGS IN NEUROSCIENCE RESEARCH

Biopsychophysiologists agree that the structure and function of the brain and spinal cord act in coordination for the sensory input of all body systems. Neuroscientists suggest the brain encompasses a much larger universe than just an organ that resides inside the cranium. Historically, neuroscience studies have used experimental designs and neuro-methodology with primarily White male participants in controlled environments to measure the basic psychological and physiological reactions of human emotions. Earlier neuroscientists utilized more invasive studies with animals, generalizing these experimental results to human populations. However, this task was difficult because the neurological mechanisms as well as the conscious-unconscious cognitions, thoughts, and emotions within the human brain are more complex. As a result of earlier researchers in the 1970s, the specialties of neurology and neuropsychology emerged in treating traumatic brain injuries (TBIs) and helping to provide standardized assessments, diagnosis, and treatment with the intention of rehabilitating the individual to their maximum medical improvement.

The field of psychoneuroimmunology, a word coined by Ader (1990), began as a discipline that provided new insights into how people's thoughts, emotions, and cognitions influenced their total psychophysiology. The problem with expanding research at the time was the unavailability of technology to test newer hypotheses such as stated in today's neuroscience research. Accordingly, psychoneuroimmunology researchers had a difficult task because, as Sapolsky (1998) has asserted, people's emotions—particularly during the stress response—have their own unique physiological arousal patterns of magnitude, frequency, and intensity. This distinctiveness results, in part, because individuals differ in how they turn on their stress response in relation to other emotions within the core structures of the brain. Some have hypothesized that people's emotional experiences manifest in other neurologically complex ways because of their different personality traits and states, behavioral response patterns, and motivational states (Mayne & Ramsey, 2001).

NEUROSCIENCE RESEARCH FOR THE 21ST CENTURY

Neuroscience in the 21st century has gone well beyond what is observed in the clinical laboratory and neurorehabilitation hospital unit. The expanding field in neuroscience, at times, presents strong philosophical and theoretical differences in how the brain functions at the quantum or multiverse level. This variance is due, in part, to the specific area of neuroscience that is driving the research agenda (i.e., experimental neuropsychology, neurobiology, biochemistry). Therefore, to understand the complex nature of the human brain, researchers had to expand to various disciplines over the years, such as psychology, biomedicine, computer science, mathematics, electrical and chemical engineering, as well as other well-defined areas of neurocognitive sciences.

Earlier research tended to highly depend on behavioral observation, self-report, standardized psychological measures, and basic physiological response patterns as measured by 20th-century technology. Thus, it was difficult to test modern neuroscience research hypotheses because of the lack of available technology. Today's standard neuroscience research protocols and designs utilize technology that can measure neurochemical and electrical impulses with a variety of brain imaging techniques (i.e., resting-state functional connectivity magnetic resonance imaging, functional magnetic resonance imaging; Tracy & Randles, 2011). Advancements in noninvasive neuroimaging and stimulation techniques are now commonly utilized in clinical experimental laboratories. Technology—such as functional magnetic resonance imaging, near-infrared spectroscopy, magnetoencephalography, single-photon emission computed tomography, and transcranial magnetic stimulation (TMS)—requires significant start-up funding (Raji et al., 2015). The typical university or college experimental psychology lab cannot afford the resources and personnel to fund such projects. As a result, much of the funding goes to government agencies, private corporations, not-for-profit organizations, and other well-connected entities with attachments to political insiders.

Overall, a more comprehensive biopsychosocial understanding of stress, trauma, and its impact on the mind, body, and spirit of service members and veterans is required to move forward with a research agenda in military neurosciences. Partnering civilian and military neuroscience research projects offers greater opportunities for (a) developing neurobiopsychosocial screening and assessment instruments, (b) decreasing combat operational stress and PTSSs in service members and veterans, and (c) facilitating medical and mental health treatments as well as neurocounseling approaches that are military specific.

NEUROBIOLOGICAL EXPRESSION OF STRESS AND TRAUMA

Brain development has been evolving for quite some time. Perhaps theories of evolution underlie the ideological and philosophical difference among neuroscience researchers. The most widely accepted scientific theory of evolution (Out of Africa) suggests that the roots of human ancestors can be traced back to Africa between 200,000 and 60,000 years ago (Cann et al., 1987). Current genomic studies suggest that human ancestors were a mix of Neanderthals who bred with modern humans from the European, East Asian, and Sub-Saharan African continents (Sankararaman et al., 2014). A common core of human biology across all cultures is that 99.9% of people's DNA is the same (Genome News Network, 2003; Weil, 1995). Even a .01%–.09% difference in DNA creates variances in eye, hair, and skin color; physical shape and appearance; and the distinct genetic code that predisposes people to certain chronic illnesses or diseases.

Although the function and structure of the brain of human ancestors may have been similar to those of modern humans, the complexity in its response to patterns of communication, learning complex and detail-oriented tasks, conscious-intentional and unconscious-unintentional thoughts and feelings, behavioral coping styles, and problem-solving abilities is much different today. Still, there is no one else on the planet exactly like "You," when considering the .01%–.09% individual differences in our DNA. Our individual uniqueness is expressed by our behavior, personality traits and states, and cognitive interpretation of life; it is also conveyed by how we perceive our environment, bring meaning to how we live, as well as the way in which we communicate verbally and nonverbally. How we turn on our stress response and the unique biopsychosocial mechanisms that prompt this variability are highly individualized.

For some service members and veterans, exposure to extraordinary stressful and traumatic events creates habitual, chronic, and persistent patterns that are well organized and can be mapped neurobiologically. Thus, emotions, stress, and trauma are mapped into the neurobiological and neurocognitive processes of the brain (Lazarus, 1999). Accordingly, understanding the perceptual-cognitive-emotional expression of everyday stress and traumatic stress is critical during therapeutic interactions with service members and veterans. Since the mid-1960s, neuroscientists have hypothesized that certain basic emotions (i.e., anger, fear, sadness, happiness, disgust) are neurobiological in nature. Each emotion arises from a distinctive part of the brain that can be measured from neurochemical and electrical impulses with a variety of brain imaging technology (Raji et al., 2015; Tracy & Randles, 2011).

Counter to the basic emotions theory of the brain, experimental studies have shown that specific emotions, located within the salience network of the brain, do not exist within the core structure of the human brain (Touroutoglou et al., 2015). Rather, in the "conceptual act" theory, emotions arise from the individual's perception, experience, and intensity of the emotion itself. Basic emotions do not arise from a separate neural network. Rather, they are constructed from a combination of activity in the core brain system that performs functions such as memory, sensory perception, as well as receptive and expressive language. In the conceptual act theory of emotions, neuroscientists predict that the same intrinsic networks engage during a variety of emotions exhibited by individuals.

Pessoa (2014) has argued that the "network" perspective of brain function should be replaced by the more common view of examining different regions of the brain. For instance, the most parsimonious view of the brain from a neuroscience perspective is to map a specific region of the brain (i.e., the visual cortex as it relates to visual perception). However, other regions of the brain do not have this specific one-to-one mapping relationship because it becomes more complex as to which areas of the brain are engaged (i.e., cognitive, perceptual, motor, emotional).

THE IMPACT OF COMBAT OPERATIONAL STRESS ON THE BRAIN

To comprehensively describe and understand the complex nature of extraordinary stressful and traumatic events among combat operators, Lieberman et al. (2016) designed a study that viewed the effects of real-world stress as opposed to laboratory-induced stress. Their hypothesis suggests that as a result of psychologically stressful activities associated with military training and combat operations, the service members' physiological reactions have a distinct signature. This signature can be measured in terms of cognitive functioning, types and levels of stress hormones released in the body, heart-rate variability, as well as the body's need for nutritional intake and some of the metabolic changes that occur in real-world combat operational stress.

To test this hypothesis, Lieberman et al. (2016) studied the impact of severe acute stress while assessing a wide array of psychological, physiological, and biochemical markers among U.S. Army active-duty soldiers going through the Survival, Evasion, Resistance, and Escape (SERE) training school. This advance training school is required for U.S. military personnel who may be deployed to regions that are at high risk for enemy capture. The training lasts for about 3 weeks, and military service members are taught the SERE techniques that will save their lives and the lives of their fellow troops. Simulated enemy capture, mock interrogations, and other techniques are used to subject service members to real-world experiences of severe and intense physical, emotional, and psychological distress. The hypothesis for SERE training is based on stress-inoculation research suggesting that service members' performance is likely to improve during stressful scenarios by simulating exposure to combat operations and extraordinary traumatic events. Theoretically, some military neuroscience researchers have suggested that prior exposure to traumatic stressors enhances warfighters' coping and resiliency skills during and after trauma exposure (Morgan et al., 2000, 2001).

As a result of SERE training, Lieberman et al. (2016) found that acute and chronic stress, modest physical demands, and food deprivation in this intensive training program substantially degraded service members' mental and psychological functioning. This finding was derived from the administration of multiple cognitive tests and mood scales. From biophysiological measures taken, the catabolic hormone cortisol increased, and the anabolic hormone testosterone decreased noticeably. Lieberman et al. further reported that because of stress-induced sympathetic nervous system arousal, there were substantial elevations in epinephrine, norepinephrine, and heart rate.

The key findings in this and other military research (Lieberman et al., 2005; Morgan et al., 2000, 2001) have significant implications for military medical and mental health providers. Combat service personnel have significant neurobiological and psychological challenges while engaging enemy combatants. This reaction is mapped in the brain and cannot be simulated in civilian life or in an experimental laboratory. Those service members who are underfed or who have poor nutritional intake while engaged in combat operations show extremely high levels of stress with depressed mood and impulsive anger. Additionally, because of sleep deprivation and continuous exposure to extraordinary and traumatic stressors, the neurobiological and psychological functioning decreases the warfighters' focus, concentration, and memory. From a neurobiological perspective, many warfighters are fighting for survival.

From a psychological perspective of observable patterns of behavior and self-report, paradoxically the warfighter "appears" in control and somewhat balanced. Overall, prior and repeated combat exposure and longer deployments can lower the service member's ability for coping and resiliency even with low-stress tasks. From a neurobiological and psychological perspective, rebooting the brain back to the "old normal" has minimal capability because the "new normal" has been mapped in the physiology of the brain for chronic and persistent patterns of unhealthy thoughts, feelings, experiences, and behaviors.

There appears to be inconclusive evidence regarding the long-term effects of military combat exposure and combat training (i.e., SERE). Stress inoculation may or may not improve overall optimal physiological and psychological function and performance. For the most part, the brain can be mapped for survival, which benefits military personnel by decreasing combat operational stress experienced during live combat missions. However, survival has no benefits for veterans who want to "reboot their hard drive" for optimal neurocognitive and neuropsychological functioning. Continuous exposure to stress and traumatic stress creates chronic and persistent patterns of neurobiological and psychological functioning that limits mental, physical, and cognitive capacity.

NEUROPATHOPHYSIOLOGY OF THE MILITARY BRAIN

Why do some military service members develop long-term chronic symptoms of posttraumatic stress disorder (PTSD) and others do not? The answer to this question has eluded and challenged neuroscientists and clinical researchers for quite some time. However, at this moment in neuroscience history, theory and application have advanced because of new imaging techniques. Current theoretical understanding and clinical research have given birth to newer experimental designs that have the capabilities of measuring real-world stress in military life. Inviting various disciplines into the neuroscience field has cultivated elegant experimental designs for application in clinical practice. This research is critical in treating TBI and complex PTSD.

Despite this mini revolution in neuroscience, there is still much to learn about the impact that stress and traumatic stress have on the various body systems. From a PTSD and TBI or blast injury perspective, mental health and neurocounseling practitioners are eager to understand the applications of neuroscience for service members' and veterans' brain health. The application for clinical military counseling is important in treating affect, mood regulation, maladaptive behaviors, learning, memory, and cognitions as well as in addressing issues related to overall mental and physical well-being. Other areas of practical application include comprehending the "dark matter" or unconscious portion of the brain, which has the potential to reveal deeper understanding and meaning underlying an individual's emotions, thoughts, cognitions, and behaviors.

THE NEUROSCIENCE OF COMPLEX PTSD AND TBI

From a neurocognitive and clinical mental health counseling perspective, PTSSs largely reflect the brain's maladaptive associative learning mechanisms during and after a traumatic event. PTSD blended with TBI complicates diagnosis and treatment. For instance, the sequence of events that occurs with PTSSs—such as reexperiencing and avoiding trauma triggers as well as negative alterations in cognitions, mood regulation, affect, and hyperarousal and reactivity—is complicated by the impaired neuroconnections seen in TBI. This impairment, in combination with a poorly regulated sympathetic-parasympathetic response found in PTSD, complicates the diagnostic and treatment options for the patient. The symptomatology of PTSD and TBI converge at some points in terms of residual functional capacity; however, PTSD and TBI are rarely distinguished in therapy because medical professionals diagnose and treat the physiological and structural aspects of TBIs, whereas mental health professionals diagnose and treat PTSD. Perhaps one of the most critical factors in working with service members and veterans with PTSD and TBI is the lack of coordination between the medical and mental health professionals after the patient with TBI is discharged from the acute care brain injury rehabilitation unit.

The co-occurring conditions of complex PTSD and TBI are of significant interest in the military neurosciences because of the complicated diagnostic and treatment options required for healing the individual's medical and mental health aspects. Prominent learning theorists have suggested that critical events related to PTSSs initiate a cycle of associative learning. The person learns maladaptive coping and defense mechanisms that become the new normal. Rebooting the system preenlistment or preinjury is not possible at this point in the military brain. The neurobiological and neuropsychological expression of PTSSs is mapped in the service member's conscious and unconscious. For some combat veterans, every situation looks like a provocation (e.g., driving in traffic, shopping in a crowded grocery store) because their thoughts, feelings, and behaviors are overgeneralized into the associative learning part of the brain. The TBI overlay impairs the person's ability to "read" environmental cues, regulate mood and anxious behaviors, process experiences that may be confusing or vague in nature, use their rational-emotive-behavioral processes, reduce inhibitions or impulsive reactions, and have a felt sense of safety and security (Homan et al., 2019; Lissek & Van Meurs, 2015). Thus, theories of associative learning are key in understanding, predicting, tracking, and decreasing the severity of PTSSs that can be complicated by TBI.

The biophysiological markers of PTSD can be measured through the region of the emotional brain known as the amygdala. The amygdala appears to be the locus of associative learning in the brain and has been linked to chronic and persistent PTSSs (Schiller et al., 2008). The amygdala plays a key role in threat detection as well as the fear learning and fear expression response. This region of the brain also regulates the manifestation of anger as well as many other emotions expressed in PTSSs and co-occurring clinical mental health symptoms (Lin et al., 2017).

Homan et al. (2019) has suggested that size, structure, and volume do matter when it comes to the amygdala. There are indeed structural changes that occur in this area as a result of traumatic stress. Other researchers have shown similar findings in which stress and trauma have created abnormalities such as atrophy of the neural connections within various structures of the brain (Sapolsky, 1998; Vasterling & Brewin, 2005; Vasterling & Verfaellie, 2009). Several studies that used tissue samples of animal and human populations revealed an increase in oxidative stress, chronic inflammation, and extracellular glutamate, which demonstrates direct evidence of biochemical deficits in the brain (Prasad & Bondy, 2015). These deficits have been exhibited by brain imaging scans and neuropsychological test performances in which individuals exhibiting PTSSs have neurocognitive limitations in memory, concentration, focus, and activities of daily living.

In a sophisticated neuroscience study, Homan et al. (2019) combined computational, morphological, and functional analyses to investigate latent markers of associative learning in PTSSs of combat veterans. One finding was that a smaller amygdala volume correlated with more severe symptoms of PTSD. Indeed, structural changes occur in the brain after extraordinary stressful and traumatic events, even in the absence of closed- or open-head trauma. As a result of pathophysiology in the brain, PTSSs can worsen.

Some veterans with high levels of combat exposure can achieve reversal learning and have greater physiological adjustment. There are complicating factors, however, in mapping and measuring veterans' pathophysiology because of the chronic and persistent mental health symptoms related to combat exposure. Confounding this problem in neuroscience is TBI and how the brain expresses traumatic symptoms both consciously and unconsciously.

The essential aspects of neuroimaging present clinical researchers with opportunities to show the patient an image (picture) of what pathophysiological events appear within their brain (Raji et al., 2015). There has been an increased interest in distinguishing the pathophysiology of PTSD and TBI. For instance, the default mode network, as seen in brain neuroimaging scans, shows hyperperfusion in patients diagnosed with PTSD and hypoperfusion in those with TBI (Buckner et al., 2008). *Hyperperfusion* is defined as a major increase in atrial blood pressure or ipsilateral cerebral blood flow that exceeds the metabolic demands of brain tissue. If this condition is not treated, it can lead to edema, intercranial pressure, brain bleed, and possible death. *Hypoperfusion* is a reduction in the amount of blood flow in the brain, which can be seen in TBI and other conditions. The default mode network allows neurologists to see the inferior orbital frontal cortex, anterior cingulate gyrus, posterior cingulate gyrus, hippocampus, precuneus, superior parietal lobe, and angular gyrus, which are important for diagnosis and treatment of complex PTSD and TBI.

The neurological significance of neuroimaging may assist in explaining contradictory results found during neuropsychological testing and clinically administered PTSD scales and may ultimately clarify treatment options. This clarification is particularly important when the patient has both TBI and PTSD. Accurate diagnostics are key and can have life-threatening consequences when implementing appropriate treatment options. For example, the use of TMS when treating PTSD can be dangerous in patients with TBI because TMS can cause seizures. Thus, when clinical uncertainty exists, having accurate imaging and biomarkers that distinguish each condition (TBI, PTSD) is critical.

NEUROSCIENCE AND MILITARY MENTAL HEALTH

Optimal mental and physical health are critical when performing the essential job functions of any military occupational specialty. So why are some military personnel more resilient than others when confronted with critical events (e.g., deployments, divorce) during their service? Why do service members participating in the same event (e.g., jumping out of an airplane, fighting enemy combatants) perceive these activities significantly differently? Some service members and veterans thrive, whereas others are totally debilitated by their military experiences.

It is first important to understand the complex interactions that take place between an individual's neurobiological and neuropsychological functioning that may determine how they react to stress, traumatic stress, and adversity. The early work of Frankl (1963) helped clarify this system when he proposed that it may not necessarily be the nature of trauma itself that predicts a person's response. Rather, it is their perception and attitude toward the traumatic event. Because certain emotions and experiences are mapped and integrated in people's neurobiology, then perhaps they can alter their mind, body, and spirit through attitudinal and perceptual change. Thus, how people activate and deactivate the sympathetic-parasympathetic response may assist in their reaction to daily stress and traumatic stress.

One key is being able to control and predict one's environment, especially during warfighting. Service members who have a good internal-external locus of control may perform better in the heat of the battle. Remapping the military brain to reconnect healthier neuropathways can be established, for example, by the practices of neurocognitive or biofeedback, mindfulness meditation, stress reduction, positive psychology, and resiliency training. These mind-body approaches attune the sympathetic-parasympathetic response and assist individuals to bring unconscious thoughts, feelings, and experiences to consciousness. Overall, when one's physical, cognitive, and mental health are stable, then generally concentration, attention, and focus all help with the critical aspects of operation tempo.

Sapolsky (1998), Van Der Kolk (2014), and others have eloquently described the emotional brain during an acute stress reaction. Initially, when people perceive an event to be highly stressful, their body goes into a fight or flight mode that activates their sympathetic nervous system. Because of previous combat training and combat exposure, the military brain appears to be mapped differently than the brain of civilians. This difference occurs because the sympathetic "flight" mechanism is generally turned down, whereas the "aggress-not-stress" or "fight" mode is turned up. Basic physiology explains that the sympathetic-parasympathetic response begins in the brain and reaches out into every organ, blood vessel, hormone, and gland in the body. This same physiological reaction is turned on even when people anticipate or believe something bad is going to happen, such as a possible enemy combatant hiding over a dune with a rocket-propelled grenade launcher or the fear of being captured, which for many warfighters is worse than the fear of being killed in action.

As a result of the perception of danger, the emotional brain releases the hormones epinephrine and norepinephrine (the British refer to these as adrenaline and noradrenaline). These hormones are secreted into the body so that a person can mobilize energy rapidly and react to a stressful or critical event (i.e., enemy combatants). Whereas the sympathetic nervous system speeds up heart rate and blood flow and releases adrenaline, the parasympathetic system slows the body down so that people are not always in a state of warfighting. One can easily see how these mechanisms become worn neuropathways in service members, and many veterans cannot switch off this process during reintegration to civilian life.

Many researchers have described how the immune system also plays a significant role in the impact that stress and traumatic stress have on a person's body (McCoyd et al., 2012; Sapolsky, 1998; Stebnicki, 2017; Van Der Kolk, 2014; Weil, 1995). As basic physiology has shown, the primary task of the immune system is to defend the body against infectious agents such as viruses, bacteria, fungi, and parasites. The system is quite complex because it has the task of remembering every cell in a person's body (i.e., brain, heart, muscle, lung, and sensory nerve cells) and being able to sort out and assign these cells to the various organs and body systems. The immune system also has a job to do because it must differentiate between normal and abnormal cell structures by recording and memorizing the distinctive cellular signature of each cell structure (referred to as *immunologic memory*). The core structure of the immune system is to defend against attacks from viruses, bacteria, or other infectious anomalies.

Clinical studies have shown how some individuals who are in a constant state of hyperarousal because of high and intense levels of stress exposure have developed significant health problems (Goleman, 2003; Kabat-Zinn, 1990; Saplosky, 1998; Wachen et al., 2013). For some, chronic stress and anxiety can become a persistent pattern involving their physical, mental, emotional, and cognitive state of being. After the biochemical reactions in the emotional brain are mapped because of intense and high levels of chronic stress exposure, an increase may be found in oxidative stress, tissue inflammation, and nitric oxide synthase; in addition, multiple stress hormones can be released, which creates an enduring neurological pattern resulting in multiple mental health conditions (Prasad & Bondy, 2015). When physical injury occurs (e.g., TBI, amputation, spinal cord injury), the individual is placed into a whole other risk category for multiple mental health conditions (e.g., major depression, anxiety disorders, substance use disorders, chronic pain conditions).

A prime example of the mind-body connection to stress, traumatic stress, and illness is the newer disorder acquired during the Gulf War labeled as Gulf War illness (GWI) or chronic multisymptom illness (CMI). This chronic condition affects about 25%–32% of the 697,000 veterans who fought in the 1991 Gulf War and is associated with fatigue, joint pain, sleep disturbance, gastrointestinal problems, headaches, skin rashes, and cognitive complaints (Janulewicz et al.,

2017; White et al., 2016). One of the largest epidemiological studies to date has reported significantly higher mental and physical health conditions as a result of GWI/CMI (Dursa et al., 2016). Gulf War veterans continue to report high levels of cardiopulmonary, neurological, and gastrointestinal diseases. Interestingly, the incidence remains high among Gulf War veterans irrespective of deployment to combat operations. Accumulating evidence suggests a strong connection between chemical exposure to nerve agents used in the Gulf War during combat deployments and GWI/CMI. However, there are limitations in the neuropsychological and neurobiological studies of GWI/CMI because of research designs, studying populations of veterans who were not deployed exhibiting similar symptoms, small sample sizes, as well as other problems in methodology (Janulewicz et al., 2017). Despite some controversy in GWI/CMI, the incidence and prevalence of mental and physical health conditions exist with combat and noncombat exposure.

It should come as no surprise that untreated intense levels of emotional, psychological, and physiological stress can become a risk factor for developing PTSD and other co-occurring mental and physical health conditions. For some service members, self-reporting medical and mental health conditions during pre- and postdeployment fitness for duty exams may place their military career and promotions in jeopardy. Overall, there is a physical, emotional, cognitive, and neurobiological cost to chronic and persistent sympathetic arousal that causes the heavy secretion of glucocorticoids and other toxins released in the nervous system. High levels of glucocorticoids along with other elements toxic to the body are markers for depression and anxiety disorders (Sapolsky, 1998). Accordingly, if the service member constantly engages in sympathetic nervous system arousal and cannot turn this down, then there is a metabolic cost that causes a cascade of neurobiological actions, ultimately impairing good mind-body health, which diminishes protective factors and resources.

The amygdala-cortical pathway in the brain is the key neural circuitry that underlies emotions and is positively correlated with increases in negative mood and affect (Barrett et al., 2007; Brother, 1989). LeDoux (1998, 2014) and others have extensively studied the emotions of fear and anxiety as a predisposing factor that triggers the frequency and intensity of how these emotions are turned on and off within the amygdala. Brain imaging has indicated that the amygdala orchestrates the most intense electrical activation when reading, interpreting, or trying to understand the emotions of self and others. Over time, the individual's inability to express or suppress emotions such as stress, grief, or trauma appears to have a neurobiological, physiological, emotional, psychological, social, and interpersonal communications cost. The emotional experience of fear and anxiety tends to become stuck in a feedback loop, particularly when engaging all the body systems. Chronic activation of the emotional brain and habitual repression of emotions can compromise the immune system and lower resistance to infections, chronic illness, and diseases (Pert et al., 2005; Sapolsky, 1998; Weil, 1995).

Some researchers have reported that there are important cultural differences in how emotions such as stress and trauma are expressed and experienced (Kitayama et al., 1995; Kohrt & Hruschka, 2010; Mauro et al., 1992). Some psychobiological factors in the cultural expression of emotions appear to be the direct result of how the individual interacts with their environment. This outcome may be because there are specific relational meanings that lead an individual to express specific emotions. Thus, within the existing culture, each emotion has its own relational meaning or core relational theme (Lazarus, 1999). This finding may suggest that the essence of emotions within the military culture may depend on (a) how others within the culture express stress and traumatic stress, (b) how emotions are appraised by others within the culture, and (c) other moderating variables that change the service member's perception and expression of stress and traumatic stress.

REMAPPING THE MILITARY BRAIN

The impact that the mind, body, and spirit have on one's emotional and physical well-being has been well documented throughout time by archaeological and historical records, ancient texts communicated through world religions and spiritual leaders, and ritual healing practices by indigenous cultures across the globe (Brennan, 1988; Eden, 1998; Harner, 1990; Mehl-Madrona, 1997; Moodley & West, 2005; Rainbow Eagle, 2003; Stebnicki, 2016; Weil, 1995; Wilber, 1996). Qualitatively, there is evidence for healing posttraumatic stress and other co-occurring conditions through complementary and integrative health approaches, as discussed in Chapter 14. One example is sweat lodge ceremonies used by many American Indian tribes for healing PTSD and other invisible wounds. Traditional non-Western indigenous healing modalities are utilized frequently by service members and veterans. One study found that the majority (80%) of service members and veterans participated in the use of at least one complementary and integrative health approach, such as yoga, herbal supplements, massage, Reiki, and acupuncture (Ysasi et al., 2016).

Indeed, there is a complex interplay among one's neurobiological, psychological, social, emotional, and cultural health that cannot be measured by neuroscience, medical technology, or mental health screening and assessment. Neuroscience cannot totally explain how prayer can work miracles, how diseases have been cured by spontaneous remission, why some veterans connect better emotionally with animals than with people, how nonverbal expressive arts increase healing potential more than talk therapy, or why family and cultural support are more effective than group psychotherapy.

Tart's (2000) classical work offers structure to understanding the different states of consciousness (self-awareness, thought, imagination); altered states of consciousness; and the transpersonal psychology of the mind, body, and spirit. There is direct application that may contribute to the neuroscience of stress and trauma. Tart suggested that there is elegance in the complexities of the mind, body, and spirit that can theoretically and experientially be enhanced in multidimensional ways. He offered a model that may be useful for coping strategies, mediating internal-external stimuli to create new realities, and entering altered states of consciousness for seeking answers to difficult problems in life. The intention is for individuals to transform previously held perceptions, cognitions, and feelings and to replace them with newfound meanings and exceptional human experiences. In Western counseling and psychology practices, emotions, thoughts, and experiences are measured by self-report, behavioral observation, and historical records. The healing potential of unconscious emotions prompted by a change in one's physical or geographic environment, guided imagery, meditation, or shamanic journey cannot be fully understood. For example, sensory deprivation has some beneficial effects on decreasing traumatic triggers in the mind and body. Reducing or eliminating unhealthy thoughts, feelings, and experiences may be a way of starving the sensory input of the brain's processing centers.

Person-centered therapeutic interactions may heal some veterans but not others. Developing self-awareness; meaning; healthy emotions, cognitions, and experiences; as well as creative problem solving is a shared responsibility outside the 53-minute psychotherapy session. Newer studies in psychotherapy show the importance of attending to clients' verbal and nonverbal communication. Empathy in particular has been well documented as an essential element of the therapeutic process. The level and quality of empathy can be measured from a physiological perspective. For example, Marci et al. (2007) looked at 20 client-therapist pairs being treated for mood and anxiety disorders. They specifically focused on the therapeutic relationships that were formed during psychotherapy sessions. Physiological measures were taken of the client and therapist as well as the client's perceived level of empathy as expressed and facilitated by the therapist. They measured electrical skin conductance, heart rate variability, voice dynamics, and body movement. They found that when high positive emotions and empathy were expressed by the therapist, then a similar physiological response was experienced by the client and therapist. This particular study supports the notion that a strong working alliance and earning the circle of trust have potential for remapping the military brain because of nonexpressed emotions.

Empathy not only has implications for cultivating the therapeutic relationship but also may bring promise to how the emotional brain can be developed in those critically affected by extraordinary stressful and traumatic events. Having a heightened sense of emotional awareness builds capacity for empathy and is closely associated with measuring the emotional intelligence of children, adolescents, and adults (Bar-On & Parker, 2000; Goleman, 2003). Thus, becoming attuned to one's thoughts, feelings, emotions, and behaviors is central to healing the mind, body, and spirit. The neuroscience of studying the emotional brain and its different states of consciousness can provide opportunities for remapping the military brain for good mental and physical health both during and after service.

CONCLUDING REMARKS

The neuroscientific paradigm within the military culture has expanded significantly within the last 10 years. The synthesis of a multidisciplinary approach offers improved medical and mental health care. It begins with understanding the etiology and epidemiological significance of the impact that military stress and traumatic stress have on the service member and veteran. The unhealthy brain has far-reaching negative implications for long-term medical, physical, and mental health conditions that potentially can debilitate well-being. Understanding the brain's profound capacity for healing itself through various complementary and integrative health approaches offers potential opportunities for service members and veterans to gain optimal living practices during and after military life. Cultivating compassion and empathy is essential for forming healthy intimate and social relationships, refining career development opportunities as a veteran, regulating moods and emotions, as well as recognizing other prospects for personal growth.

REFERENCES

Ader, R. (1990). *Psychoneuroimmunology* (2nd ed.). Academic Press.

Bar-On, R., & Parker, J. D. (2000). *The handbook of emotional intelligence: Theory, development, assessment, and application at home, school, and in the workplace.* Jossey-Bass.

Barrett, L. F., Bliss Moreau, E., Duncan, S. L., Rauch, S. L., & Wright, C. I. (2007). The amygdala and the experience of affect. *Social Cognitive Affect in Neuroscience, 2*(2), 73–83. https://doi.org/10.1093/scan/nsl042

Brennan, B. A. (1988). *Hands of light: A guide to healing through the human energy field.* Bantam Books.

Brother, L. (1989). A biological perspective on empathy. *American Journal of Psychiatry, 146*(1), 10–19. https://doi.org/10.1176/ajp.146.1.10

Buckner, R. L., Andrews-Hanna, J. R., & Schacter, D. L. (2008). The brain's default network: Anatomy, function, and relevance to disease. *Annals of the New York Academy of Sciences, 1124*(1), 1–38. https://doi.org/10.1196/annals.1440.011

Cann, R. I., Stoneking, M., & Wilson, A. C. (1987, January 1). Mitochondrial DNA and human evolution. *Nature, 325*(6099), 31–36. https://doi.org/10.1038/325031a0

Dursa, E. K., Barth, S. K., Schneiderman, A. I., & Bossarte, R. M. (2016). Physical and mental health status of Gulf War and Gulf era veterans: Results from a large population-based epidemiological study. *Journal of Occupational and Environmental Medicine, 58*(1), 41–46. https://doi.org/10.1097/JOM.0000000000000627

Eden, D. (1998). *Energy medicine.* Tarcher/Putman.

Frankl, V. E. (1963). *Man's search for meaning.* Pocket Books.

Genome News Network. (2003, January 15). *Genome variations.* http://www.genomenewsnetwork.org/resources/whats_a_genome/Chp4_1.shtml

Goleman, D. (2003). *Healing emotions: Conversations with the Dalai Lama on mindfulness, emotions, and health.* Shambhala.

Harner, M. (1990). *The way of the shaman.* HarperSanFrancisco.

Henry, M., Fishman, J. R., & Youngner, S. J. (2007). Propranolol and the prevention of post-traumatic stress disorder: Is it wrong to erase the "sting" of bad memories? *The American Journal of Bioethics, 7*(9), 12–20. https://doi.org/10.1080/15265160701518474

Homan, P., Levy, I., Feltham, E., Gordon, C., Hu, J., Li, J., Pietrzak, R. H., Southwick, S., Krystal, J. H., Harpaz-Rotem, I., & Schiller, D. (2019). Neural computations of threat in the aftermath of combat trauma. *Nature Neuroscience, 22*(3), 470–476. https://doi.org/10.1038/s41593-018-0315-x

Howell, A. (2017). Neuroscience and war: Human enhancement, soldier rehabilitation, and the ethical limits of dual-use frameworks. *Millennium: Journal of International Studies, 45*(2), 133–150. https://doi.org/10.1177/0305829816672930

Janulewicz, P. A., Krengel, M. H., Maule, A., White, R. F., Cirillo, J., Sisson, E., Heeren, T., & Sullivan, K. (2017). Neuropsychological characteristics of Gulf War illness: A meta-analysis. *PLoS One, 12*(5), Article e0177121. https://doi.org/10.1371/journal.pone.0177121

Kabat-Zinn, J. (1990). *Full catastrophe living: Using the wisdom of your body and mind to face stress, pain, and illness.* Dell.

Kaku, M. (2014). *The future science of the mind: The scientific quest to understand, enhance, and empower the mind.* Anchor Books.

Kitayama, S., Marcus, H. R., & Matsumoto, H. (1995). Culture, self, and emotion: A cultural perspective on "self-conscious" emotions. In J. P. Tangney & K. W. Fischer (Eds.), *Self-conscious emotions: The psychology of shame, guilt, embarrassment, and pride* (pp. 439–464). Guilford Press.

Kohrt, B. A., & Hruschka, D. J. (2010). Nepali concepts of psychological trauma: The role of idioms of distress, ethnopsychology and ethnophysiology in alleviating suffering and preventing stigma. *Cultural Medicine Psychiatry, 34*(2), 322–352. https://doi.org/10.1007/s11013-010-9170-2

Kosal, M. E., & Huang, J. Y. (2015). Security implications and governance of cognitive neuroscience: A ethnographic survey of researchers. *Politics and the Life Sciences, 34*(1), 93–108. https://doi.org/10.1017/pls.2015.4

Lazarus, R. S. (1999). *Stress and emotions: A new synthesis.* Springer.

LeDoux, J. (1998). *The emotional brain: The mysterious underpinnings of emotional life.* Touchstone.

LeDoux, J. E. (2014). Coming to terms with fear. *Proceedings of the National Academy of Sciences of the United States of America, 111*(8), 2871–2878. https://doi.org/10.1073/pnas.1400335111

Lieberman, H. R., Bathalon, G. P., Falco, C. M., Kramer, F. M., Morgan, C. A., & Niro, P. (2005). Severe decrements in cognition function and mood induced by sleep loss, heat, dehydration, and undernutrition during simulated combat. *Biological Psychiatry, 57*(4), 422–429. https://doi.org/10.1016/j.biopsych.2004.11.014

Lieberman, H. R., Farina, E. K., Caldwell, J., Williams, K. W., Thompson, L. A., Niro, P. J., Grohmann, K. A., & McClung, J. P. (2016). Cognitive function, stress hormones, heart rate and nutritional status during simulated captivity in military survival training. *Physiology & Behavior, 165,* 86–97. https://doi.org/10.1016/j.physbeh.2016.06.037

Lin, T., Gilam, G., Raz, G., Or-Boricheve, A., Bar-Haim, Y., Fruchter, E., & Hendler, T. (2017). Accessible neurobehavioral anger-related markers for vulnerability to post-traumatic stress symptoms in a population of male soldiers. *Frontiers in Behavioral Neuroscience, 11,* Article 38. https://doi.org/10.3389/fnbeh.2017.00038

Lissek, S., & Van Meurs, B. (2015). Learning models of PTSD: Theoretical accounts and psychobiological evidence. *International Journal of Psychophysiology, 98*(3), 594–605. https://doi.org/10.1016/j.ijpsycho.2014.11.006

Marci, C., Ham, J., Moran, E., & Orr, S. (2007). Physiologic correlates of perceived therapist empathy and social-emotional process during psychotherapy. *Journal of Nervous and Mental Disease, 195*(2), 103–111. https://doi.org/10.1097/01.nmd.0000253731.71025.fc

Mauro, R., Sato, K., & Tucker, J. (1992). The role of appraisal in human emotions: A cross-cultural study. *Journal of Personality and Social Psychology, 62*(2), 301–317. https://doi.org/10.1037/0022-3514.62.2.301

Mayne, T. J., & Ramsey, J. (2001). The structure of emotion: A nonlinear dynamic systems approach. In T. J. Mayne & G. A. Bonanno (Eds.), *Emotions: Current issues and future directions* (pp. 1–37). Guilford Press.

McCoyd, J. L. M., Walter, C. A., & Lopez Levers, L. (2012). Issues of loss and grief. In L. Lopez Levers (Ed.), *Trauma counseling: Theories and interventions* (pp. 77–97). Springer.

Mehl-Madrona, L. (1997). *Coyote medicine: Lessons from Native American healing*. Fireside.

Moodley, R., & West, W. (2005). *Integrating traditional healing practices into counseling and psychotherapy*. Sage.

Morgan, C. A., III, Hazlett, G., Wang, S., Richardson, E. G., Schnurr, P., & Southwick, S. M. (2001). Symptoms of dissociation in humans experiencing acute, uncontrollable stress: A prospective investigation. *American Journal of Psychiatry, 158*(8), 1239–1247. https://doi.org/10.1176/appi.ajp.158.8.1239

Morgan, C. A., III, Wang, S., Mason, J., Southwick, S. M., Fox, P., Hazlett, G., Charney, D. S., & Greenfield, G. (2000). Hormone profiles in humans experiencing military survival training. *Biological Psychiatry, 47*(10), 891–901. https://doi.org/10.1016/S0006-3223(99)00307-8

Pert, C. B., Dreher, H. E., & Ruff, M. R. (2005). The psychosomatic network: Foundations of mind-body medicine. In M. Schlitz, T. Amorok, & M. Micozzi (Eds.), *Consciousness and healing: Integral approaches to mind-body medicine* (pp. 61–78). Elsevier.

Pessoa, L. (2014). Understanding brain networks and brain organization. *Physics of Life Review, 11*(3), 400–435. https://doi.org/10.1016/j.plrev.2014.03.005

Prasad, K. N., & Bondy, S. C. (2015). Common biochemical defects linkage between post-traumatic stress disorders, mild traumatic brain injury (TBI) and penetrating TBI. *Brain Research, 1599*, 103–114. https://doi.org/10.1016/j.brainres.2014.12.038

Rainbow Eagle. (2003). *Native American spirituality: A walk in the woods*. Rainbow Light and Company.

Raji, C. A., Willeumier, K., Taylor, D., Tarzwell, R., Newberg, A., Henderson, T. A., & Amen, D. G. (2015). Functional neuroimaging with default mode network regions distinguishes PTSD from TBI in a military veteran population. *Brain Imaging and Behaviors, 9*(3), 527–534. https://doi.org/10.1007/s11682-015-9385-5

Rippon, G., & Senior, C. (2010). Neuroscience has no role in national security. *American Journal of Behavioral Neuroscience, 1*(2), 37–38. https://doi.org/10.1080/21507741003699322

Rosenberg, L., & Gehrie, E. (2007). Against the use of medical technology for military and national security interests. *American Journal of Bioethics, 7*(5), 22–24. https://doi.org/10.1080/15265160701290330

Sankararaman, S., Mallick, S., Donnemann, M., Prufer, K., Kelso, J., Paabo, S., Patterson, N., & Reich, D. (2014, March 20). The genomic landscape of Neanderthal ancestry in present-day humans. *Nature, 507*(7492), 354–357. https://doi.org/10.1038/nature12961

Sapolsky, R. M. (1998). *Why zebras don't get ulcers: An updated guide to stress, stress-related diseases, and coping*. W. H. Freeman and Company.

Schiller, D., Levy, I., Niv, Y., Le Doux, J. E., & Phelps, E. A. (2008). From fear to safety and back: Reversal of fear in the human brain. *Journal of Neuroscience, 28*(45), 11517–11525. https://doi.org/10.1523/JNEUROSCI.2265-08.2008

Stebnicki, M. A. (2016). Integrative approaches in counseling and psychotherapy: Foundations of the mind, body, and spirit. In I. Marini & M.A. Stebnicki (Eds.), *The professional counselor's desk reference* (2nd ed., 593–604). Springer.

Stebnicki, M. A. (2017). *Disaster mental health counseling: Responding to trauma in a multicultural context*. Springer.

Tart, C. T. (2000). *States of consciousness*. iUniverse.com.

Touroutoglou, A., Lindquist, K. A., Dickerson, B. C., & Feldman Barrett, L. (2015). Intrinsic connectivity in the human brain does not reveal networks for "basic" emotions. *Social Cognitive and Affective Neuroscience, 10*(9), 1257–1265. https://doi.org/10.1093/scan/nsv013

Tracy, J. L., & Randles, D. (2011). Four models of basic emotions: A review of Ekman and Cordaro, Izard, Levenson, and Panksepp and Watt. *Emotion Review, 3*(4), 397–405. https://doi.org/10.1177/1754073911410747

Van Der Kolk, B. (2014). *The body keeps the score: Brain, mind, and body in the healing of trauma*. Penguin Books.

Vasterling, J. J., & Brewin, C. R. (2005). *Neuropsychology of PTSD: Biological, cognitive, and clinical perspectives*. Guilford Press.

Vasterling, J. J., & Verfaellie, M. (2009). Introduction—Posttraumatic stress disorder: A neurocognitive perspective. *Journal of the International Neurobiological Society, 15*(6), 826–829. https://doi.org/10.1017/S1355617709990683

Wachen, J. S., Shipherd, J. C., Suvak, M., Vogt, D., King, L. A., & King, D. W. (2013). Posttraumatic stress symptomatology as a mediator of the relationship between warzone exposure and physical health symptoms in men and women. *Journal of Traumatic Stress, 26*(3), 319–328. https://doi.org/10.1002/jts.21818

Weil, A. (1995). *Spontaneous healing*. Ballantine Publishing Group.

White, R. F., Steele, L., O'Callaghan, J. P., Sullivan, K., Binns, J. H., Golomb, B. A., Bloom, F. E., Bunker, J. A., Crawford, F., Graves, J. C., Hardie, A., Klimas, N., Knox, M., Meggs, W. J., Melling, J., Philbert, M. A., & Grashow, R. (2016). Recent research on Gulf War illness and other health problems in veterans of the 1991 Gulf War: Effects of toxicant exposures during deployment. *Cortex, 74*, 449–475. https://doi.org/10.1016/j.cortex.2015.08.022

Wilber, K. (1996). *A brief history of everything*. Shambhala.

Ysasi, N. A., Graf, N., Brown, A. D., & Sharma, R. (2016). Receptiveness toward complementary and alternative medicine by veterans and military servicepersons: Implications for counseling professionals. *Military Behavioral Health, 4*(1), 32–46. https://doi.org/10.1080/21635781.2015.1093977

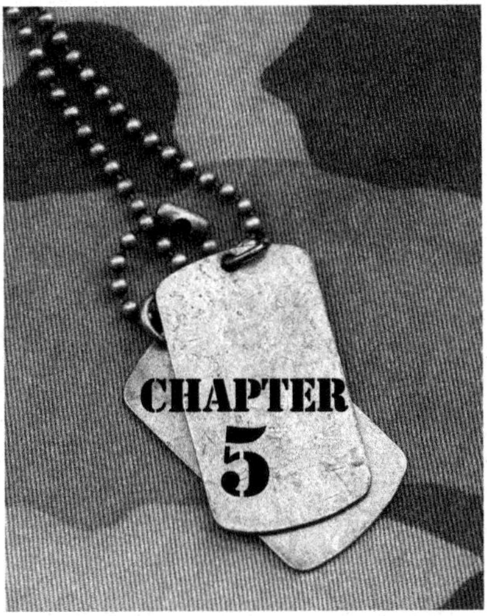

PSYCHOSOCIAL ASPECTS OF MILITARY SUICIDE

No easy day . . .

—Common military expression of combat veterans

★ ★ ★

Since the start of Operation Enduring Freedom and Operation Iraqi Freedom, the incidence of military suicide has risen dramatically across all branches of the U.S. Armed Forces and among active-duty service members, veterans, reservists, and National Guard soldiers. In this chapter, I discuss the epidemiological significance of military suicide, the mental health risk factors associated with suicide, the effects on military families, suicide assessment, and suicide prevention and treatment approaches within a psychosocial framework.

For military families, the psychosocial aspects of death resulting from veteran suicide are much different than when a loved one is killed in action. For instance, service members who are killed in action are honored and recognized for their bravery by the military. However, when a veteran commits suicide, some military families perceive and grieve this act as shameful. While the service member is on a combat deployment, it is anticipated that bad things could happen, such as medical, physical, and psychological injuries or the possibility that they may be killed in action. After the individual separates from service and transitions to civilian life, many military families feel a sense of relief. The threat of combat injury or casualty is no longer at the forefront of marital conflict or parental distress. However, combat veterans with underlying medical, physical, and mental health conditions are at higher risk for self-harm. Thus, the service member dying in combat operations is a much different bereavement event for family members than a veteran dying as a result of a suicide completion. It is excruciatingly difficult for family members to make sense and meaning of their loved one's military service.

EPIDEMIOLOGY OF MILITARY SUICIDE

Historically, suicide has been the second leading cause of death in the military and is largely due to the increase in mental and physical health disorders acquired during military service (LeardMann et al., 2013; Matarazzo et al., 2014; Reger et al., 2015; I. H. Stanley et al., 2018; Sterling et al., 2017). The cumulative impact of more than 20 years of war; the frequent and intense level of service-related medical, physical, and mental health conditions; the stigma of seeking mental health counseling; and the low acceptance of suicide prevention programs among military personnel all create a combination of factors leading to suicidal ideation, lethal attempts, and completions.

When addressing issues of epidemiology in military suicide research, one must differentiate between incidence and prevalence. Most parsimoniously expressed, *incidence* is the measure of the frequency of newly diagnosed cases of a disease or illness or, in this instance, the morbidity of suicide. Epidemiologists use the term *crude incidence*, which is the number of new cases of military suicide during the year expressed in terms of new cases that occur per 100,000 within the military population. It is calculated by simply dividing the total number of new suicides within a given time period by the total number of military personnel. *Prevalence* is the total number of cases of a disease, illness, or—in this instance—suicide morbidity that exist within a given population.

One problem that arises in military suicide epidemiology research is that the number of suicides expressed is the total average rate of military suicides. Thus, some studies do not account for other correlates and confounding factors. Most studies in peer-reviewed journal articles account for these differences in the "limitations and confounding results" section. Some military research studies do not differentiate well between intended and unintended suicide deaths. For example, in one study, Cox et al. (2017) looked at misclassification of suicide rates and found multiple recording errors (i.e., possible suicide, probable suicide, definite suicide). Outside of any statistical miscalculations, the human cost to military families, friends, and unit members can be psychologically debilitating. Statistical recording errors and investigations within military mental health research and forensics may also significantly affect death benefits that military families receive regarding possible, probable, or definite suicide completion; service-connected disability ratings; and discharge status (i.e., honorable, less than honorable).

Many studies on military suicide have reported data acquired from the U.S. Department of Veterans Affairs (VA) system of health care. Thus, these statistics are skewed toward those receiving ongoing medical and mental health care for their chronic conditions. Limitations with this data collection method do not account for veterans using health care providers outside the VA system. Hence, these veterans may not be tracked or surveilled. Therefore, this area of study is complex. However, data collection, interpretation, and reporting of results can all affect decision makers who develop suicide prevention and treatment programs.

What are the data collection sources for military suicide statistics? The U.S. Department of Defense (DoD; 2019) and other governmental and nongovernmental organizations actively partner in collecting surveillance data, performing research analysis, and providing clinical interventions and program evaluations. This is done on a quarterly and annual basis. The Centers for Disease Control and Prevention (CDC) National Violent Death Reporting System (https://www.cdc.gov/violenceprevention/datasources/nvdrs/index.html), the DoD Medical Mortality Registry (Gardner et al., 2000), the DoD Suicide Event Report (https://www.dspo.mil/Prevention/Data-Surveillance/DoDSER-Annual-Reports/), and the Military Suicide Research Consortium (https://msrc.fsu.edu/) create new opportunities for a variety of suicide research, prevention, and treatment-related projects. Some organizations, such as the Military Suicide Research Consortium, were established to enhance the military's ability to rapidly identify and promote evidence-based prevention and intervention programs for service members and veterans.

Clearly, there are significant challenges in the epidemiology of military suicide research regarding data collection, monitoring, validation of distinct measures, risk assessments, and the characterization of suicide risk and protective factors (Ringer et al., 2018). Traditionally, it has been hypothesized that 85% of suicide deaths occur in men who are younger because they are higher risk takers, behave more aggressively, act more violently to assert themselves, exhibit higher levels of anger with low impulse control, and tend to use firearms more frequently than their female counterparts. This area in military suicide research is also ambiguous because studies are limited as to why men are at higher risk than women. One paradoxical factor is that there are equal numbers of men and women who reside in short- and long-term psychiatric and substance abuse programs as a result of their suicidal behaviors (Sterling et al., 2017).

Currently, one of the most significant challenges in military suicide research is the other paradox that exists between the incidence and prevalence of combat versus noncombat exposure and the crude incidence rate of suicide completions. Historically, combat deployments have been associated with significantly higher levels of mental health problems and suicidality (e.g., posttraumatic stress disorder [PTSD], major depressive disorder, anxiety disorders, and substance use disorders; Harmon et al., 2016; Kline et al., 2016; LeardMann et al., 2013; Mansfield et al., 2011). However, this association is no longer the case. Many studies have attempted to characterize the unique risks and protective factors in military suicide completions (Ringer et al., 2018). Accordingly, there is growing consensus among researchers that (a) suicidal behaviors among combat versus noncombat personnel indicate a statistical significance but are small in magnitude and show little difference (I. H. Stanley et al., 2018); (b) killing exposure may magnify suicidal ideation and is considered a predisposing risk factor to suicide completion, but the relationship is not clear (Kline et al., 2016); (c) documented mental health conditions before deployment (e.g., PTSD, depression, anxiety, substance use disorders) place service members at a significantly higher risk for suicide attempts and completions than nondetected mental health conditions (Leard-Mann et al., 2013); and (d) many studies rely on records review to collect data, creating a variance by raters in the interpretation and documentation of the data. Overall, the epidemiology of military suicide is a complex area for analysis; yet, it is critically important for decision makers motivated to provide quality suicide prevention and treatment programs.

VETERAN SUICIDE

The real risk of suicidal behaviors increases after medical separation from military service. The absolute number of suicides is highest among veterans 55–74 years old, who account for 38% of all veteran deaths by suicide (VA, 2019). In 2019, the VA released the *National Veteran Suicide Prevention Annual Report*. The interested reader may want to consult this full report, which combines current findings in the three groups affected by suicide: active-duty service members, veterans, and former National Guard soldiers and reservists. The results suggest that suicide prevention is a national priority for the VA and partnering medical and mental health clinics. The report addresses a comprehensive approach to veteran health with the intention to halt the progression of suicidality in military populations. Key results of the VA's (2019) report are statistically highlighted as follows:

- The number of veteran suicides exceeded 6,000 deaths per year from 2008 to 2017 or 15.9 veteran suicides per day in 2005 and 16.8 in 2017.
- In 2017, 45,390 nonveteran adults and 6,139 veterans in the United States died from suicide completions, representing proportionately that veterans had 1.5 times the suicide rate.
- The number of suicide deaths among the general population in the United States increased by almost 44% during 2005–2017, whereas there was a 6% increase in the number of suicide deaths in the veteran population during this same reporting period.
- Suicide completion by firearms resulted in almost 71% of all male veteran deaths and 43% of female veteran deaths in 2017.
- Approximately 59% of veterans who died by suicide (between 2016 and 2017) recently were undergoing mental health and substance abuse treatment from the VA health care system. Suicide rates among veterans receiving VA services were highest among those diagnosed with bipolar and opioid use disorders.
- Although major depressive disorder is a significant risk factor among veteran suicides, the suicide rate decreased from 2005 to 2017 from 70.2 per 100,000 to 63.4 per 100,000.

The data collected in this report utilize results from partnering organizations. The intention is to develop key initiatives and priorities for (a) suicide crisis services (i.e., veterans' crisis lines); (b) research and innovative projects; (c) forming community resources, outreach, and partnerships; (d) forming clinical partnerships for mental health providers with coordination of care and evidence-based treatment approaches; (e) expansion of the integration of primary medical and mental health care as well as universal screening measures; and (f) specially focused veteran programs for military sexual trauma (MST) and women's health care.

MILITARY SUICIDE RISK FACTORS

Military suicide researchers oftentimes rely on mental health risk factors as reported by the American Psychiatric Association's practice guidelines for the assessment and diagnosis of suicidality (Harmon et al., 2016). The following general risk factors are associated with suicidal behaviors:

- One or more diagnosed or undiagnosed mental health conditions, such as major depressive disorder, anxiety, PTSD, or substance use disorders;
- Communication of a suicide threat or a previous suicide attempt;

- Exposure to past or current sexual assault, physical trauma, or critical incidents involving violence;
- Exposure to past or current critical life events and other psychosocial stressors (e.g., loss of a loved one or friend, divorce, legal issues, life-threatening illness or disability, homelessness, unemployment);
- Formulation of a specific plan and the means (weapons) to harm oneself;
- Little or no support system, coping skills, or resources to assist in a crisis; and
- Ages that represent younger (18–34 years) and older (55–74 years) men.

Suicide rates among active-duty service members have reached unprecedented levels and have nearly doubled in the U.S. Army and U.S. Marine Corps (Skopp et al., 2016). The rates for U.S. Air Force suicide completions also doubled during 2019. Suicide is particularly high among individuals with infantryman and combat engineer military occupations (Kessler et al., 2015; May & Klonsky, 2016). Traditionally, suicide rates in the military have been lower than in the civilian population (Eaton et al., 2006) despite the repeated exposure to military training exercises and combat deployments (Harmon et al., 2016). However, military suicide is now the second leading cause of death in military life and has surpassed the suicide rates within the general civilian population (Matarazzo et al., 2014; Reger et al., 2015; I. H. Stanley et al., 2018; Sterling et al., 2017). Overall, the research shows that 37% of active-duty service members who died from a suicide completion exhibited premeditation of deliberate self-harm and had a plan of action that led to their death.

Interestingly, combat deployments alone are not directly associated with the increased rates of deliberate self-harm or suicide completions because at least half of all suicide completions involved active-duty service members who were never deployed to a combat theater (Kessler et al., 2015; Kline et al., 2016; Reger et al., 2015). Indirect combat exposure, or supporting combat operations, has been shown to increase the risk for more intense suicidal behaviors that could potentially lead to lethal attempts or completions (Fontana & Rosenheck, 1995). Some researchers have suggested that killing enemy combatants and noncombatant civilians may create a type of moral injury that has the greatest deleterious psychological impact on service members. This finding is particularly relevant for those who have preexisting psychological conditions who have never received any type of mental health treatment (Kline et al., 2016).

SUICIDE RISK FACTOR OF MST

The mental health consequences of non-MST have been discussed in the civilian literature for years and have contributed to the development of the assessment, diagnosis, prevention, and treatment of sexual assault. Most researchers and clinicians agree, in both military and nonmilitary mental health, that sexual assault survivors acquire significant mental health problems, increasing the risk of suicidal ideation, lethal attempts, and completions. The consequences of MST also pose a risk, secondary to PTSD, in the development of suicidal behaviors (Sexton et al., 2018).

For example, 22%–45% of female veterans and 1%–2% of male veterans have had unwanted sexual advances, harassment, abuse, and assault such as rape while serving. Female veterans with a history of MST who identify as sexual and gender minorities have nearly twice the rate of suicide attempts compared with other veterans seeking treatment for military trauma–related symptoms (Sexton et al., 2018). Given the amplified rate of suicide attempts for this group, there is still a lot to understand in terms of assessment, diagnosis, and treatment approaches to decrease the risk of future suicidal behaviors among high-risk military populations.

A qualitative analysis of data gathered from large-scale military suicide surveillance systems—such as the DoD Suicide Event Report and the CDC National Violent Death Reporting System—indicates that the most common precipitating critical incident related to active-duty suicide completions is intimate partner problems (i.e., violence, abuse, neglect). Overall, one of the unique differences between sexual assaults in military versus civilian life is that most women who have experienced MST continue to live and work near their perpetrator. Some perpetrators of sexual assault are higher ranking officers, which creates significant difficulties in reporting such critical incidents and has career implications for the victim. As a result of MST and other multiple traumas that may occur in military life, many individuals develop complex PTSD and co-occurring mental health disorders requiring treatment for depression, anxiety, and substance use disorders.

OTHER SUICIDE RISK FACTORS IN MILITARY LIFE

Other high-risk factors among military populations have been studied. For example, regarding gender, suicide attempts were greatest among female soldiers who had never been married and active-duty men who had been recently demoted because of a Uniform Code of Military Justice violation (Skopp et al., 2016). Researchers found that military service members and veterans who identify as lesbian, gay, bisexual, and transgender (LGBT) are at increased risk for suicide completions (Matarazzo et al., 2014). Historically, the civilian literature has shown an increased risk of suicide among individuals who self-identify as LGBT. More specifically, gay and bisexual men have a fourfold increased risk and lesbian and bisexual women have a threefold increased risk of attempting suicide.

Besides mental health and substance use disorders, there are clinically significant psychosocial factors related to deliberate acts of self-harm among service members and veterans, which include critical areas in military life such as job-related financial stress, incarceration, and dishonorable discharge from military service because of legal issues (Skopp et al., 2019).

One area rarely discussed involves the spouses and dependents of service members who have committed suicide. This deficiency is because the DoD did not release data on military family suicide until 2017 (Jowers, 2019). The DoD data, which partly depend on data supplied by the CDC, indicate that the overall suicide rate among family members was 6.8 per 100,000 within the population. The military spouse rate of suicide was 11.5 per 100,000, and the rate among dependents was 3.8 per 100,000. Adjusting for age and gender, the suicide rates within the civilian population were comparable to those in military families. As in other data on the incidence and prevalence of military suicide, there are some limitations and confounding problems, such as determining whether the military spouse who committed suicide was a civilian, active-duty service member, or veteran. Overall, it is essential that treatment efforts involve both the individual service member and their significant family members. This task becomes difficult particularly when more than half of the 20 million veterans nationwide do not use Veterans Health Administration services, making identification of suicide risk factors challenging (France & Hallows, 2019).

MILITARY SUICIDE ASSESSMENT

Military suicide screening and assessments can be utilized for all levels of primary, secondary, and tertiary prevention. These instruments are met with some degree of cynicism in terms of their effectiveness and predictability, primarily because many are self-report instruments. Realistically, active-duty personnel understand the negative stigma associated with seeking mental health treatment and its consequences for their career and promotions (Arbisi et al., 2013). Unfortunately, mental health conditions underlying suicidality that go unrecognized, unreported, untreated, or undertreated can have severe consequences in the life of military veterans as the mental health symptoms become more chronic and persistent.

The challenge in suicide screening, assessment, and prevention is to identify those military personnel and veterans who are at risk, yet not clinically suicidal. A priority in military mental health is reducing the number of suicidal behaviors that may result in death. One of the critical issues in military suicide is the primary medical and mental health provider's ability to assess the degree of lethality in service members and veterans. Research indicates that (a) some suicide screening methods do not lend themselves to consistent administration, scoring, and follow-up treatment; (b) approximately 25% of military personnel who die by suicide had a medical appointment within 30 days of their death; (c) military enlistees often falsify information related to mental and behavioral health concerns that could place them in a higher risk category; and (d) the warning signs associated with the level and degree of lethality are not recognized by providers during screening, so treatment is not pursued (Griffith & Bryan, 2018).

Indeed, early identification and detection of suicidality provide the greatest opportunity for prevention of suicide attempts or completions. Clinical suicide risk assessments that assign a level of risk (i.e., low, moderate, high) unfortunately do not offer an absolute means to prevent suicide attempts or completions (VA & DoD, 2013). Because suicide assessment is not static, the individual's level of risk should be viewed on a continuum of low, moderate, and high risk. Other important biopsychosocial factors for service members and veterans also influence the level of suicidality:

- Sociocultural group as it relates to one's mental health and mental health treatment;
- Level of social support to assist in stabilizing mood, affect, and behavioral lifestyle;
- Coordination of treatment between primary care and mental health providers;
- Clinically significant critical life events that have presented within the last 30 days or so (e.g., separation; divorce; death of a spouse, family member, or friend; incarceration; legal or financial issues; chronic life-threatening illness or disability; loss of occupation or career);
- Perception and attitude toward a critical life event as communicated by the individual;
- Diagnosis of major depressive disorder, anxiety, trauma disorder, substance use disorder, or bipolar disorder;
- Communication of the intent to harm self or others;
- Communication of a plan to harm self or others; and
- Previous suicidal ideation, threats, attempts, or lethal attempts of deliberate self-harm.

Multiple brief suicide screenings and assessments facilitated by primary care medical and mental health providers evaluate stressful life events along a continuum of low, moderate, and high (Bryan et al., 2014; Griffith & Bryan, 2018; Rosellini et al., 2017; Sterling et al., 2017). Important areas for evaluating suicide risk along the continuum are offered next; each item may be formed into open- and closed-ended questions:

- Changes in any social or intimate relationships (i.e., loss of spouse, intimate partner, family members, friend),
- Starting or ending a job by the individual or family member (i.e., unemployment, fired, quit, less-than-honorable discharge),
- Starting or ending educational opportunities by the individual or family member (i.e., dropping out of school because of poor academics, maladaptive behaviors, loss of interest in future),
- Legal issues incurred by the individual or family member (i.e., driving under the influence, lawsuit, upcoming court hearing or mediation),
- Financial status changes for the individual or family member (i.e., loss of income, reduced disability benefits, credit card or gambling debt),
- Change in drinking habits (i.e., more frequent, binge drinking, level of alcohol by volume),
- Changes in mood and affect (i.e., feeling more down, fatigued, lack of interest, not motivated to engage in activities at or outside of home, low self-esteem or self-image), and
- Gun ownership (i.e., purchase of new firearms, means of storing weapons, last time weapon was fired).

The literature on suicide assessment in the military offers multiple items to consider when evaluating the level of threat or risk (Harmon et al., 2016; VA, 2019; VA & DoD, 2013). The interested reader should consult the reference list for other appropriate screenings, assessments, algorithms for the assessment and management of suicide, as well as other prevention and treatment resources. Accordingly, competent clinical military counselors should

- Choose assessments that consider multiple factors in evaluating the service member's, veteran's, and family member's level of suicidality or threat;
- Apply clinical judgment based on a comprehensive clinical assessment that informs appropriate interventions along the continuum of low, moderate, or high threat;
- Consider the level of threat and other factors that relate to high-risk populations (e.g., women and minority women with a history of MST or intimate partner violence, service members and veterans identifying as LGBT, individuals deployed to special operation missions);
- Recognize salient aspects of the military culture and that they may not disclose or communicate feelings, thoughts, and behaviors associated with suicide;

- Recognize that service members' self-disclosure of psychologically distressing events and clinically significant mental health symptoms affects their fitness for duty, perceived ability to lead, job roles, and career and promotions;
- Identify the cultural stigma of mental health treatment seeking in and out of the military;
- Monitor one's professional attitude and perception toward gun ownership and weigh this opinion with the weapons training requirement as being part of the military occupation; and
- Recognize service members' and veterans' positive attributes, coping and resiliency skills, unit support acting as extended family members, and other unused opportunities to assist in deescalating a mental health crisis and decrease suicide threat levels.

Overall, suicidal thoughts and behaviors can be evaluated in multiple clinical settings and at various levels of low, moderate, or high suicide threat. The fact remains that most service members and veterans who are on the threat continuum do not have a suicide completion.

MILITARY SUICIDE PREVENTION AND TREATMENT

Several epidemiological studies of civilian suicide with large sample sizes have led military researchers to apply some of the clinical and demographic characteristics, risk and protective factors, as well as prevention and treatment approaches for military populations (France & Hallows, 2019; Griffith & Bryan, 2018; Johnson et al., 2014; Leard-Mann et al., 2013). Military and nonmilitary mental health research groups have teamed up to thoroughly understand the unique clinical characteristics that contribute to suicidality within the U.S. military. From a suicide prevention perspective, it is helpful to understand intervention, prevention, and treatment strategies. These strategies are typically communicated in epidemiology within three levels: primary, secondary, and tertiary. When discussing epidemiological medical and mental health concerns, each level has a distinctive purpose, strategy, approach, and intention for prevention. These three levels are most parsimoniously defined as follows:

Primary prevention: This level of prevention focuses on the number of new cases of suicidal ideation, lethal attempts, and completions. It also delineates the associated risk factors. The intention at this level is psychoeducation to promote awareness and knowledge of military suicide risk and protective factors. Informing key constituents at the primary prevention level provides opportunities for connecting with community-based medical and mental health partners. In the military, primary prevention includes a broad-based approach communicated through the command structure, engaging service members with online and live training sessions. The emphasis is typically on increasing optimal health and influencing good mental and behavioral health (i.e., nutrition, exercise, peer counseling, regular medical checkups). Medical and mental health clinicians are also assets in primary prevention efforts who can partner with unit commanders as well as veteran treatment facilities and clinics.

Secondary prevention: This level of prevention aims to reduce the progression of suicidality through early detection, identification, and interventions. Primary medical and mental health care providers who can identify service members or veterans who float on the suicide risk continuum are the key to this level of prevention. Intervention is facilitated to mitigate the progression of the mental health symptoms that lead to suicidality.

Tertiary prevention: This level of prevention attempts to reduce the severity of the mental symptoms associated with suicide. Some efforts involve mandatory substance abuse and mental health treatment, whereas other efforts focus on fitness-for-duty evaluations. Tertiary prevention tends to serve higher risk military populations who have exhibited a history of negative mental health behaviors and consequences related to their suicidality.

Most suicide prevention efforts within the DoD are aimed at primary prevention programs (Ramchand et al., 2014). It has been my clinical experience that many younger enlistees are not fully influenced by primary prevention programs aimed at stress inoculation and good mental health hygiene. These active-duty personnel sometimes are "strongly recommended" by base medical providers to seek a mental health provider off base for more confidential and long-term treatment. Despite the strong recommendations to seek mental health counseling, many active-duty service members do not make a first appointment for fear of peer or unit reprisal, loss of security clearances, and lack of job and rank promotions. There have been some successes that recognize mental health symptoms and early warning signs of suicidality with the strategies and interventions of professional and peer support such as found in the following programs: Comprehensive Soldier and Family Fitness, Comprehensive Airman Fitness, Sailor Assistance and Intercept for Life, and Combat Operational Stress Control (Griffith & Bryan, 2018). Accordingly, some comprehensive programs equip military personnel with specific information and tools that indirectly decrease significant mental health symptoms associated with suicidality. Many of these programs assist service members with (a) identifying the clinically significant mental health symptoms related to combat operational stress, (b) increasing good cognitive behavioral functioning, and (c) locating tools and resources for effective stress coping and resiliency.

Nonmilitary community-based clinicians, hospitals, and clinics also play a key role in preventing suicide completions. These medical and mental health providers can partner with base clinics (e.g., U.S. Naval hospitals, U.S. Army clinics) for integrated and coordinated patient care. The VA clinics have also provided leadership in forming partnerships, expanding access to mental health screening, prevention, and treatment with military service members, veterans, and families (France & Hallows, 2019).

On the basis of salient characteristics in military suicidology and the related literature on military suicide prevention and treatment, the following recommendations are offered:

- A positive correlation exists between suicidal behaviors and specific critical life events that occur in and out of military life, such as combat operational stress and trauma, MST, intimate partner violence, financial and legal issues, as well as separation and divorce. Thus, prevention and treatment approaches have the potential to address suicide and mental health risk factors by forming well-matched treatment groups of service members and veterans on and off military base.
- Clinicians should weigh the level of their active-duty client's lethality with protecting the service member's career. If suicidality is not addressed early on, the mental health symptoms soon become apparent to self, unit peers, and military families and worsen in some cases. Thus, therapeutic opportunities may be lost to save a life if prevention and intervention strategies are ignored.
- All phases of the deployment cycle have unique stressors associated with how successfully one transitions through each phase (i.e., social support, healthy intimate relationships, economic stability, mood regulation and stabilization). Addressing mental health issues and symptoms early on as they relate to acute stress and adjustment disorders has the potential to reduce the level and intensity of military life.
- Approaches such as mindfulness-based stress reduction, breathing meditation, yoga, and other complementary and integrative health approaches have shown improvement in the reduction of the mental health symptoms associated with acute stress, anxiety, low mood and affect, alcohol and tobacco misuse, and process addictions.
- Structured programs that offer peer support; accountability to self and others; and a list of other multiple resources in religious, faith-based, and spiritual communities are effective.
- A critical component of suicide prevention within the military culture utilizes coping and resiliency training to facilitate activities that promote optimal wellness throughout the life span of service members and veterans.
- Therapeutic and process groups matched by gender, racial, and ethnic characteristics are effective. Some examples include female service members and veterans, minorities, LGBT individuals, and other racial and ethnic groups.

- Stress debriefings facilitated by mental health professionals triaging at-risk groups for more intensive interventions are essential for both prevention and treatment approaches.
- The use of the Veterans Crisis Line (1-800-273-8255; press 1) as well as local community mental health providers can save the life of a service member or veteran. The VA's Patient Safety Plan is also critical in six important areas (i.e., warning signs, internal coping strategies, people and social settings that provide distraction, people who can offer help, professionals and agencies to contact, and making a safe environment; B. Stanley & Brown, 2008).

Interested readers should consult the reference list for specific details on suicide prevention and treatment programs across the various branches of the military. It is critical that all medical and mental health care providers remain vigilant with screening, assessment, prevention, and treatment of suicidal behaviors across the risk continuum. Partnering with military installations and community-based providers is a shared responsibility.

PSYCHOSOCIAL ASPECTS OF MILITARY SUICIDE

Although medical and mental health researchers and practitioners stand ready to handle the epidemiological concerns of military suicide, it requires an attitudinal and leadership shift by the DoD to implement policies that advocate for good mental health hygiene among service members and veterans. The medical and mental health of the military is only as good as the leadership itself who can organize, plan, implement, and advocate for optimal functioning within military life as well as during reintegration and transition. However, online education and training regarding good mental health hygiene do not appear to effectively address issues of suicidality. For many service members, it does not appear relevant because they typically do not experience more chronic, persistent, and intense mental health symptoms related to suicidality until they separate from the military.

Tick (2014), in his work with veterans' moral injury, stated that "no society is healthy without a healthy, functioning elder warrior class leading the way into a future of hope, responsibility, true security, and peacemaking based on the transformational wisdom and healing gained from an ordeal" (p. xix). The essential point regarding the psychosocial aspects of military suicide is that the environment itself can be part of the problem. Good mental health functioning does not totally reside within the individual service member and veteran. It is critical to reduce the stigma and disincentives associated with mental health treatment seeking by providing good access to screening, prevention, and treatment without consequences to the service member's promotion and career. The moral injury of war comes with a profound psychosocial cost to a service member's or veteran's mental, physical, and spiritual health. Some are positively transformed by their warfighting or military life experiences, whereas others are defeated. Accordingly, unique psychosocial adjustment and mental health characteristics test the service member's ability to reintegrate and transition successfully. Tick has suggested that being in combat itself and killing others is an abnormal experience. Accordingly, restoring the soul after war is strongly needed. The invisible wounds of war are a natural artifact of warriorhood. The natural consequence of exposure to high levels of stress, trauma, and violence that result from warfighting is the threat of suicide along the continuum of risk and lethality.

Many practitioners have suggested that some veterans feel betrayed by their military service. These veterans become isolated and detached from society because most civilians do not understand the mental, physical, spiritual, and existential challenges of military life. Perhaps one of the greatest challenges in the psychosocial adjustment of transitioning is the persistent complex bereavement that occurs as the result of trauma exposure and the frequent loss of life (Stebnicki, 2018). For instance, the nature of the suicide death itself affects both military families and those who served within the deceased member's unit. In a sense, the family system (biological and extended military family members) feels a sickness and vulnerability to the mental health virus of suicide that has claimed the life of their loved one. For many, survivor guilt prompts symptoms of complex and persistent grief and bereavement.

Grief and loss in the military can be ambiguous in nature. The suicide virus within the military family is a multidimensional phenomenon because of the range of symptoms, risk factors, and mental health conditions associated with the death event itself. From a psychodynamic perspective, competent clinicians can clearly observe healthy and unhealthy grief responses as well as good and poor coping and resiliency skills in their military clients. Some in the military express little emotion after a combat-related casualty or suicide completion, whereas others are overwhelmed by the experience. Many times, we look to others in our family and culture to determine how we should express and experience grief, what we should feel and think, and how to respond. In chronic and persistent grief, the following risk factors are important considerations during grief counseling with military families, friends, or unit members:

- The type and nature of the relationship that the service member or veteran had/has to the deceased;
- The type of death experienced (i.e., combat, suicide, natural causes) and whether the death was witnessed by any of the survivors;

- Where the survivor was physically and geographically when the death occurred (i.e., within the continental United States, outside the continental United States, same mission, in country but different mission);
- Anniversary dates, holidays, or past celebrations with the deceased, which ultimately place survivors at risk for feeling vulnerable and fragile (increasing the potential for self-harm);
- Grief and loss that accentuate the individual's current medical, physical, and mental functioning (e.g., the survivor's major depressive disorder may intensify and become more severe), placing the survivor in a more vulnerable mental or cognitive state;
- Level of acknowledgment and expression of the death and associated losses;
- Level of psychosocial adjustment, social and professional support, or any resources that the survivor can access to heal their mind, body, and spirit;
- Clinically significant mental health symptoms that have occurred since the time of death (e.g., flashbacks, night terrors, emotional or social detachment, isolation, avoidance or intrusive thoughts related to the death experience, cognitive and emotional feelings of numbness, detachment, confusion, intense levels of bitterness, anger, hostility, feelings of hopelessness and helplessness); and
- Presence and level of any suicidal ideation as well as history of ideation or attempts.

In many models of grief and bereavement therapy, there is a growing acceptance that attachment, remembering, and continuing the bonds with the deceased are both natural and healthy (Koblenz, 2016; Worden, 2009). The following grief therapy approaches are offered to assist survivors in continuing the bonds in their work:

- Connecting with the deceased by making efforts to locate them (e.g., in heaven, in another dimension in time and space, in the wind or water);
- Experiencing the deceased in dreams, daily thoughts, and prayers;
- Communicating with the deceased by speaking with them through silent thoughts, verbal expression, and gravesite visitation;
- Remembering the deceased in a conscious way through intentional rituals and ceremonies; and
- Using a variety of objects for attachment (e.g., clothing, jewelry, dog tags, medals, patches, home videos).

Therapeutic benefits with these "remembering" therapeutic strategies assist survivors in clarifying and bringing meaning to the relationship they had with the deceased. They also assist survivors with (a) decreasing any ambiguity with the death, (b) recognizing the reality of the death and associated losses, (c) addressing any unresolved feelings and thoughts, (d) strengthening the bond with the deceased, and (e) honoring the memory of a fallen unit member.

Overall, there are multiple opportunities for mental health professionals to prepare for, plan, and intervene in a variety of critical incidents in military life. The grief associated with combat casualties and suicide is an emerging area of interest but has rarely been addressed in the research. This lack of research is particularly the case regarding symptomatology associated with persistent complex bereavement conditions and complex PTSD.

CONCLUDING REMARKS

The epidemiological significance of military suicide demands clinicians' complete and full attention to the appropriate resources for screening, assessment, prevention, and treatment. Even one suicide is tragic to the service member's family members, loved ones, and military family. Most service members and veterans do not experience suicidality. The negative societal stigma and perception regarding veteran mental health and suicide lethality can negatively reinforce veteran self-care efforts. Military suicidality also presents other problems with difficulties finding jobs, educational opportunities, careers, and forming social and intimate relationships. Suicide assessment needs to be viewed across the continuum of suicide lethality. Suicide prevention and mental health treatment works most effectively when it is endorsed by all military health systems. Shifting the attention to identification and prevention will change the conversation from living with the stigma of a "diagnosis" to coping and resiliency skills that can provide opportunities for optimal personal growth.

REFERENCES

Arbisi, P. A., Rusch, L., Polusny, M. A., Thuras, P., & Erbes, C. R. (2013). Does cynicism play a role in failure to obtain needed care? Mental health service utilization among returning U.S. National Guard soldiers. *Psychological Assessment, 25*(3), 991–996. https://doi.org/10.1037/a0032225

Bryan, C., Blount, T., Kanzler, K. A., Morrow, C. E., Corso, K. A., Corso, M. A., & Ray-Sannerud, B. (2014). Reliability and normative data for the Behavioral Health Measure (BHM) in primary care behavioral health settings. *Families, Systems, & Health, 32*(1), 89–100. https://doi.org/10.1037/fsh0000014

Cox, K. L., Nock, M. K., Biggs, Q. M., Bornemann, J., Colpe, J., Dempsey, C. L., Heeringa, S. G., McCarroll, J. E., Ng, T. H., Schoenbaum, M., Ursano, R. J., Zhang, B. G., & Benedek, D. M. (2017). An examination of potential misclassification of Army suicides: Results from the Army Study to Assess Risk and Resilience in Servicemembers. *Suicide and Life-Threatening Behavior, 47*(3), 257–265. https://doi.org/10.1111/sltb.12280

Eaton, K. M., Messer, S. C., Garvey Wilson, A. L., & Hoge, C. W. (2006). Strengthening the validity of population-based suicide rate comparisons. *Suicide and Life-Threatening Behavior, 36*(2), 182–191. https://doi.org/10.1521/suli.2006.36.2.182

Fontana, A., & Rosenheck, R. (1995). Attempted suicide among Vietnam veterans: A model of etiology in a community sample. *American Journal of Psychiatry, 152*(1), 102–109. https://doi.org/10.1176/ajp.152.1.102

France, D., & Hallows, J. (2019, October 29). Suicide prevention strategies with the military-affiliated population. *Counseling Today, 62*(5), 42–47. https://ct.counseling.org/2019/10/suicide-prevention-strategies-with-the-military-affiliated-population/

Gardner, J. W., Cozzini, C. B., Kelley, P. W., Kark, J. A., Peterson, M. R., Gackstetter, G. D., & Spencer, J. D. (2000). Department of Defense Medical Mortality Registry. *Military Medicine, 165*(Suppl. 2), 57–61. https://doi.org/10.1093/milmed/165.suppl_2.57

Griffith, J., & Bryan, C. J. (2018). Preventing suicides in the U.S. military. *Psychological Services, 15*(3), 251–261. https://doi.org/10.1037/ser0000225

Harmon, L. M., Cooper, R. L., Nugent, W. R., & Butcher, J. L. (2016). A review of the effectiveness of military suicide prevention programs in reducing rates of military suicides. *Journal of Human Behavior in the Social Environment, 26*(1), 15–24. https://doi.org/10.1080/10911359.2015.1058139

Johnson, L. L., O'Connor, S. S., Kaminer, B., Jobes, D. A., & Gutierrez, P. M. (2014). Suicide-focused group therapy for veterans. *Military Behavioral Health, 2*(4), 327–336. https://doi.org/10.1080/21635781.2014.963762

Jowers, K. (2019, September 26). Here's what first-ever data shows about military family suicides. *Military Times*. https://www.militarytimes.com/2019/09/27/heres-what-first-ever-data-shows-about-military-family-suicides/

Kessler, R. C., Stein, M. B., Bliese, P. D., Bromet, E. J., Chiu, W. T., Cox, K. L., Colpe, L. J., Fullerton, C. S., Gilma, S. E., Gruber, M. J., Heeringa, S. G., Lewandowski-Romps, L., Millikan-Bell, A., Naifeh, J. A., Nock, M. K., Petukhova, M. V., Rosellini, A. J., Sampson, N. A., Schoenbaum, M., . . . Ursano, R. J. (2015). Occupational differences in US Army suicide rates. *Psychological Medicine, 45*(15), 3293–3304. https://doi.org/10.1017/S0033291715001294

Kline, A., Weiner, M. D., Interian, A., Shcherbakov, A., & St. Hill, L. (2016). Morbid thoughts and suicidal ideation in Iraq war veterans: The role of direct and indirect killing in combat. *Depression and Anxiety, 33*(6), 473–482. https://doi.org/10.1002/da.22496

Koblenz, J. (2016). Growing from grief: Qualitative experiences of parental loss. *OMEGA, 73*(3), 203–230. https://doi.org/10.1177/0030222815576123

LeardMann, C. A., Powell, T. M., Smith, T. C., Bell, M. R., Smith, B., Boyko, E. J., Hooper, T. I., Gackstetter, G. D., Ghamsary, M., & Hoge, C. W. (2013). Risk factors associated with suicide in current and former US military personnel. *Journal of the American Medical Association, 310*(5), 496–506. https://doi.org/10.1001/jama.2013.65164

Mansfield, A. J., Bender, R. H., Hourani, L. L., & Larson, G. E. (2011). Suicidal or self-harming ideation in military personnel transitioning to civilian life. *Suicide and Life-Threatening Behavior, 41*(4), 392–405. https://doi.org/10.1111/j.1943-278X.2011.00039.x

Matarazzo, B. B., Barnes, S. M., Pease, J. L., Russell, L. M., Hanson, J. E., Soberay, K. A., & Gutierrez, P. M. (2014). Suicide risk among lesbian, gay, bisexual, and transgender military personnel and veterans: What does the literature tell us? *Suicide and Life-Threatening Behavior, 44*(2), 200–217. https://doi.org/10.1111/sltb.12073

May, A. M., & Klonsky, E. D. (2016). What distinguishes suicide attempters from suicide ideators? A meta-analysis of potential factors. *Clinical Psychology: Science and Practice, 23*(1), 5–20. https://doi.org/10.1111/cpsp.12136

Ramchand, R., Eberhart, N. K., Guo, C., Pedersen, E. R., Savitsky, T. D., Tanielian, T., & Voorhiers, P. (2014). Developing a research strategy for suicide prevention in the Department of Defense: Status of current research, prioritizing areas of need, and recommendations for moving forward. *Rand Health Quarterly, 4*(3), Article 16. https://europepmc.org/articles/PMC5396216;jsessionid=91B6924317319D70CE9F66AC6DE70BAB

Reger, M. A., Smolenski, D., Skopp, N. A., Mezger-Abamukang, M. J., Kang, H. K., Bullman, T. A., Perdue, S., & Gahm, G. A. (2015). Risk of suicide among US military service members following Operation Enduring Freedom or Operation Iraqi Freedom deployment and separation from the US military. *JAMA Psychiatry, 72*(6), 561–569. https://doi.org/10.1001/jamapsychiatry.2014.3195

Ringer, F. B., Soberay, K. A., Rogers, M. L., Hagan, C. R., Chu, C., Schneider, M., Podlogar, M. C., Witte, T., Holm-Denoma, J., Plant, E. A., Gutierrez, P. M., & Joiner, T. E. (2018). Initial validation of brief measures of suicide risk factors: Common data elements used by the Military Suicide Research Consortium. *Psychological Assessment, 30*(6), 767–778. https://doi.org/10.1037/pas0000519

Rosellini, A. J., Stein, M. B., Benedek, D. M., Bliese, P. D., Chiu, W. T., Hwang, I., Monahan, J., Nock, M. K., Petukhova, M. V., Sampson, N. A., Street, A. E., Zaslavsky, A. M., Ursano, R. J., & Kessler, R. C. (2017). Using self-report surveys at the beginning of service to develop multi-outcome risk models for new soldiers in the U.S. Army. *Psychological Medicine, 47*(13), 2275–2287. https://doi.org/10.1017/S003329171700071X

Sexton, M. B., Davis, M. T., Anderson, R. E., Bennett, D. C., Sparapani, E., & Porter, K. E. (2018). Relation between sexual and gender minority status and suicide attempts among veterans seeking treatment for military sexual trauma. *Psychological Services, 15*(3), 357–362. https://doi.org/10.1037/ser0000207

Skopp, N. A., Holland, K. M., Logan, J. E., Alexander, C. L., & Floyd, C. F. (2019). Circumstances preceding suicide in U.S. soldiers: A qualitative analysis of narrative data. *Psychological Services, 16*(2), 302–311. https://doi.org/10.1037/ser0000221

Skopp, N. A., Smolenski, D. J., Sheppard, S. C., Bush, N. E., & Luxton, D. D. (2016). Comparison of suicide attempters and decedents of the U.S. Army: A latent class analysis. *Suicide and Life-Threatening Behavior, 46*(4), 413–426. https://doi.org/10.1111/sltb.12227

Stanley, B., & Brown, G. K. (2008). *Patient safety plan template.* https://suicidepreventionlifeline.org/wp-content/uploads/2016/08/Brown_StanleySafetyPlanTemplate.pdf

Stanley, I. H., Rogers, M. L., Hanson, J. E., Gutierrez, P. M., & Joiner, T. E. (2018). PTSD symptom clusters and suicide attempts among high-risk military service members: A three-month prospective investigation. *Journal of Consulting and Clinical Psychology, 87*(1), 67–78. https://doi.org/10.1037/ccp0000350

Stebnicki, M. A. (2018). Psychosocial counseling aspects of grief, death, and dying. In I. Marini & M. A. Stebnicki (Eds.), *The psychological and social impact of illness and disability* (7th ed., pp. 245–256.). Springer.

Sterling, A., Bakalar, J. L., Perera, K. U., DeYoung, K. A., Harrington-LaMorie, J., Haigney, D., & Ghahramanlou-Holloway, M. (2017). Perspectives of suicide bereaved individuals on military suicide decedents' life stressors and male gender role stress. *Archives of Suicide Research, 21*(1), 155–168. https://doi.org/10.1080/13811118.2016.1166087

Tick, E. (2014). *Warrior's return: Restoring the soul after war.* Sounds True.

U.S. Department of Defense. (2019). *Department of Defense (DoD) Annual Suicide Report: Calendar Year (CY) 2018.* https://www.airforcemag.com/PDF/DocumentFile/Documents/2019/2018_ASR_External_Briefing_092619.pdf

U.S. Department of Veterans Affairs. (2019, September). *2019 National Veteran Suicide Prevention Annual Report.* https://www.mentalhealth.va.gov/docs/data-sheets/2019/2019_National_Veteran_Suicide_Prevention_Annual_Report_508.pdf

U.S. Department of Veterans Affairs & U.S. Department of Defense. (2013, June). *VA/DoD clinical practice guideline for assessment and management of patients at risk for suicide.* https://www.healthquality.va.gov/guidelines/MH/srb/VADODCP_SuicideRisk_Full.pdf

Worden, J. W. (2009). *Grief counseling and grief therapy: A handbook for the mental health practitioner* (4th ed.). Springer.

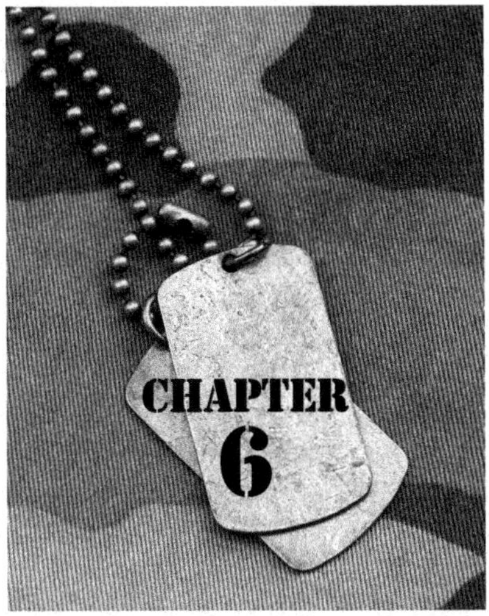

PSYCHOSOCIAL ASPECTS OF CHRONIC ILLNESS AND DISABILITY IN VETERAN HEALTH

The defining characteristics of most chronic illnesses and disabilities are the individual's perception and attitude of the event itself and how it relates to their residual functional capacity and ability to transcend such an experience.

—Mark A. Stebnicki, 2020

★ ★ ★

In this chapter, I explore and discuss veteran health care issues and the impact that chronic illness and disability have on veteran transition to civilian life. Many veterans have been exposed to Coronavirus (COVID-19) and need testing, medications to control symptoms, and medical equipment (e.g., ventilators). At the time of this writing, a COVID-19 vaccination is under development that may be available to help veterans in late 2020 and beyond. If developed, this vaccine will help deter second- and third-wave infections. Thus, the U.S. Department of Veterans Affairs (VA; 2020b) has ramped up their telemedicine or telehealth programs during periods of mandated social distancing and social isolation to deal with nonurgent care evaluating symptoms through VA Video Connect.

Indeed, there are multiple roles and responsibilities of government and private health care providers to maintain and increase optimal medical, physical, and mental health functioning. A model of psychosocial adjustment and adaptation to disability is offered that will assist clinicians to anticipate and predict the various psychosocial phases that are important for successful veteran reintegration and transition. Guidelines are presented for prevention and treatment to deal with the multiple complex challenges in veteran medical, physical, and psychological health; vocational and social adjustment; as well as environmental functioning.

Some veterans are at considerable risk for chronic health conditions that may result in permanent and total disability. Comprehensive and quality care for persons with chronic illnesses and disabilities requires appropriate education, training, and professional experiences to work optimally with the individual (Smart, 2016). To move forward with this mission, it is vital that veterans receive the highest quality of health care.

MONITORING THE HEALTH NEEDS OF VETERANS

Community-based outpatient clinics and inpatient rehabilitation treatment facilities (e.g., to treat traumatic brain injury [TBI], spinal cord injuries, substance abuse) play an important role in the VA and Veterans Health Administration (VHA) service delivery system and are essential for providing optimal medical and mental health care for more than 3 million veterans. Comprehensive and quality medical and mental health treatment continue to be a priority for veterans throughout the life span. However, the concerns related to veterans' health care as identified by the U.S. Department of Defense (DoD), U.S. Congress, and various veteran organizations are numerous and wide ranging.

Veterans' health care needs are not addressed for multiple reasons. Military researchers have suggested that few veterans seek mental health treatment because of social and self-stigma (Hitt & Massi Lindsey, 2019; Skopp et al., 2012). Female veterans with military sexual trauma (Campbell & Raja, 2005; Zinzow et al., 2015) and members of the LGBT veteran community have poorer health outcomes because of concerns of safeguarding their privacy and social stigma (Johnson & Federman, 2013; Stebnicki et al., 2015). Veterans in rural communities (Ysasi & McDaniels, 2018), minority veterans (Pittman et al., 2019; Tsai et al., 2014), and veterans with disabilities (Baker & Cormier, 2015) all tend to have less access to health care treatment, rendering these groups as vulnerable and at risk for chronic medical and mental health conditions.

In the VA and DoD Joint Executive Committee strategic plan for 2019–2021 (VA & DoD, 2019), robust priorities have been proposed for optimizing the mental and physical health needs of veterans. Four strategic goals are provided in this report that center on (a) high-quality, patient-centered health care access with increased patient satisfaction outcomes; (b) providing comprehensive services and benefits that are patient centered and integrated within the veteran's community; (c) provision of effective and efficient delivery of services in the planning and operations of the VA's national health care system; and (d) creating a seamless transition from active duty to veteran life in which patient care is integrated and health care decision-making metrics are maximized (e.g., more timely VA disability determination ratings and eligibility, carry through on medical plans and treatment).

As a result of these strategic goals and efforts driven by Section 702 of the National Defense Authorization Act for Fiscal Year 2017, the Defense Health Agency is reorganizing the way in which military hospitals and clinics are managed in terms of departments, administrations, and regional military treatment facilities. The goal of the Defense Health Agency is to create a more integrated, efficient, and modern system of managed care that will improve the quality of treatment that veterans receive (Military Health System Communications Office, 2020).

The U.S. Government Accountability Office (2018) provides oversight and monitoring of the nation's 168 VA medical centers and 733 community-based outpatient clinics. In 2016, these clinics provided health care to more than 3 million veterans at a cost of $3.5 billion. Although most community-based outpatient clinics (632 of 733 clinics) are owned and operated by the VHA, 14% (n = 101) are operated by non-VHA health care organizations that contract with the federal government. The U.S. Government Accountability Office has cited long-standing concerns regarding quality of treatment, inaccurate and incomplete reporting of data regarding patient outcomes, lack of guidance and training for staff, as well as other issues that potentially compromise the medical, physical, and mental health care of U.S. veterans. Consequently, these current challenges and deficits within the health care system need to be addressed because veterans are one of the highest risk groups in the United States regarding medical, physical, and mental health treatment.

Most mental health practitioners who completed graduate coursework in traditional counselor education or psychology programs received training primarily in the biomedical model of treatment. This model is characterized by "professionals" who assess, diagnosis, and treat the "patient's mental health disorder" with a substantial focus on the psychopathology of the individual. Facilitating treatment within the biopsychosocial model focuses on person-informed and person-centered therapeutic approaches. Thus, the clinician partners with the client, who is empowered by health care choices and responsibilities.

Competent clinical military counselors understand that providing services to persons with chronic illnesses and disabilities is hindered by negative societal attitudes and stigma that influence personal self-esteem and self-concept. Skilled practitioners also facilitate therapeutic interactions within a multicultural context, attuning therapeutic practices to the identity of the client while considering the unique cultural attributes that eventually assist in building rapport and earning the circle of trust. Competent clinicians are also mindful of issues related to social justice, such as disability rights legislation that protects and promotes access to housing, transportation, jobs, and other privileges afforded to all Americans. In addition, many other essential elements are needed to provide optimal quality of care and to ensure that the needs of individuals are met (Marini & Stebnicki, 2018).

HEALTH DISPARITIES AMONG VETERANS

Goals for improving health disparities among veterans are outlined in the VA and VHA plans for a comprehensive and quality health care service delivery system. The disparities in veteran medical, physical, and mental health care are well understood and elucidated within various governmental and veteran organizational reports. Health disparities among minority groups have been well documented for quite some time in the civilian epidemiology literature. In military epidemiology, health disparities among minority veterans are visually depicted on health surveillance maps that reflect reduced utilization, lower quality of care, and negative patient health outcomes (Kondo et al., 2017; Ysasi & McDaniels, 2018).

One critical area of concern involves veterans who get left behind after separation from service and become homeless. Veteran homelessness negatively affects medical, physical, and mental health care outcomes and creates a major group of veterans affected by health disparities. The estimated number of homeless veterans in the United States has declined since 2010. Yet, in January 2019, there were still 37,085 veterans who remained homeless (VA, 2019). Compared with civilians, veterans are at a significantly higher risk for homelessness because of numerous risk factors that include, but are not limited to, (a) low socioeconomic status; (b) lower pay grade (E1–E4) at the time of separation from service; (c) separation from service with a general or less-than-honorable discharge; (d) exposure to combat operational stress that prompts higher levels of posttraumatic stress, depression, anxiety, substance use, psychotic disorders, and suicidal ideation; (e) preenlistment medical and mental health conditions and other characteristics that were negatively affected by military life; and (f) misuse of opioids initially prescribed because of muscular skeletal pain conditions (Bachhuber et al., 2015; Hayden, 2018). Other substantial risk factors have arisen among homeless veterans previously deployed to Afghanistan and Iraq who sustained medical, physical, and psychological injuries during combat operations (e.g., TBI, posttraumatic stress disorder [PTSD]). This group is particularly challenged during reintegration and transition because of the lack of career options resulting from lower job skills and complications from mental and physical disabilities.

Other gaps in health care services include treating chronic and persistent medical conditions that manifest long after the service member has been discharged. This occurrence becomes problematic for veterans with conditions of unknown etiology that mimic symptoms from groups of other diseases that may be undiagnosed, misdiagnosed, or undertreated by veteran health care providers. A prime example is the newer chronic medical condition referred to as Gulf War illness (GWI) or chronic multisymptom illness (CMI). This chronic condition affects about 25%–32% of the 697,000 veterans who fought in the 1991 Gulf War and is associated with chronic fatigue, joint pain, wake-sleep disorders, gastrointestinal problems, headaches, skin rashes, and cognitive complaints (Janulewicz et al., 2017; White et al., 2016).

One of the largest epidemiological studies to date has reported significantly higher mental and physical health conditions as a result of symptoms associated with GWI/CMI (Dursa et al., 2016). Gulf War veterans continue to report high levels of cardiopulmonary, neurological, and gastrointestinal diseases. Interestingly, the incidence remains high among Gulf War veterans irrespective of whether they were deployed to combat operations. Accumulating evidence suggests a strong association between exposure to chemicals, such as nerve agents used during combat deployment, and the symptoms reported. Despite the reported clinically significant symptoms of GWI/CMI, the literature in military medicine reports limitations and confounding results in research studies. Some of these shortcomings include errors in research methodologies, the use of veteran populations from other wars exhibiting similar symptoms, studies with small sample sizes, and other design issues that fail to validate this medical condition (Janulewicz et al., 2017). One factor that stands out is the similar incidence and prevalence of GWI/CMI in mental and physical health conditions regardless of combat exposure or support of combat operations.

At the time of this writing, the VA has implemented aggressive public health measures to ensure the health of veterans during the COVID-19 pandemic (VA, 2020a). Testing is available to veterans, clinical screenings can be made through telemedicine approaches, health care providers are working in coordination to ensure that protective medical equipment and procedures are in place, and education is being disseminated to veterans to contain the spread of COVID-19. This approach has created both deficits and opportunities for partnering TRICARE mental health providers to offer treatment using telemental health approaches. Usage of such services is at an all-time high for veterans requiring ongoing treatment and first-time mental health services. The DoD has also received millions of dollars in funding from the U.S. Congress to assist in testing, prevention, and treatment of active-duty service members, reservists, and National Guard soldiers, particularly those who have been deployed overseas in global pandemic hot spots.

VETERANS LIVING WITH CHRONIC ILLNESSES AND DISABILITIES

The World Health Organization (n.d.) has reported that about 1 billion persons worldwide live with a disability. Many of these disabilities are caused by motor vehicle accidents; falls causing catastrophic injury; acts of physical, sexual, and intimate partner violence; and war. The serious injuries typically acquired during these incidents include TBI, traumatic amputation, spinal cord injury, as well as muscular skeletal and chronic pain conditions.

Statistically, most persons in the United States will spend the last 12 years of their life in a state of decreased physical, neurocognitive, or psychological functioning because of chronic health conditions (Eisenberg et al., 1999; Falvo, 2017). Military service members who were exposed to extraordinary stressful and traumatic events are in a higher risk category for long-term chronic health conditions that may not show up for years but will eventually limit residual functional capacity (Livneh & Antonak, 2018; Marini & Stebnicki, 2018; Stebnicki, 2001, 2016, 2017).

MILITARY TBI

TBIs and blast injuries, known as the signature medical concerns of Operation Iraqi Freedom (OIF) and Operation Enduring Freedom (OEF), are discussed at length in Chapter 8. In terms of veteran health initiatives, the incidence and prevalence of TBI is substantial in both veterans and civilians. Proportionately, military service members acquire TBI at a higher frequency than civilians. Between 2000 and 2018, more than 383,947 U.S. service members worldwide sustained a TBI (Defense and Veterans Brain Injury Center, 2020). Approximately 10%–20% of veterans deployed to the Iraq (OIF) and Afghanistan (OEF) wars sustained a TBI, making it one of the most disabling and frequently occurring injuries of OIF and OEF (Elder, 2015; Hoge et al., 2008). Although more than 80% of all military TBIs are reported as mild, much of the attention medically has focused on treating moderate and severe TBIs. Long-term adverse health conditions are associated with all TBIs, specifically dementias and chronic traumatic encephalopathy. Unfortunately, between 2003 and 2006, many military service members with mild TBI went either unreported or underreported, causing this serious condition to be untreated or undertreated (Chase & Nevin, 2015).

Psychosocial adjustment to chronic illness and disability among service members takes on unique cultural characteristics that differ from civilians because of how the illness or disability was acquired (Buck, 2012; Stebnicki, 2017). For instance, many military personnel acquired their TBI after being "blown up" during combat operations, which is not typical among civilians. After acquiring a TBI or blast injury in the military, service members are at higher risk for multiple neurological deficits, muscular skeletal or orthopedic injuries (e.g., chronic pain syndromes, traumatic amputation, multiple joint or ball-and-socket injuries), sensory deficits (i.e., medically determinable hearing and vision loss, loss of feeling and sensation), soft tissue injuries, traumatic amputations, and burns. A major consequence of TBI is the increased incidence of PTSD. As a result of co-occurring medical, physical, and mental health conditions acquired during military life, the term *complex PTSD* signifies the multidimensional nature of these health conditions.

OTHER CHRONIC HEALTH CONDITIONS

During the initial stages of most acute and traumatic injuries, the service member may be evacuated out of harm's way and flown to an acute care military treatment facility. In the case of TBI, after medical stabilization, the service member would be transferred to a military neurorehabilitation unit where they would spend weeks or months receiving intensive speech, occupational, and physical therapies, along with other treatments by allied health specialists. Depending on the person's medical stability, as well as neurocognitive and physical improvement, they may be discharged to complete therapy through outpatient services back in the United States at an appropriate military clinic on or off base. The status of their residual functional capacity will be determined at some point, which may be a year postinjury, where the medical community will indicate whether they have reached maximum medical improvement. Meanwhile, the service member is dealing with the psychosocial adjustment across multiple life areas. This adjustment includes—but is not limited to—work and educational settings; social, emotional, and interpersonal demands; recreational activities; as well as family-relational and independent living. Overall, when maximum medical improvement is reached, it typically results in medically and psychologically determinable impairments that require a medical separation from the military in which the service member is granted a disability rating with earned disability benefits.

Psychosocial adjustment to chronic illness and disability is an ongoing struggle that often follows the veteran throughout their lifetime. Following this paragraph, I present a list of frequently reported and clinically significant veteran health symptoms that are well documented in the literature and require ongoing medical care (Lehavot et al., 2013; Wachen et al., 2013). The list is divided into specific body systems followed by the most frequently occurring symptoms as reported by veterans to their health care provider. Competent practitioners understand that veterans are at high risk and require more comprehensive and frequent medical, physical, and mental health treatment. It is important to understand that many medical symptoms often have a psychological component. For instance, panic attacks and high levels of anxiety can mimic symptoms of chest pain. Anxiety particularly has been linked to the health of the gastrointestinal system. Stressful life events and traumatic experiences manifest in dermatological skin disorders and migraine headaches. The medical community, not surprisingly, treats such conditions at times from the biomedical model, prescribing various medications to treat the primary symptoms rather than addressing the etiology. Overall, the following body systems and medical symptoms are frequently reported as significant problems by veterans and their medical providers:

- Cardiovascular: chest pain
- Dermatological: skin disorders (e.g., rashes, eczema, psoriasis, unexpected hair loss, scalp problems)
- Gastrointestinal: frequent diarrhea, recurrent abdominal pain, recurrent nausea
- Genitourinary: sexual difficulties or discomfort, loss of bowel and bladder control
- Musculoskeletal: loss of strength, joint and muscle pain, joint stiffness
- Neurological: recurrent migraines, numbness, difficulty speaking, tinnitus, eye and vision problems
- Pulmonary: wheezing, coughing, shortness of breath, frequent coughing

As a result, mental health practitioners should consider the following guidelines as they relate to the development of a comprehensive plan of medical, physical, and mental health treatment for veterans:

- Encourage veterans to consult their medical providers for assessment, evaluation, and diagnosis of any related medical conditions;
- Understand the mind-body connection as it relates to extraordinary stressful and traumatic experiences of veteran health;
- Coordinate a plan of care with your veteran's medical providers through the release of information, disclose medical and psychological treatments and compliance, and develop ongoing health evaluation points critical for mind-body issues;
- Approach veteran medical and mental health care from a behavioral lifestyle perspective, encouraging integrative health strategies—such as healthy nutrition, exercise, movement throughout one's daily

activities, healthy intimate and interpersonal relationships, as well as therapeutic recreational activities that can be accommodated and tailored for the veteran's interests, aptitudes, and personality traits—and reinforcing resiliency approaches;

- Combine the veteran's structured plan of care with natural supports, being mindful of the impact that the environment has on mental and physical health and resources;
- Explore the veteran's preenlistment behavioral lifestyle habits, risk behaviors, physical health characteristics, personality traits, coping and resiliency skills, mental health hygiene, and other vital life areas to enhance strengths and attributes; and
- Identify and recognize the unique cultural attributes that may predispose the veteran to poorer medical, physical, and mental health concerns while combining the veteran's indigenous or cultural belief system of healing the mind, body, and spirit.

PSYCHOSOCIAL ADJUSTMENT TO CHRONIC ILLNESS AND DISABILITY

As a result of life-saving medical advances and technology, more military service members from OIF and OEF have survived traumatic injuries than from all other wars (Cooper et al., 2018). In fact, more than 52,000 U.S. service members have been injured, with more than 7,000 casualties the result of OIF and OEF. As of February 2020, Operation Inherent Resolve, which commenced in August 2014, resulted in 88 active-duty service members, reservists, and National Guard soldiers killed in action and 175 injured in combat (Defense Casualty Analysis System, n.d.). Despite a significant reduction in casualties and injuries, the United States is still at war, and the mission creep does not have a timetable.

A considerable volume of research in psychosocial rehabilitation pertains to adaptation and adjustment to acquired disability. In the traditional counseling and psychology literature, psychosocial rehabilitation has been a difficult topic to discuss and provide guidelines for application. Most studies are nonmilitary related and are within the discipline of rehabilitation counseling. From a developmental psychology perspective, there are critical life stages of social and emotional development, as well as other predictable and anticipated phases, that the individual transitions through during their life span. However, early developmental theorists did not consider the impact that chronic illness and disability have during early childhood, adolescence, and adulthood (Marini, 2018). Persons with mental and physical disabilities do not have opportunities to experience critical life junctures along the developmental continuum. More specifically, they experience social stigma and stereotypes at much higher rates than persons without disabilities. Additionally, persons with disabilities have significantly elevated rates of unemployment, unavailability of quality health care, substandard independent living situations, transportation difficulties, and restricted access to public accommodations because of accessibility issues. For instance, the environment itself can be a barrier to full participation for a person in a wheelchair or an individual who has had both legs amputated.

Psychosocial adjustment, adaptation, and response to chronic illness and disability are a complex interplay of the individual's medical, physical, psychological, social, emotional, spiritual, educational, vocational, and environmental functioning. Illness and disability affect the physical and mental health of veterans in profound ways, complicating reintegration and transition to civilian life. Psychosocial adjustment issues affect military families and may begin during the deployment cycle; they are often accentuated after medical separation from military service (Basham, 2013; Pincus et al., 2020). Overall, the culture of disability in military life has both similarities and differences with that of persons who did not serve. Some common characteristics associated with psychosocial adjustment to chronic illness and disability (Falvo, 2017; Livneh & Antonak, 2018; Marini & Stebnicki, 2018; Stebnicki, 2001) include—but are not limited to—the person's

- Unique experiences of how they acquired their illness or disability (e.g., motor vehicle accident, an improvised explosive device attack, playing sports);
- Additional cultural attributes of race, ethnicity, gender, gender orientation, spiritual beliefs, country of origin, as well as other salient characteristics;
- Degree of residual functional capacity and the impact that the illness or disability has on independent daily functioning;
- Attitude and perception of their own disability and related factors, such as body image, level of independence, self-efficacy, and internal-external locus of control;
- Comparison of self with others who appear normal or able-bodied and the assimilation of what the biomedical model of health refers to as a disorder, psychopathology, or diagnosis that diminishes and separates the person from societal expectations of what normal should look and act like;
- Level of coping and resiliency skills; pre- and postdisability experiences of handling loss, grief, and extraordinary stressful and traumatic events; and the specific meaning and significance assigned to the major life changes resulting from living with a physical or mental health condition;
- Natural support systems—such as family, friends, and social organizations—and the level of motivation to reach out for help when needed;

- Prolonged course of medical or mental health treatment that requires ongoing evaluation, treatment, use of medication and medical equipment, and ongoing adjustment to the plan of care (there may also be needs for accommodation at work, school, home, or public places);
- Uncertain or ambiguous diagnosis and prognosis of a specific medical condition and the medical community's ability to competently and effectively provide treatment; and
- Constant and intense psychosocial stressors and the overall impact that they have on the family dynamics.

There are difficulties moving forward in treatment planning without comprehensive medical information. Thus, a good medical record provides all therapeutic partners with information regarding the (a) stability, (b) progressive nature, (c) episodic nature, (d) degenerative nature, and (e) periods of exacerbation and remission of the client's health condition.

The knowledge, awareness, and skills to work competently with your client's chronic illness or disability are essential as they relate to treatment strategies over time. Here are a few case illustrations:

- Persons with TBI generally reach maximum medical improvement in about a year, after which there is a period of stability. Assisting your client with the appropriate accommodations to maximize their cognitive abilities, physical capacity, accessibility requirements, as well as mental and behavioral health needs is vital.
- Aging has a significant impact on chronic illness and disability. There is a decline in physical, mental, and cognitive function. The physical and architectural environment may require accommodation across multiple life areas. The person may exhibit deteriorating cognitive abilities; decline in energy level; chronic fatigue; as well as ambulation, balance, and strength issues requiring a personal care assistant.
- Persons with traumatic amputation require ongoing monitoring of their skin integrity on their stump. Common medical management of persons with traumatic amputation is for self-monitoring of pressure sores. Multiple prosthetic devices are required throughout one's lifetime. Assisting your client with accessibility issues, body image, mental health symptoms, and ongoing need for medical equipment is essential to maintain optimal levels of independent functioning and overall health.
- Persons with back or other orthopedic injuries (e.g., degenerative disc disease, stenosis of spinal cord) require pain management interventions. As their muscular skeletal system becomes compromised in older age, the degenerative nature and severity of their injury may become more intense to manage. Thus,

ongoing use of therapeutic modalities is critical to maintain optimal physical and mental health functioning (e.g., physical therapy, home exercises, use of heat, acupuncture, managing pain medications). Skin integrity is essential to manage to prevent pressure sores. Personal care assistance may be required for daily activities.

The intention of these four case illustrations is to show that the clinician may have to adjust their client expectations across the life span regarding the progressive nature of the illness, disease, or disability. Implied within the construct of psychosocial rehabilitation is that individuals may traverse along a continuum of disability. At one end of the continuum, the person may not feel physically or psychologically "disabled." Adjustment and adaptation to illness and disability are multidimensional and can relate to possessing a positive attitude and perception regarding their physical and mental health conditions. People who have appropriate accommodations (i.e., medical equipment, technology for independent functioning) have improved opportunities for independent living in the least restrictive environments, whereas—on the other end of the disability continuum—other people may have critical and intense needs for physical or psychological care. The person may relapse, placing them back into the hospital for another surgery, requiring further rehabilitation and other intensive treatments. As a result of a medical crisis, the individual is at risk for a psychological relapse and may regress to earlier phases of their acute injury (e.g., blown up, lost a limb, sustained a TBI).

Implied in the construct of psychosocial rehabilitation is that persons with chronic illnesses and disabilities have multiple losses of mental, physical, cognitive, social, emotional, and psychological functioning. The ability to sustain their career, education, relationships, and independent functioning has been compromised. Competent clinical military counselors understand that veterans with chronic illnesses and disabilities may experience multiple losses:

- Loss of one's identity as a solider, sailor, Marine, airman, or Coastie;
- Loss of military career, educational opportunities, and any other meaningful future vocational or career opportunities;
- Loss of control over one's decision-making capacity and independence, which leads to reliance on external sources of support and total dependence on family members for care;
- Loss of a sense of fairness and justice, which leads to questioning the meaning of their military service;
- Loss of emotional, cognitive, and mental health abilities to regulate thoughts, behaviors, mood, and affect; and
- Loss of physical capacity, body image, and the ability for sexual or intimate relationships.

Psychosocial adjustment to chronic illness and disability within the biopsychosocial model views the individual as a "survivor" rather than a "victim," which is a critical point for practitioners to understand. Metaphorically, practitioners can empower survivors by focusing on "operation survivor" or "operation self-care" within the therapeutic environment. A survivor is focused on the "mission" of coping, resiliency, regulation of mood and affect, and cultivating optimal levels of health and well-being. Experienced therapists who have listened to testimonials of veteran survival understand which of their clients are survivors and which are not. Therapists can assist veterans by constructing meaning in their traumatic experiences. They can provide the motivation for change and cultivate feelings and cognitions of hope and resiliency to transcend the multiple losses that veterans have experienced in their military life. Therapists can teach resiliency skills and provide opportunities to open doors to cultivate other integrative health and healing resources outside of session. Alternatively, viewing veterans from a victim perspective takes on the characteristics of learned helplessness and hopelessness. It disempowers veterans for achieving optimal physical and psychological health.

Competent clinical military counselors who understand both the veteran and disability culture have a veteran-empowered base to focus their therapeutic efforts. For instance, multiple other areas within the biopsychosocial model of disability need to be evaluated, such as (a) what meaning does the person ascribe to their disability? (b) how does the person evaluate their own adjustment and adaptation to their disability? and (c) does the person pathologize their experience of disability or do they see themselves as no different than others? Thus, a comprehensive clinical evaluation considers more than mental health–related factors. Consideration is given to the client's issues of psychosocial adjustment for coping and resiliency.

General standardized measures of adaptation to chronic illness and disability have existed for quite some time and offer psychometrically sound assessments that measure the individual's adjustment to chronic illness, acceptance of physical disability, perception of their impaired health status, and psychological and emotional reactions to impairment and disabling conditions. The interested reader should refer to Livneh and Antonak's (1997) comprehensive discussion of multiple measures of adjustment to disability. A sample of the subscales and content items measuring adjustment and adaptation to illness and disability includes the person's

- Attitude and perception of the physical and mental health care they receive,
- Home environment (how physically and architecturally accommodating it is for optimal independent functioning) and level of assistance and support,

- Quality of supportive family and extended family relationships,
- Level and quality of sexual and intimate healthy relationships in their life,
- Quality of social relationships and involvement in therapeutic activities,
- Psychological and emotional stressors in their life that exacerbate existing mental health conditions (e.g., PTSD, anxiety, depression, and substance use disorders),
- Levels of self-esteem and body image,
- Sleep hygiene and resting habits,
- Nutritional and eating habits that promote a positive behavioral lifestyle, and
- Reaction to their impairment or disability as it relates to the eight psychosocial scale items within models of psychosocial adjustment (i.e., shock, anxiety, denial, depression, internalized anger, externalized hostility, acknowledgment, and adjustment).

PSYCHOSOCIAL STAGE MODELS OF DISABILITY

Several stage models have been offered in the literature regarding psychosocial adaptation to disability, trauma, crisis, grief, and loss (Antonak & Livneh, 1991; Garfield, 1979; Kubler-Ross, 1969; Livneh, 2001; Livneh & Antonak, 2018; Shontz, 1975; Smart & Smart, 2018). These models emphasize that the (a) prolonged course of treatment, (b) often uncertain prognosis, (c) constant intense psychological-emotional stressors, (d) limited daily functioning, and (e) psychological impact on family and friends all combine to create complications in adjustment and adaptation to extraordinary stressful and traumatic events.

Stage models of psychosocial adjustment and adaptation also make it clear that (a) there is no universal experience or response to chronic illness, trauma, and disability; (b) a state of final adjustment (sometimes referred to as resolution, acceptance, assimilation, or reintegration) is not always achievable by the individual; and (c) on the basis of the available clinical and empirical evidence, psychological recovery does not follow an orderly sequence. Thus, individuals may experience phases of adjustment on a continuum, regress to an earlier phase, skip one or more phases, or overlap with other phases (Livneh & Antonak, 1997). Overall, it is suggested that each stage of adaptation and adjustment to disability (a) requires different coping patterns; (b) can be both maladaptive and adaptive; and (c) is associated with a variety of emotional triggers that hinder the survivor's ability to adapt to their experience of trauma, loss, or disability.

The overall purpose of stage models of disability is to assist mental health practitioners with a conceptual clinical perspective of how the individual transitions through their illness or disability. They can also assist mental health practitioners in treatment planning and deciding what course of action is appropriate within the rehabilitation process.

Livneh and Antonak (2018) offered a stage model based on more than 30 years of research. This model provides a comprehensive overview of the psychosocial reaction and experiences of individuals living with a chronic illness or disability. Although considerations were not given to the military culture specifically, the model does consider persons with acquired traumatic experiences as well as other physical and psychological conditions. Ultimately, this model can assist clinical military counselors in conceptually understanding the personal adjustment needs associated with the psychosocial rehabilitation process.

First, several common assumptions of this psychosocial stage model need to be identified. These assumptions, which are based on the various other stage models of adaptation and adjustment to illness and disability, include the following:

1. Adaptation is a dynamic and individualized process whereby the person's premorbid or preinjury level of functioning may determine how well they deal with the loss and grief associated with their illness or disability.
2. The adaptation process is not a linear progression; rather, the individual may regress to an earlier phase or skip one or more phases altogether.
3. The duration of each phase of adaptation depends on factors such as age of onset, premorbid personality, prior experience with crisis situations, nature and severity of the illness or disability, extent of social support, and the human and financial resources available to the person.
4. Successful transition through the phases of adaptation should produce increased psychological growth and maturity as observed by the person's coping mechanisms.
5. Not all individuals reach the theoretical endpoint of adaptation and adjustment.

A brief description of Livneh and Antonak's (2018) psychosocial stage model is offered next. Unique aspects in each phase of this stage model and its application need to be examined for the military and veteran culture. I have adapted this model to include some salient aspects that may differentiate civilians versus veterans with disabilities.

Shock and initial impact are generally perceived as the individual's initial or emergency reaction to the onset of a sudden and severe physical injury or psychological trauma. It is a reaction resulting from the impact of an overwhelming extraordinary stressful event during exposure to a specific critical incident, such as combat operations or posttraumatic stress. This stage is characterized by psychic numbness, depersonalization, cognitive disorganization, and often dramatic loss of communication abilities. First responders, medics, and emergency medical personnel are typically not recognized or remembered by the service member as they are being evacuated out of a combat zone.

Anxiety is viewed as a panic reaction typically experienced after the initial sensing of the magnitude of the physical or psychological traumatic event. Typical reactions to anxiety are signified by confused thinking, cognitive overload, numerous physiological responses, panic reaction, and hyperreactivity. At this stage, the service member's sympathetic nervous system is in overdrive. They are cognitively irrational, physiologically fighting for survival.

Denial is observed as the painful realization of the extent, duration, and future implications of the chronic illness or disability. It involves the individual (a) reacting resistively or defensively or (b) minimizing the chronicity of their disabling condition. Denial often includes an irrational and unrealistic expectancy of recovery by developing a distorted picture of reality. Depending on the severity, the service member will likely be "med boarded" out of the service. Medical separation from service and transition to civilian life invites a cascade of other unhealthy emotions and behaviors that the service member will have to deal with eventually.

Depression is a reaction often observed among most persons with an acquired physical or psychological disability. Symptomatology will vary depending on the disability. Some issues that become a source of depression include the impact and perceived loss associated with the individual's physical, social, emotional, and psychological functioning; career; independence; and financial stability. Depending on the person's personality characteristics before the disability, past reactions to stressors and trauma, and other biological and neurochemical attributes, they often feel helpless, hopeless, isolated, or self-depreciated. This stage becomes a critical area for the veteran's life, and they may exhibit behaviors of suicidality.

Anger and hostility represent self-directed resentment and bitterness and are often associated with feelings of self-blame. Feelings of self-guilt and survivor guilt are also often observed, as are self-injurious and suicidal ideation. If the service member had unit buddies die during battle, the feelings of survivor guilt are intensified. This reaction is most evident in veterans who have a first level of awareness and realization that their impairment may be a permanent and chronic condition. This stage is also viewed as the veteran's attempt to retaliate against other family members or health care professionals. This phase is characterized by aggressive verbally and physically threatening behaviors, antagonistic and overly critical responses to others, and passive-aggressive behaviors. Depending on other critical events happening around the veteran (e.g., multiple surgeries, extended physical rehabilitation, divorce, substance use disorder, or opioid addiction), they may become homicidal or be at risk for suicidality.

Acknowledgment is regarded as the first awareness that the veteran has cognitively reconciled or accepted the permanency of their physical or psychological condition. The future implications that result in major life changes, such as military reintegration and transition, will also be realized. Veterans in this stage attempt to gain a new sense of acceptance and self-concept. They reappraise their life values, actively seek new meanings, and initiate goals that will lead them to the final theoretical stage of adjustment, integration, and growth.

Adjustment, integration, and growth are theoretically conceptualized as the final stage or phase of the adaptation process. This phase involves multiple factors that support the veteran's total awareness and meaning (affectively and cognitively) of the functional limitations or barriers imposed by the chronic physical or psychological disability. Persons may partially or fully assimilate into their new life space and successfully adapt to the civilian environment around them. Veterans who reach this phase reestablish a positive self-worth, realizing the existence of their residual functional capacity and newly discovered potentials. They retain their status and identity as a veteran and identify other veterans who may need emotional support and assistance. Despite the veteran's permanent or chronic condition, they actively initiate, pursue, and implement good healthy self-esteem and social connections; interpersonal and intimate relationships; educational, career, and vocational endeavors; as well as other goals that lead to optimal health and wellness.

Overall, an abundance of personal, social, emotional, and natural supports can be cultivated by veterans because of their extended military families. The veteran's capability for healthy coping and resiliency skills depend on multiple factors, such as their attitude and perception regarding their military life. Their level of social, family, spiritual, environmental, and financial support as well as their internal-external resources all influence the outcome of their psychosocial health and well-being.

COPING STRATEGIES

Coping strategies and stress appraisal have been studied for decades by classical theorists and stress researchers (e.g., Frankl, 1963; Kabat-Zinn, 1990; Lazarus, 1999; Lazarus & Folkman, 1984; Selye, 1950). The literature specific to how the individual copes with a variety of physical and psychological conditions is quite substantial. Coping, as it relates to persons with chronic illnesses and disabilities, is viewed as a psychological strategy to decrease, modify, or diffuse the impact of stressful and critical life events (Livneh & Antonak, 2018). The defining characteristics of coping include variables such as how the person (a) exhibits and experiences coping as a state or trait; (b) controls or manipulates their coping strategies; (c) organizes their coping style on a range of internal-external characteristics; and (d) responds from an affective, cognitive, or behavioral style of coping.

Falvo (2017) described *coping strategies* in relation to persons with chronic illnesses and disabilities as subconscious mechanisms for dealing with stress. Thus, the intention of coping is natural. It is a means for the person to reduce their levels of stress and anxiety. Coping styles are particularly relevant for veterans dealing with physical and psychological conditions. This is because in psychosocial adjustment to the trauma of illness or disability, the veteran has a strong need to bring balance, normalcy, productivity, and a certain quality of life back for optimal functioning. Multiple coping strategies are examined in the literature. However, the more common ones associated with persons who have acquired chronic illnesses or disabilities are listed next. As noted in the previous section, I delineate salient characteristics of healthy and unhealthy coping and interpret them for veterans.

Denial: Extraordinary stressful and traumatic events can be extremely overwhelming for veterans and their families. Denial may be experienced by the veteran on multiple physical, cognitive, psychological, emotional, social, and spiritual levels. When an overwhelming traumatic experience results in a disabling condition (e.g., being shot at, being blown up), the individual may deny the harsh reality of their newly acquired disabling condition. Depending on the severity of the disability, the veteran's residual functional capacity and independent functioning may be reduced. Thus, denial is a natural coping process and may be expressed consciously and unconsciously; furthermore, the veteran may exhibit denial in healthy and unhealthy ways. For example, an individual with a spinal cord injury may verbalize "I need to walk and drive again so I can get back to the fight." The conscious expression of "the need to work again" is healthy because it emphasizes the service member's career identity, purpose, and meaning of the mission.

However, if the service member has acquired a permanent condition that compromises ambulation, balance, coordination, and strength to be an able-bodied warfighter, then the service member may not have a realistic grasp of their permanently disabling condition requiring life-long medical treatment and rehabilitation. Denying the reality of the need for medical treatment, rehabilitation therapy, and psychological trauma is quite normal and is expected during initial phases of psychosocial adjustment and adaptation to chronic illnesses and disabilities. It is a way for the veteran to cope with the overwhelming experiences of being medically separated from service. Psychologically, the veteran is living in the past and is not focused on the here and now. If these unconscious or conscious thoughts and expressions persist for weeks and months until eventual medical separation from the service, then it is likely that the veteran is in unhealthy denial. Denial ultimately hinders their ability to progress to the point of maximum medical improvement or psychosocial adjustment.

Regression: Psychosocial response, adaptation, and adjustment to chronic illness and disability as described in this chapter can make it seem that the person transitions sequentially from one stage of adjustment to the next. After the individual successfully completes one psychosocial phase, theoretically, this achievement creates personal and psychological growth and enhanced psychosocial functioning. The individual then has the confidence, functional ability, self-concept, as well as the mental and emotional balance to achieve other necessary tasks and behaviors, which moves this person along the continuum of adjustment.

However, in regression, the veteran may return to an earlier stage of the psychosocial stage model, which signals poor adjustment and psychological growth. Regression to early stages of the psychosocial stage model is quite normal and expected, particularly with chronic and persistent physical and mental health conditions. However, if the person remains in a state of stagnation for weeks or months, it will be difficult to reach optimal levels of adjustment and integration to the mental, emotional, and social demands of civilian life. Some veterans intentionally (consciously) or unintentionally (unconsciously) may choose not to take responsibility for their overall physical and psychological health and well-being. This choice may be seen by others in the veteran's environment as poor adjustment to civilian life. The stigma attributed to poor adjustment to civilian life then spreads or is generalized to the veteran population as a whole.

Compensation: A natural artifact of having reduced physical or psychological functioning is for the individual to try out unfamiliar feelings, thoughts, and behaviors while they are attempting to achieve healthy reintegration and transition. Veterans with disabilities have multiple challenges with maintaining activities of daily living; healthy social connections; good physical, emotional, and psychological health; and maximum levels of independence. Healthy veterans become quite adept at creating accessible environments that accommodate their disability. Compensation is utilized as a coping strategy with the intention to improve life with reduced residual functional capacity. Compensation as a coping mechanism is also an attempt to achieve a higher degree of efficacy in one life area (e.g., educational and career opportunities outside the military) while sacrificing other life areas that are not attainable (e.g., physical training, shooting a rifle, driving a truck).

Veterans who use compensation behaviors and actions directed toward positive goals and outcomes are generally considered resilient. One strong indicator of resiliency is the ability to bounce back from adversity and not fear trying out new challenges (e.g., dating again, going out in public, returning to school). Compensation is observed when the individual loses functional capacity in one life area, then makes an attempt to excel in another. At times, persons with disabilities may be seen by others as "overcompensating" for their disability, which is associated with negative attributes. For instance, a person with a double amputation may want to try sky diving, scuba diving, or surfing. Others in the environment may sense that the veteran has become an overachiever. They may overcompensate as a way of proving to self and others that physical capacity has not limited their ability to function. The concept of overcompensation is not without controversy because most of the time people use their own personal values, philosophy, and beliefs to determine how others should live their lives. The primary consideration while evaluating compensation and overcompensation as a coping strategy is whether the activities or behaviors derive positive benefits to the person with a disability or whether there is harm to self and others.

Rationalization: Most individuals rationalize, justify, explain, or defend their reasoning for choosing everything from high-risk behaviors (i.e., substance use, driving fast) to intimate relationships. It is part of being human. Rationalization as a coping strategy allows the individual to find socially acceptable reasons for their behavior. It also serves to provide justification for not accomplishing a task or feeling motivated to achieve therapeutic goals. For most individuals, rationalizing feelings, emotions, thoughts, and behaviors is a personality state or trait and a normal way of being. A primary consideration for assessing the use of rationalization as a coping strategy is to look at the positive and negative effects it has on the veteran's physical and mental health. In many instances, rationalization serves as an avoidance mechanism or an irrational reaction to something that most others deem healthy.

Diversion of feelings: Many persons with disabilities feel a range of emotions related to their chronic and persistent disability. For instance, many veterans may exhibit a range of maladaptive coping behaviors regarding their mood and affect, such as irritability, anger, or hostility. These clinically significant symptoms may relate directly to their complex physical and mental health conditions (i.e., TBI, PTSD). Diverting negative emotions and behaviors toward others in the external environment (e.g., spouse, family members, health care providers) is unhealthy. Diverting feelings and behaviors internally can be self-destructive and equally unhealthy. Ultimately, the person chooses the feelings, attitudes, behaviors, and actions that allow them to grow personally and psychologically.

A natural artifact of acquired physical and psychological trauma is the struggle to find a healthy balance of feelings, thoughts, and actions that will lead toward optimal levels of psychosocial adjustment and overall well-being. Veterans who have complex physical and mental health conditions typically go through most phases of psychosocial adjustment and adaptation to their chronic illness or disability. Competent clinical military counselors understand how veterans progress through the various stages of psychosocial adjustment and know how to anticipate and plan for changes in the veteran's physical and psychological health. Veteran resiliency can be measured by the amount of psychological growth and development. Bringing meaning and purpose to one's present life situation and successfully transitioning psychosocially through the natural phases of adjustment lay the foundation for healing the mind, body, and spirit.

BEST PRACTICES FOR VETERAN PSYCHOSOCIAL ADJUSTMENT

Competent clinical military counselors understand the complex nature, interaction effects, and impact that disabilities have on the veteran's psychosocial health. Accordingly, the integration of psychosocial therapeutic treatment strategies is essential in transcending the medical model of disability. Skilled and competent therapists understand that disability may reside outside the veteran because the architectural environment may not be accessible for full participation. Skilled and competent therapists understand that societal stereotypes, stigma, and negative attitudes have a detrimental impact on the mental health and well-being of veterans and military families. To assist practitioners in working toward the psychosocial health and well-being of veterans with chronic illnesses and disabilities, I offer the following guidelines for consideration when dealing with psychosocial adjustment issues.

Recognize the person as a survivor: Viewing the person as a "trauma victim" discounts the person's survival skills. Victimhood negatively reinforces the stereotype of being helpless, hopeless, dependent, and defenseless. Facilitating therapeutic strategies as a "trauma survivor" empowers the veteran to view themselves as an individual that has good coping and resiliency skills. The military culture as a cohesive group or unit is generally more resilient than civilians who experience extraordinary stressful and traumatic events. This resiliency is primarily because the military trains individuals for multiple confrontations with enemy combatants, humanitarian mobilizations to war-torn countries, and deployments to respond to natural disasters. Some researchers have suggested that military training activities serve as a protective factor and inoculate the individual against traumatic stress.

Treat the individual, not the disability: Veterans with chronic illnesses and disabilities should be considered within the context of the society and environment where they live. Disability is a multidimensional construct. It is an interaction of how the person perceives their functional capacity, independence, and ability to do all things that people without disabilities can do. The deaf culture is one example of a culture that has determined its own unique values, beliefs, rituals, traditions, and other salient attributes. For instance, many people who are deaf do not perceive themselves as "a person with a disability."

Rather, society assigns and projects this identity onto the deaf culture itself. Persons who are deaf are different than those who are hard of hearing. The deaf community primarily comprises those individuals who acquired their deafness at birth or in early childhood. Members of the deaf culture are unique because they have their own mode of communication and language (e.g., American Sign Language), their own arts (e.g., National Theater of the Deaf), and their own system of higher education (e.g., Gallaudet University, Washington, DC). Likewise, members of the military culture are also unique because they have their own language, rituals, customs, organizational system, ranks, and many other cultural attributes. Veterans determine their own cultural identity and assign specific meaning that is connected to their military and civilian life.

Accept that extraordinary stressful and traumatic events are real and legitimate: Veterans involved in extraordinary stressful and traumatic events such as warfighting can benefit from physical and psychological therapeutic interventions. Research indicates that generally between 30% and 60% of veterans most affected by their traumatic military experiences will require long-term physical and mental health services. Some veterans deployed in noncombat units—who may have been close to but not at the epicenter of the combat theater of operations—may report the same level, degree, and frequency of stress and trauma. Some medical and mental health practitioners view this finding as paradoxical. However, all people turn on their stress mechanisms differently. Stress is the person's perception and attitude toward different critical events. Some veterans may have feelings of survivor guilt, may be emotionally weak, and may not be able to move beyond the horrors of warfighting. Trauma may be acquired by direct exposure, witnessing the critical event(s), learning or hearing about the trauma through a close friend or family member, or experiencing repeated trauma exposure. It has been shown that the body keeps a record of trauma within the various structures of the brain. The physiological and psychological effects associated with extraordinary stressful and traumatic events are a normal response to an abnormal event. Military trauma is not a somatoform disorder. Complex trauma experienced by veterans places them in a higher risk category for military suicidality.

Preenlistment mental health conditions predict postdeployment, reintegration, and transition reactions: Preexisting physical and psychological health can predict posttrauma recovery. Researchers have suggested that service members with preenlistment mental health conditions (e.g., depression, anxiety, trauma, substance use disorders) are most vulnerable among their ranks when confronted with the challenges of military life. This vulnerability is particularly an issue during trauma exposure. It is important to recognize that previous untreated trauma predisposes service members and veterans to the intensification of clinically relevant symptoms, which becomes a basis for treating complex trauma. Accordingly, untreated or undertreated physical and psychological conditions—as well as other critical life events (e.g., death of a family member, divorce, unit buddy's suicide completion)—all create disabling effects that render the person with an acceleration of chronic and persistent health symptoms. The combination and synergistic effects of preexisting physical and mental health conditions intensify vulnerability to critical and traumatic events. Thus, exposure to extreme stressors and trauma exposure act as "trigger events" that may exacerbate current physical and mental health functioning.

Preenlistment coping and resiliency skills predict postdeployment, reintegration, and transition success: Exposure to extraordinary stressful and traumatic events places service members and veterans at risk for long-term physical and psychological health problems, including moral injury. The mind, body, and spirit of individuals within the military culture are strong and resilient at the onset of enlistment, particularly given the intense commitment to the military as an occupation or career choice. Stress and trauma exposure may occur within one's military career. However, not all service members and veterans who have encountered trauma exposure acquire long-term physical or psychological conditions. Although extraordinary stressful and traumatic events can result in debilitating health conditions, researchers have clearly shown that not all service members or veterans exposed to traumatic stressors have the long-term complications of PTSD. Skilled and competent clinical military counselors know the importance and significance of their military client's ability to transcend trauma. Practitioners also recognize their client's coping and resiliency skills. They understand how to cultivate unused healing opportunities and facilitate opportunities for growth in one's mind, body, and spirit.

Earning the circle of trust is essential with military clients: Skilled and competent clinical military counselors understand the unique individual, sociocultural, and environmental attributes of their military clients. They understand how to analyze the individual's strengths and challenges and to cultivate an optimal rapport, with the intention of creating trust before implementing the use of therapeutic interventions. Earning the circle of trust is an ongoing goal for therapy. Rapport building itself is therapeutic and is a pathway to the working alliance. Thus, cultivating an authentic approach in a deeply intense therapeutic environment takes time but has rewards when dealing with complex physical and psychological health conditions in military life.

Empowering service members and veterans with natural support systems has long-term benefits: Family, friends, unit members, faith-based communities, veteran organizations, as well as other support groups can be pivotal in coping, recovery, and psychosocial adaptation to extraordinary stressful and traumatic health conditions. Natural support systems, by definition, are positive influences found within the individual's natural environment and are readily available when called on as a healing resource. Natural supports change and evolve over time. The natural supports that service members or veterans utilize today may not exist tomorrow. It may be that the individual or support system itself has geographically relocated to another base, has been deployed or mobilized, has separated from service or retired, or has been changed in other ways. Thus, skilled and competent clinical military counselors recognize the military client's need for ongoing natural support systems and assist them with cultivating similar resources within new environments. The intention of cultivating natural support systems with clients is to promote independence; self-motivation; self-responsibility; as well as optimal psychological, social, and emotional growth. Mostly, natural supports can be an extension of the therapeutic environment. Thus, it is critical for the individual and therapist to partner in cultivating natural resources.

Survivors of extraordinary stressful and traumatic events heal at different rates: The service member's or veteran's ability to cope, bounce back, or cultivate resiliency and hardiness with their psychosocial adjustment to a physical or mental health condition varies significantly. Many times, psychosocial adjustment to chronic illness, disability, and trauma does not fit neatly into a theoretical stage model. Victor E. Frankl (1963) summed up this point by suggesting that it is not necessarily the nature of the trauma itself that will affect one's ability to cope psychologically with its consequences. Rather, it is the person's own attitude and perception toward the trauma. Placing expectations and conditions on trauma survivors for meeting goals, moving along, or coming out of a depressive state requires the practitioner to view the person qualitatively as a unique individual who is composed of many attributes and characteristics. Society as a whole particularly places an overemphasis on when persons "should be done grieving" or when they "should be moving along in their grief." Thus, skilled and competent clinical military counselors understand the unique and complex grief and trauma that service members and veterans must manage. Overall, competent professionals recognize and understand (a) how each military client heals at their own pace; (b) how clients may relapse and regress to earlier phases of psychosocial adaptation and adjustment; and (c) that healing the mind, body, and spirit from trauma is a journey, not a destination.

CONCLUDING REMARKS

The literature on psychosocial adjustment issues is replete with theories and models of treatment primarily for nonmilitary populations. Translating psychosocial adjustment approaches to the military culture is essential for healing the mind, body, and spirit of veterans. The long-term physical and psychological health conditions of veterans have been discussed, and guidelines have been offered to clinical military counselors with the intention of addressing the holistic needs of veterans and family members. Psychosocial health and healing extraordinary stressful and traumatic events acquired during military life require a different understanding that includes a unique set of strategies to facilitate brief, immediate, and long-term interventions.

REFERENCES

Antonak, R. F., & Livneh, H. (1991). A hierarchy of reactions to disability. *International Journal of Rehabilitation Research, 14*(1), 13–24. https://journals.lww.com/intjrehabilres/citation/1991/03000/a_hierarchy_of_reactions_to_disability.2.aspx

Bachhuber, M. A., Roberts, C. B., Metraux, S., & Montgomery, A. E. (2015). Screening for homelessness among individuals initiating medication-assisted treatment for opioid use disorder in the Veterans Health Administration. *Journal of Opioid Management, 11*(6), 459–462. https://doi.org/10.5055/jom.2015.0298

Baker, L. R., & Cormier, L. A. (2015). *Disasters and vulnerable populations: Evidenced-based practice for the helping professions.* Springer.

Basham, K. K. (2013). Facilitators and barriers in effective clinical practice with postdeployment military couples and families. *Military Behavioral Health, 1*(22), 22–30. https://doi.org/10.1080/21635781.2012.721061

Buck, R. P. (2012). The impact of war on military veterans. In L. Lopez Levers (Ed.), *Trauma counseling: Theories and interventions* (pp. 434–453). Springer.

Campbell, R., & Raja, S. (2005). The sexual assault and secondary victimization of female veterans: Helping-seeking experiences with military and civilian social systems. *Psychology of Women Quarterly, 29*(1), 97–106. https://doi.org/10.1111/j.1471-6402.2005.00171.x

Chase, R. P., & Nevin, R. L. (2015). Population estimates of undocumented incident traumatic brain injuries among combat-deployed US military personnel. *Journal of Head Trauma Rehabilitation, 30*(1), 57–64. https://doi.org/10.1097/HTR.0000000000000061

Cooper, L. N., Holiday, R. P., Holder, N. D., Jackson, J., North, C., & Suris, A. M. (2018). Working with trauma-related mental health problems among combat veterans of the Afghanistan and Iraq conflicts. In I. Marini & M. A. Stebnicki (Eds.), *The psychological and social impact of illness and disability* (7th ed., pp. 311–342). Springer.

Defense and Veterans Brain Injury Center. (2020, May 11). *DoD worldwide numbers for TBI.* http://dvbic.dcoe.mil/dod-worldwide-numbers-tbi

Defense Casualty Analysis System. (n.d.). *Operation Inherent Resolve (OIR).* https://dcas.dmdc.osd.mil/dcas/pages/casualties_oir.xhtml

Dursa, E. K., Barth, S. K., Schneiderman, A. I., & Bossarte, R. M. (2016). Physical and mental health status of Gulf War and Gulf War era veterans: Results from a large population-based epidemiological study. *Journal of Occupational and Environmental Medicine, 58*(1), 41–46. https://doi.org/10.1097/JOM.0000000000000627

Eisenberg, M. G., Glueckauf, R. L., & Zaretsky, H. H. (1999). *Medical aspects of disability: A handbook for the rehabilitation professional.* Springer.

Elder, G. A. (2015). Update on TBI cognitive impairment in military veterans. *Current Neurology and Neuroscience Reports, 15*(10), Article 68. https://doi.org/10.1007/s11910-015-0591-8

Falvo, D. R. (2017). *Medical and psychosocial aspects of chronic illness and disability* (6th ed.). Jones & Bartlett Learning.

Frankl, V. E. (1963). *Man's search for meaning.* Pocket Books.

Garfield, C. A. (1979). *Stress and survival: The emotional realities of life-threatening illness.* Mosby.

Hayden, S. C. (2018). Supporting veterans experiencing homelessness through a theoretically-based career development group. *Journal of Military and Government Counseling, 6*(4), 215–255.

Hitt, R., & Massi Lindsey, L. L. (2019). Military members' perceptions of social norms about mental health for combat stress. *Military Behavioral Health, 8*(2), 181–190. https://doi.org/10.1080/21635781.2019.1630039

Hoge, C. W., McGurk, D., Thomas, J. L., Cox, A. L., Engel, C. C., & Castro, C. A. (2008). Mild traumatic brain injury in U.S. soldiers returning from Iraq. *New England Journal of Medicine, 358*(5), 453–463. https://doi.org/10.1056/NEJMoa072972

Janulewicz, P. A., Krengel, M. H., Maule, A., White, R. F., Cirillo, J., Sisson, E., Heeren, T., & Sullivan, K. (2017). Neuropsychological characteristics of Gulf War illness: A meta-analysis. *PLoS One, 12*(5), Article e0177121. https://doi.org/10.1371/journal.pone.0177121

Johnson, L., & Federman, E. J. (2013). Pathways and barriers to care for LGBT veterans in the U.S. Department of Veterans Affairs (VA). *Journal of LGBT Issues in Counseling, 7*(3), 218–235. https://doi.org/10.1080/15538605.2013.812928

Kabat-Zinn, J. (1990). *Full catastrophe living: Using the wisdom of your body and mind to face stress, pain, and illness.* Dell.

Kondo, K., Low, A., Everson, E., Gordon, C. D., Veazie, S., Lozier, C. C., Freeman, M., Motuápuaka, M., Mendelson, A., Friesen, M., Paynter, R., Friesen, C., Anderson, J., Boundy, E., Saha, S., Quiñones, A., & Kansagara, D. (2017). Health disparities in veterans: A map of the evidence. *Medical Care, 55*(Suppl. 2), S9–S15. https://doi.org/10.1097/MLR.0000000000000756

Kubler-Ross, E. (1969). *On death and dying.* Macmillan.

Lazarus, R. S. (1999). *Stress and emotions: A new synthesis.* Springer.

Lazarus, R. S., & Folkman, S. (1984). *Stress, appraisal, and coping.* Springer.

Lehavot, K., Der-Martirosian, C., Simpson, T. L., Shipherd, J. C., & Washington, D. L. (2013). The role of military social support in understanding the relationship between PTSD, physical health, and healthcare utilization in women veterans. *Journal of Traumatic Stress, 26*(6), 772–775. https://doi.org/10.1002/jts.21859

Livneh, H. (2001). Psychosocial adaption to chronic illness and disability: A conceptual framework. *Rehabilitation Counselor Bulletin, 44*(3), 151–160. https://doi.org/10.1177/003435520104400305

Livneh, H., & Antonak, R. F. (1997). *Psychosocial adaptation to chronic illness and disability.* Aspen Publishers.

Livneh, H., & Antonak, R. F. (2018). Psychological adaptation to chronic illness and disability: A primer for counselors. In I. Marini & M. A. Stebnicki (Eds.), *The psychological and social impact of illness and disability* (7th ed., pp. 77–90). Springer.

Marini, I. (2018). Theories of adjustment and adaptation to disability. In I. Marini & M. A. Stebnicki (Eds.), *The psychological and social impact of illness and disability* (7th ed., pp. 91–119). Springer.

Marini, I., & Stebnicki, M. A. (Eds.). (2018). *The psychological and social impact of illness and disability* (7th ed.). Springer.

Military Health System Communications Office. (2020, January 30). *DHA stands up first four health care markets.* Health.mil. https://health.mil/News/Articles/2020/01/30/DHA-stands-up-first-four-health-care-markets

National Defense Authorization Act for Fiscal Year 2017, Pub. L. 114–328 (2016, December 23). https://www.congress.gov/114/plaws/publ328/PLAW-114publ328.pdf

Pincus, S. H., House, R., Christenson, J., & Adler, L. E. (2020). *The emotional cycle of deployment: Military family perspective.* Military.com. http://www.military.com/spouse/military-deployment/dealing-with-deployment/emotional-cycle-of-deployment-military-family.html

Pittman, J. O. E., Baer, J., Everett, J., Dozier, M. E., Almklov, E., & Afari, N. (2019). Post-9/11 Latino veteran mental health service utilization. *Military Behavioral Health, 7*(4), 414–425. https://doi.org/10.1080/21635781.2019.1595228

Selye, H. (1950). Stress and the general adaptation syndrome. *British Medical Journal, 1*(4667), 1383–1392. https://doi.org/10.1136/bmj.1.4667.1383

Shontz, F. C. (1975). *The psychological aspects of physical illness and disability.* Macmillan.

Skopp, N. A., Bush, N. E., Vogel, D. L., Wade, N. G., Sirotin, A. P., McCann, R. A., & Metzger-Abamukong, M. J. (2012). Development and initial testing of a measure of public and self-stigma in the military. *Journal of Clinical Psychology, 68*(9), 1036–1047. https://doi.org/10.1002/jclp.21889

Smart, J. F. (2016). Counseling individuals with disabilities. In I. Marini & M. A. Stebnicki (Eds.), *The professional counselor's desk reference* (2nd ed., pp. 417–421). Springer.

Smart, J. F., & Smart, D. W. (2018). Models of disability: Implications for the counseling profession. In I. Marini & M. A. Stebnicki (Eds.), *The psychological and social impact of illness and disability* (7th ed., pp. 49–67). Springer.

Stebnicki, M. A. (2001). The psychosocial impact on survivors of extraordinary, stressful, and traumatic events: Principles and practices in critical incident response for rehabilitation counselors. *Directions in Rehabilitation Counseling, 12*(6), 57–71.

Stebnicki, M. A. (2016). Military counseling. In I. Marini & M. A. Stebnicki (Eds.), *The professional counselor's desk reference* (2nd ed., pp. 499–506). Springer.

Stebnicki, M. A. (2017). *Disaster mental health counseling: Responding to trauma in a multicultural context.* Springer.

Stebnicki, M. A., Grier, P. J., & Thomas, J. F. (2015). Best practices in the healthcare of LGBT military service members, partners, and families. *Journal of Military and Government Counseling, 3*(3), 150–171.

Tsai, J., Desai, M. U., Cheng, A. W., & Chang, J. (2014). The effects of race and other socioeconomic factors on health service use among a nationally representative sample of U.S. veterans. *Psychiatry Quarterly, 85*(1), 35–47. https://doi.org/10.1007/s11126-013-9268-0

U.S. Department of Veterans Affairs. (2019, November 18). *Homeless veterans.* https://www.va.gov/HOMELESS/pit_count.asp#:~:targetText=This%20national%20snapshot%20of%20Veteran%20homelessness%20showed%20that%3A&targetText=37%2C085%20veterans%20experienced%20homelessness%20in,through%20the%20HUD%2DVASH%20program

U.S. Department of Veterans Affairs. (2020a, May 12). *Novel Coronavirus disease (COVID-19).* https://www.publichealth.va.gov/n-coronavirus/?utm_source=Homepage&utm_campaign=Coronavirus

U.S. Department of Veterans Affairs. (2020b, March 25). *Using VA Video Connect to guard against infection.* https://www.blogs.va.gov/VAntage/72994/using-va-video-connect-guard-infection/

U.S. Department of Veterans Affairs & U.S. Department of Defense. (2019, March 18). *Joint strategic plan: Fiscal years 2019–2021.* https://prhome.defense.gov/Portals/52/Documents/VA-DoD%20FY%202019-2021%20JSP%20(signed%20March%2018%202019).pdf

U.S. Government Accountability Office. (2018, April). *VA health care: Actions needed to improve oversight of community-based outpatient clinics.* https://www.gao.gov/assets/700/691221.pdf

Wachen, J. S., Shipherd, J. C., Suvak, M., Vogt, D., King, L. A., & King, D. W. (2013). Posttraumatic stress symptomatology as a mediator of the relationship between warzone exposure and physical health symptoms in men and women. *Journal of Traumatic Stress, 26*(3), 319–328. https://doi.org/10.1002/jts.21818

White, R. F., Steele, L., O'Callaghan, J. P., Sullivan, K., Binns, J. H., Golomb, B. A., Bloom, F. E., Bunker, J. A., Crawford, F., Graves, J. C., Hardie, A., Klimas, N., Knox, M., Meggs, W. J., Melling, J., Philbert, M. A., & Grashow, R. (2016). Recent research on Gulf War illness and other health problems in veterans of the 1991 Gulf War: Effects of toxicant exposures during deployment. *Cortex, 74*, 449–475. https://doi.org/10.1016/j.cortex.2015.08.022

World Health Organization. (n.d.). *Injury-related disability and rehabilitation.* http://www.who.int/violence_injury_prevention/disability/en/

Ysasi, N. A., & McDaniels, B. W. (2018). Challenges faced by veterans residing in rural communities. In D. A. Harley, N. A. Ysasi, M. L. Bishop, & A. R. Fleming (Eds.), *Disability and vocational rehabilitation in rural settings: Challenges to service delivery* (pp. 139–150). Springer.

Zinzow, H. M., Britt, T. W., Pury, C. L., Jennings, K., Cheung, J. H., & Raymond, M. A. (2015). Barriers and facilitators of mental health treatment-seeking in U.S. active duty soldiers with sexual assault histories. *Journal of Traumatic Stress, 28*(4), 289–297. https://doi.org/10.1002/jts.22026

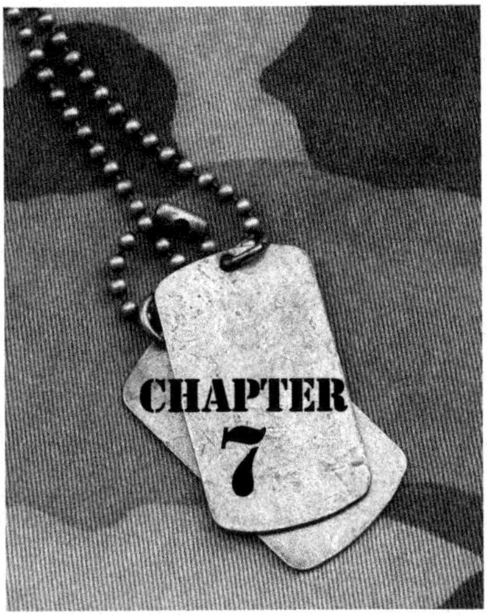

PSYCHOSOCIAL ASPECTS OF CHRONIC PAIN AND OTHER MEDICAL CONDITIONS IN MILITARY LIFE

Pain is just weakness leaving the body . . . Suck it up . . .
—Common military expression

★ ★ ★

This chapter addresses the medical and psychosocial aspects of chronic pain and other types of medical conditions, such as spinal cord injury (SCI) and traumatic amputation, that are associated with chronic pain conditions in military life. The primary focus of this chapter is on the unique, yet complex, experience of chronic pain in the military as it relates to physical and psychological conditions. The psychosocial impact on military occupation and independent functioning is also discussed. Guidelines for the screening, treatment, and prevention of chronic pain are offered to clinical military counselors.

Pain is one of the most frequently reported physical complaints in both military and civilian medical settings. Researchers have suggested that acute and chronic pain conditions affect between 100 and 126 million people in the United States (Institute of Medicine, 2011; Nahin, 2017). Poorly managed chronic pain conditions in civilian medical practices cost an estimated $560–$635 billion annually, considering all health care expenses (e.g., medications, physical therapy, surgeries, acute hospitalizations, physician visits; Brundage & Rubertone, 2014; Nahin, 2017).

Both acute and chronic pain conditions occur from nociceptive and neuropathic pain and are typically idiopathic in nature. Consequently, many medical practitioners find it challenging to evaluate the underlying conditions associated with the patient's report of acute and chronic pain. Psychogenic pain, or psychologically based pain, is also common among military service members and veterans. This condition is due to the military career itself, which has a higher incidence of posttraumatic stress and other co-occurring mental health disorders than in civilian life.

PREVALENCE AND INCIDENCE OF CHRONIC PAIN IN THE MILITARY

From a psychological point of view, somatic complaints of pain are difficult for medical and mental health providers to evaluate and treat. This issue arises when the medical records have an unknown etiology for the patient's complaints of pain. To complicate matters, the most frequent form of medical treatment for chronic pain symptoms, in both civilian and military medical treatment facilities, is medications prescribed to reduce the sensation and intensity of pain—particularly, the use of opioids. As a result, an increased risk of opioid use disorders has become the "Achilles' heel" of veteran medical and mental health care.

Among military veterans, chronic pain is the most common physical complaint, with more than 50% of men and 76% of women reporting chronic pain conditions to their health providers (Blakey et al., 2018; Kearns & Heapy, 2016). Overall, it is estimated that chronic pain conditions among active-duty service members and veterans range between 50% and 82% (Blakey et al., 2018; Brintz et al., 2020; Miller et al., 2017).

The etiology of chronic pain conditions in the military from a biophysiological point of view seems clear. It begins in boot camp, where extreme physical-exertional and psychological demands are placed on the individual's muscular skeletal system, joints, tendons, and muscles. This repetitive motion and heavy exertion begins the cascade of high-risk injuries (e.g., sprains, strains, tears, dislocations, spinal disc herniation, protrusion), which can lead to deteriorating conditions later in life. Some individuals can sustain this high level of physical activity, whereas others cannot. Specific medical conditions—such as blast injuries, traumatic brain injuries (TBIs), amputations, and burns—are also known to cause higher rates of chronic pain (Ruff et al., 2009; Runnals et al., 2013). After separation from military service, at least half of veterans will be awarded disability benefits on the basis of various well-documented physical and psychological conditions, with chronic pain being pronounced, resulting in reduced functional capacity (Gatchel et al., 2009).

Veterans have a significantly higher utilization of physical and mental health services, with chronic pain topping the list of medical complaints. The National Institutes of Health's National Center for Complementary and Integrative Medicine has reported that nearly two thirds of veterans are seen by medical providers for chronic pain conditions (Nahin, 2017). In a large sample size of veterans (N = 67,696), researchers reported that veterans were more likely than nonveterans to report back (33%) and joint (42%) pain (Nahin, 2017). In the category of "severe" chronic pain conditions, the prevalence was significantly higher in veterans than nonveterans. Veterans seeking medical treatment for severe pain conditions reported severe pain in their back (22%), jaw (38%), and neck (28%) as well as severe migraines (19%). Other studies have reported a higher incidence of severe chronic pain conditions. For instance, in a study of individuals deployed in support of Operation Iraqi Freedom (OIF) and Operation Enduring Freedom (OEF), more than 47% of veterans sought medical treatment for severe back and neck pain (Center for Deployment Psychology, n.d.; Reisman, 2016).

Posttraumatic stress symptoms typically co-occur with chronic pain conditions. Some studies have indicated that 97% of veterans seeking treatment for posttraumatic stress disorder (PTSD) also reported experiencing a chronic pain condition (Miller et al., 2017). The growing epidemic of opioid use disorders creates complex treatment decisions for medical providers. Overall, the psychological distress, poorer psychosocial functioning, and disabling conditions associated with chronic pain are pervasive among military service members and veterans. One of the most worrisome statistics indicates that chronic pain conditions predispose veterans to significantly higher rates of veteran suicidal ideation, lethal attempts, and completions (Blakey et al., 2018; Calati et al., 2015; Ilgen et al., 2010).

CLASSIFICATION AND ASSESSMENT OF PAIN

Pain is a multidimensional and multidetermined phenomenon and is defined by multiple sources and specialty areas. One of the more widely published definitions of pain is by the International Association for the Study of Pain (2011), which describes pain as an unpleasant sensory and emotional experience associated with actual or potential tissue damage or described in terms of such damage. However, M. Cohen et al. (2018) have proposed that pain is a mutually recognizable somatic experience that reflects a person's apprehension of threat to their bodily or existential integrity. Common assumptions within most definitions of pain include (a) a mind-body component based on an unpleasant sensory and emotional experience; (b) subjective universal ratings of pain typically measured on a scale ranging from 0 to 10; (c) measurable and observable conditions related to external and internal tissues, body systems, organs, and function and structure within the muscular skeletal system; and (d) a distinction made between acute and chronic pain.

Acute pain is typically the result of an injury or inflammation. Some of the most common sources of acute pain are infections, burns, untreated dental conditions, broken bones, surgical interventions, invasive medical procedures, and childbirth. *Chronic pain* is considered a pathological condition that serves no useful purpose and persists beyond the expected period of healing and typically lasts longer than 3–6 months (S. P. Cohen & Raja, 2016). Chronic pain conditions are also typically associated with impairments related to phantom limb pain, migraines, and fibromyalgia. These conditions are normally accompanied by both physical and psychological stress. Some of the most common sources of chronic pain originate from headaches and migraines, arthritis and joint pain, fibromyalgia, endometriosis, intestinal tract issues, trauma or postsurgical pain, muscular skeletal disorders, shingles, sickle cell disease, cancer, stroke, and diabetes. Several pain syndromes are considered "generalized pain" conditions, such as peripheral neuropathy, radiculopathy, causalgia, and reflex dystrophies. These conditions are now classified by the medical community as *complex regional pain syndromes* (International Association for the Study of Pain, 2011).

Because pain is typically rated by self-report, it is considered subjective. Subjective universal ratings of pain are measured on a scale of ranging from 0 (*no pain at all*) to 10 (*worst possible pain, requiring emergency medical treatment*). Most pain rating scales include content areas for evaluating the patient's physical, social, behavioral, and mental health. The individual's experience and response to pain is multidetermined and is based on their perception, threshold, and tolerance of pain (Falvo & Holland, 2018; Winterowd & Sims, 2016). Other factors have been noted as important considerations in the psychosocial assessment of chronic pain. These factors include mood and affect disorders, personality traits, addictive-type disorders, family relationships, environment, culture, spirituality, and daily stress (LeShan, 1979; McCarberg et al., 2012; Milks, 2012; Stebnicki, 2017).

Varieties of standardized, functional screening, and assessment tools measure the service member's and veteran's experience of pain. For example, the Pain Assessment Screening Tool and Outcomes Registry (PASTOR) is a 20- to 30-minute comprehensive self-report survey that provides a measure of the patient's experience of chronic pain (Defense & Veterans Center for Integrative Pain Management, n.d.). This assessment instrument was developed as a result of the National Defense Authorization Act for Fiscal

Year 2010 to improve the assessment and treatment of chronic pain among military service members and veterans. PASTOR uses items and content from other instruments developed by the National Institutes of Health, such as the Patient-Reported Outcomes Measurement Information System (https://commonfund.nih.gov/promis/index). This system uses computerized adaptive testing technology to administer the fewest number of questions to precisely obtain the most accurate measurement of pain. PASTOR also incorporates items from the Defense and Veterans Pain Rating Scale (Defense & Veterans Center for Integrative Pain Management, n.d.).

The sample questions presented next are offered to clinical military counselors as a qualitative and subjective measure of one's experience of pain. The content of these questions is derived from typical questions asked on intake interviews in pain clinics and pain management programs. Despite their subjective nature, the following self-report questions can be asked at varying intervals of treatment, which can provide a self-report of the increase or decrease in the client's pain experiences:

- Where is the location of your pain?
- How frequently do you experience pain?
- What type of pain do you have (dull ache, sharp, burning, throbbing, blunt)?
- How long does the pain typically last?
- How intense is the pain on a scale ranging from 0 (*no pain at all*) to 10 (*pain so severe that you would have to go to the emergency room*)?
- What types of activities cause the onset of your pain?
- What activities typically aggravate your pain condition?
- Are you in pain now? Describe where the pain is and what it feels like.
- What measure do you use to alleviate the pain (e.g., lay down, stretch, exercise)?
- What types of medication do you take for pain? What are the dosages? How effective is the medication at relieving the pain? Do you have any medication side effects?
- What kinds of activities are you still able to perform while in pain?
- What activities do you avoid because of the pain?
- How has pain changed what you can or cannot do in your life (at work, school, home, family, socially)?
- How does pain affect intimate or sexual relationships?
- How has pain changed your relationship with family or friends?
- How has pain changed your personality, mood, emotions, or general outlook on life?
- Are you involved in any litigation related to your pain condition?

THE PSYCHOSOCIAL ASPECTS OF PAIN IN THE MILITARY

Pain is a multidimensional and multidetermined phenomenon. All people experience some degree of pain at various points throughout their lives, such as burns on a hot stove, bee stings, broken bones, childbirth, dental work, and nonserious or non-life-threatening injuries. Pain is an indication that something is wrong in the body. The individual's response to pain varies greatly and depends on multiple factors. In this section, I discuss the growing importance of understanding the physical, psychological, emotional, social, neurocognitive, spiritual, and other relevant aspects of chronic pain that may assist practitioners in developing therapeutic pain management, treatment, and prevention programs for military clients.

Early pain researchers assessed the degree of one's pain on the basis of specific daily activities. For instance, some individuals pace themselves throughout the day so that they will not aggravate their pain condition (pacers), whereas others totally avoid activities and recline in a chair, couch, or bed (Fordyce, 1982). Other researchers have discussed pain in regard to three separate groups: (a) *pain reducers*, those who attempt to minimize and downplay their experience of pain; (b) *pain augmenters*, those who magnify their experiences of pain; and (c) *moderators*, those who neither magnify nor minimize their experience of pain (Stiller, 1975). Thus, having a good understanding of the client's perception of pain and how it restricts their independence and overall well-being is a good starting point for developing therapeutic interventions.

Pain expressed in the military is much different than in civilian life. No intrinsic rewards exist for service members who want to magnify their pain. The military as an occupation is quite physically demanding, particularly during combat deployment. Therefore, complaining about pain is not an option. The culture demands that the individual perform their job to the highest level. If a service member cannot "suck it up Buttercup," they may be perceived by others in their unit as weak, not motivated, or not committed. If a serious injury occurs, light duty work may not be possible in some military occupational specialties. Moreover, if chronic pain conditions persist and are not medically treatable, the service member may be recommended for a medical separation.

No benefits are awarded for acquired chronic pain conditions among active-duty personnel. Chronic pain conditions hinder promotion in rank and moving forward in one's military career. Furthermore, treatment options for chronic pain are limited, particularly during deployment. The use of pain medications is restricted, particularly for active-duty personnel. For example, Curthoys (2018) reported that only 6% of soldiers were taking an opioid while on active duty. This finding represented a 45% drop in the chronic use of opioids from the previous 4 years. The military medical community is discouraged from prescribing opioids, and their use by service members is restricted.

Treating chronic pain conditions in the veteran population is much different than treating them in active-duty personnel. This difference is primarily because more treatment options are available to veterans. However, complex chronic pain conditions among veterans bring a host of psychosocial and mental health issues that complicate healing. For instance, the use of prescription medications to treat the physiological symptoms of chronic pain can accentuate pain receptors (Goodwin, 2016). Opioid addiction can also develop, which complicates the veteran's physical and psychological health. The body naturally synthesizes opioid compounds and releases these substances to various parts of the brain that regulate pain perception and intensity. The modulation of pain receptors with synthetic opioids is a delicate balance between therapeutic use and opioid misuse (Sapolsky, 1998).

Researchers have shown that chronic pain can be both emotional and physical. The pathophysiological and neurobiological influences of chronic pain and depression have considerable overlap. This topic has been of interest in recent years among neuroscience researchers. In fact, it is estimated that between 30% and 85% of persons treated for chronic pain conditions are also diagnosed with a depressive or anxiety disorder (Sheng et al., 2017; Williams et al., 2003). The sensory pathways that spark chronic pain after injury share the same region of the brain involved in mood regulation. For example, norepinephrine and serotonin pathways that are present in the prefrontal cortex and limbic systems of the brain are also known to be activated in mood disorders such as depression.

Several sophisticated studies relate to the physical and emotional experiences of persons with chronic pain. These studies have shown that persons with chronic pain conditions (e.g., traumatic amputation, psychological trauma-related experiences) who had a prior diagnosis of major depressive disorder have a poorer prognosis for recovery, whereas those who have a chronic pain–only condition because of an underlying medical condition (e.g., patients with cancer or stroke who do not have a history of depression) have a better prognosis. The relationship between mental health conditions such as posttraumatic stress, depressive disorders, and chronic pain has been debated among neuroscience researchers. Multiple explanations that go beyond the scope of this chapter have been offered to unravel the mysteries of conditions such as fibromyalgia and various unknown viruses that cause chronic pain conditions.

Because the experience of chronic pain is both physical and emotional, some clients report chronic pain without the presence of any underlying medically determinable condition. In such cases, the person may have clinically significant symptoms related to a *somatic symptom disorder*. First, it is important to differentiate somatic symptom disorders from other related disorders. For example, in *factitious disorders*, the individual consciously falsifies or fabricates physical and psychological symptoms for some personal gain or external reward (e.g., getting out of work, claiming disability benefits). In addition, psychological factors affecting other medical conditions are clinically significant because of their influence on the course and prognosis of a diagnosable medical condition. For instance, the reduced mind-body health, negative perceptions and attitudes about one's physical and mental health, and overall well-being of the person can exacerbate chronic pain conditions that hinder coping abilities.

Another important point to differentiate in somatic symptom disorders is real pain from pain that is imagined, fabricated, or contrived. For example, there are some viruses of an unknown etiology that may mimic symptoms related to other medical conditions. In fact, the medical conditions of fibromyalgia and Gulf War syndrome, once thought to be falsely contrived by pain patients, now have standardized medical assessments, diagnostic criteria, and treatment protocols. Overall, medical and psychological assessments of chronic pain conditions are challenging for individuals who express chronic pain absent of any underlying physical and psychological conditions.

The clinical aspects of somatic symptom disorders are important for an expanded discussion because some mental health conditions, such as PTSD and depressive disorders, are first reported by patients as physical complaints of pain. A primary distinction made in somatic symptom disorders are complaints about chronic pain absent of any underlying medical or physical condition. Somatic complaints of chronic pain—absent of any disease, disability, or injury—are typically an unhealthy and abnormal expression of the true experience of pain. In other words, in somatic symptom disorders, the person may have complaints and worries about an illness or disease that does not exist or is not medically verifiable. These worries may present as mild, moderate, or severe. Such individuals may schedule frequent medical visits and exhibit prescription-seeking behaviors. They may also have multiple requests to be evaluated by various medical specialists.

Additionally, somatic symptom disorders have chronic and persistent levels of moderate to high anxiety. Some clients may exhibit traits of dysthymia or depressed mood. This emotional state may be accompanied by feelings of negativity, communication of unhealthy thoughts and feelings, or engagement in maladaptive behaviors. If abnormal or unhealthy thoughts, feelings, and behaviors persist—and are expressed disproportionately to the person's current physical and mental health status—this behavior may indicate a mild, moderate, or severe somatic symptom disorder.

Cumulative, chronic, and acute stress appears to be associated with higher levels of chronic pain and suffering. The impact that chronic daily stress has on the individual and their family members in military life is undisputable. The day-to-day commitment and occupational stressors associated with military life are difficult for many civilians to comprehend. Accordingly, it is of paramount importance for military medical and mental health practitioners to understand the association between chronic stress and chronic pain. It is vital that all medical, allied health, and mental health providers partner and coordinate services to competently assess, diagnose, treat, and prevent chronic pain conditions.

Stress and traumatic stress researchers, particularly in the multidisciplinary fields of psychoneuroimmunology, support the assertions that chronic stress has a profound negative and harmful impact on the mind, body, and spirit (Garfield, 1979; Kabat-Zinn, 1990; Lazarus, 1999; Moodley & West, 2005; Myers & Sweeney, 2005; Sapolsky, 1998; Schlitz et al., 2005; Tick, 2014; Van Der Kolk, 2014; Weil, 2000). The impact that chronic psychosocial stressors have on the client's ability to maintain good mental, physical, and spiritual wellness eludes some practitioners when it comes to treating the chronic pain condition. Therefore, I now present some guidelines that are based on theory, research, and the practice of treating chronic pain in both medically based as well as complementary and integrative health (CIH) settings. These guidelines are offered to clinical military practitioners as a holistic approach to the assessment, treatment, management, and prevention of chronic pain.

- Facilitate comprehensive clinical assessments, form partnerships with medical and allied health providers, and acquire a full understanding of your client's physical and psychological problems.
- A unique psychological challenge is created when patients are told by medical professionals, "You will have to learn how to live with the pain . . . there is nothing more I can do for you." Persons who accept this challenge and want to defeat their chronic pain are living life on their terms. Others may give up and suffer because the medical community stated, "There is nothing more that can be done."
- Most medical providers do not teach the patient *how* to live with chronic pain. Therefore, your mission as a therapist is to assist your client in accepting the challenge rather than accepting the diagnosis.
- Acknowledging and accepting the challenge to be healthy and living optimally may have more to do with one's attitude and perception of living fully in mind, body, and spirit. This area will be important in your comprehensive clinic assessment. Attitudinal change has a profound impact on the individual for transformational healing.

- Medical providers use pain scales ranging from 0 to 10, whereas competent therapists empower their clients by allowing them to create their own scale and choosing optimal mental, physical, and spiritual well-being.
- Psychosocial adjustment and adaptation to chronic health conditions exist on a continuum from *zero wellness* to *profound transformative experience*. Assist clients with real-world functional living along the continuum, which may be communicated by them as feeling higher levels of contentment, peace, and satisfaction as well as a felt sense of meaning or letting go. Empowering clients with "living life on their own terms" has potential to be transformational and quite empowering.
- Developing a strong sense of an internal locus of control, as opposed to an external locus, is an indicator of good psychological health and emotional resiliency. Competent therapists understand how to facilitate strategies and approaches that empower clients to choose their own thoughts, feelings, behaviors, and experiences.
- Develop a combination of behavioral lifestyle habits and evidence-based therapeutic strategies that work well with treating chronic pain conditions (e.g., cognitive behavioral therapy, mindfulness-based stress reduction [MBSR], coping strategies). In addition, provide your client with a "go bag" of therapeutic approaches to expand treatment options for different settings (e.g., home, work, school, social, recreational).
- Restoring the mind, body, and spirit back to balance is a journey, not a destination. Explore signs, symbols, meanings, and metaphors along the path that assist your client to come out of the darkness into the light.
- Appraise and explore your client's pain triggers by facilitating and coaching wellness and survivor strategies as opposed to focusing on how to "live with their pain." Understand the complex physical and psychological conditions that predispose the individual to high-risk behaviors (e.g., opioid misuse, suicidal ideation, excessive alcohol consumption).
- Carefully evaluate your client's behavioral lifestyle habits (e.g., exercise, nutrition, use of body mechanics) and mental health symptoms (e.g., mood, affect, insomnia, sleep hygiene, social and emotional well-being) that tend to aggravate or increase chronic pain.
- Assess your client's cultural beliefs (e.g., wisdom, attitudes, spirituality)—particularly their belief about healing and the use of resources—and integrate them into health and healing approaches.

OTHER MEDICAL CONDITIONS ASSOCIATED WITH CHRONIC PAIN

Multiple other disabling conditions are acquired in military life in which the physical trauma sustained creates intense levels of chronic pain co-occurring with a psychological disorder. In this section, I focus on SCI and traumatic amputation, which are common disabling conditions acquired in higher incidence by military service members since the war on terrorism began in 2001. The consequences typically result in a medical separation from military service with a 100% disability rating from the U.S. Department of Veterans Affairs (VA). Overall, long-term physical and psychological health concerns are a significant challenge for military individuals and their family members.

SCI

Approximately 238,000–332,000 civilians in the United States are living with SCI, with 17,500 new cases reported annually (National Spinal Cord Injury Statistical Center, 2017). More than half of all SCIs occur in people between 16 and 30 years old. Men account for approximately 80% of all injuries because they tend to engage in higher risk activities. SCI in civilian life primarily occurs from motor vehicle accidents (36%), falls (28.5%), violence (14.3%), and sports injuries (9%; National Spinal Cord Injury Statistical Center, 2017).

SCI acquired during military service is somewhat different than in civilian life. This difference is due in part to the nature of the military occupation itself and the cultural identity associated with being in excellent physical condition. Some studies have shown a lower incidence of SCI during OIF and OEF than reported in any other wars. This reduction is primarily because of emergency battlefield medicine and life-saving technologies. Infantry and combat personnel now have the benefit of being evacuated to a rear military trauma facility, whereas in previous wars, service members would have perished on the battlefield.

Military service members and veterans have a higher incidence of SCI, between 4.3 and 5.6 per 100,000 people, compared with civilians with SCIs, who represent less than 1% per 100,000. Presently, 11%–14% of combat veterans have acquired an SCI (Furlan et al., 2019). Unlike civilians, service members acquire their SCI because of improvised explosive device attacks, landmines, gunshot wounds, as well as helicopter and motor vehicle accidents.

The VA health care system has the largest single network of neurorehabilitation facilities in the United States. It provides comprehensive rehabilitation to more than 27,000 veterans with SCI in 25 different SCI specialty rehabilitation facilities throughout the United States (VA, 2019). The VA's neurorehabilitation team addresses patient issues related to their medical, physical, psychosocial, vocational, mental health, social, emotional, family, and independent living needs.

Successful psychosocial adaptation and adjustment to SCI are based on multiple individual, social, emotional, psychological, familial, and environmental factors (Marini, 2016; Marini & Brown, 2016). For example, persons with SCI must prepare for the long-term physical and psychological needs to increase optimal functioning and well-being. Multiple physical and architectural barriers may hinder accessibility, mobility, and independence at home and in the community. The use of assistive technology is also vital to enhancing one's independence and optimal functioning. Psychological resiliency is essential for persons with SCI because of the adverse physical and psychological issues that they must deal with daily. The financial cost of taking care of persons with SCI is insurmountable for some military families who do not have 100% financial resources to cover items such as medical equipment, assistive technology, specific medical treatments, and caregiver support.

SCI is often seen as a separate category of disability because of the catastrophic, pervasive, and—at times—life-threatening nature of this critical injury. The immediate or acute stage of traumatic SCI generally is one of physical and psychological chaos and shock for the individual and their family members. Thus, family and caregiver support is perhaps one of the most important factors in healthy recovery. The transformational challenge of SCI requires the individual to seek out and discover a new self-identity as a "person with a disability" or a "person with SCI." Some service members with SCI may take on the identity of a "wounded warrior" and gain support from the military community. The grief, loss, and trauma of SCI predispose the individual to multiple mental health issues, such as PTSD, depression, anxiety, and substance use disorders. Clinical practitioners will also want to monitor suicidality risks.

Overall, clinical military counselors have a variety of strategies, approaches, and areas to address that will benefit veterans with SCI. For example, there are many assistive technology devices available to assist persons with SCI in becoming more independent (Disabled World: http://www.disabled-world.com/; Spin Life: http://www.spinlife.com/). Multiple resources also can assist veterans with SCI with the following items: mobility and driving, transferring, adaptive sports and exercise equipment, voice recognition systems, environmental control units, and devices that interface with computers. Given the serious nature of SCI, the individual and their family members will require intensive support in the rehabilitation process with goals centered on successful adjustment, redefining quality of life, and optimal physical and mental health and well-being.

Traumatic Amputation

The newer term *traumatic amputation* refers to the severance of a body part because of an acute traumatic injury, most typically the result of an improvised explosive device attack, motor vehicle accident, or other injuries sustained during armed conflict (Falvo & Holland, 2018). In some cases, amputation is necessary when the military service member acquires thermal injuries such as burns, severe frostbite, severe peripheral vascular disease because of poor circulation (such as in diabetes), or severe infections of the bone. Amputation in this situation would be considered either a planned or urgent medical procedure.

Explosive devices and landmines were responsible for approximately 88% of all traumatic amputations among dismounted troops during OIF and OEF (Wallace, 2012). Despite declining deaths on the battlefield, traumatic amputations have increased overall since the war on terrorism began in 2001. By September 2010, 1,158 service members had sustained a traumatic amputation of at least one limb. Improved body armor, blast-resistant technology, and battlefield medicine have saved many lives in the combat theater in comparison with other wars. Much like TBI, some military literature has referred to traumatic amputations as the "signature injuries" of OIF and OEF. Statistically, those who have sustained an SCI because of being blown up or a Humvee accident likely also have a TBI.

During the critical event of traumatic amputation on the battlefield, a common emergency medical procedure is to save the upper or lower extremities that were severed. In some situations, reimplantation surgery may be attempted to reattach the severed limb. Reimplantation studies have shown that less than 50% of individuals have functional use or sensation of the affected limb. If the upper or lower extremities can be surgically repaired, the psychological outcome may be an improved quality of life for the individual. Basically, it is hypothesized that service members benefit from improved psychosocial adjustment when their body image can be preserved (Brown & Wu, 2003). However, in one small study ($N = 137$), Mitchell et al. (2019) compared those who underwent limb salvage with those who did not have reimplantation surgery, 40 months postinjury, and found no significant differences in improved psychosocial adjustment. Although the individuals with amputations in this study screened positive for PTSD (19%) and major depressive disorder (12%), Mitchell et al. noted that 64% of the individuals with amputations were either working or going to school, and 39% were involved with vigorous recreational activities. Psychosocial adjustment to military traumatic amputation has not been explored in the literature with the same frequency as TBI and PTSD. Thus, data are limited as to the psychosocial response patterns among military veterans. Clinical military counselors will want to cultivate strategies that enhance good psychosocial adjustment, such as delineated in Chapter 6. Practitioners will also want to consider other underlying medical conditions that challenge the client. Many individuals with amputations must also deal with a blast or brain injury, other orthopedic impairments, vision or hearing loss, or burns.

One clear factor in the medical research is the medical and physical complications that develop after amputation surgery, which include edema, skin ulceration, contractures, bone spurs, and scoliosis. Multiple allied health professionals (e.g., physical therapists, occupational therapists, assistive technology consultants) also assist in the physical rehabilitation of the service members. As the result of traumatic amputation, the service member's residual functional capacity is compromised, and they will typically be "med boarded" out of active-duty service.

After the service member with an amputation becomes medically stable with good skin integrity and a well-healed stump, they are fitted with a temporary prosthetic device. Eventually with more healing time, the individual will receive a more permanent prosthetic device that is fitted by a prosthetist. Prosthetic devices are commonly fabricated as a substitute for the missing body part. These artificial limbs increase independence and physical functioning for the individual and can be used for cosmetic and functional purposes. Persons who "accept" these devices function better independently. Prosthetics can also improve the veteran's quality of life and psychosocial adjustment and adaptation toward their newly acquired disability.

Phantom sensation and phantom limb pain are a common occurrence among many veterans with amputations. This chronic and severe pain is experienced in a body part that no longer exists. Phantom pain diminishes over time. However, some can be incapacitated by the severity of this atypical chronic pain condition (Knotkova et al., 2012). Multiple disciplines will be challenged when assisting veterans with amputations to deal with this unique chronic pain.

Some important goals for service members and veterans in the rehabilitation process involve increasing independent functioning. Multiple environments will challenge the service member as they transition to civilian life. Understanding that transition is a major life stressor for most service members, veterans with disabilities have even greater challenges. Many veterans with amputations will be confronted with significant physical, psychological, social, and emotional adjustments that can complicate healing efforts. Clinical military counselors can assist veterans with amputations who are transitioning to civilian life deal with issues related to body image, self-esteem, and overall psychosocial adjustment to their newly acquired disability. After the veteran with an amputation becomes physically and psychologically stable, the vocational rehabilitation specialist can assist them with educational goals, jobs, and careers. Understanding the veteran's predisability level of functioning; coping and resiliency skills; social, emotional, and interpersonal characteristics; and aptitudes and motivation for work or education can assist them in getting back to some level of "normalcy."

Tick (2014) has suggested that in Native American traditions, physical wounds were embraced and not hidden. There was a warrior pride among tribal members who fought for their culture. For many veterans, the mental and emotional wounds of war are hidden because of PTSD, depression, anxiety, and substance use disorders. However, for veterans with amputations and other visible injuries, a warrior ethos is projected. Many veterans with amputations are part of a military subculture in which their image as a wounded warrior is embraced. The body image, scars, and prosthetic devices are proudly displayed.

The apparent successful psychosocial adjustment may be, in part, because veterans with amputations have many more resources and access to technology than in any other wars. McFarland et al. (2010) have assembled a comprehensive list of resources for wounded warriors with traumatic limb loss. The interested reader will want to consult the references. Another resource available to veterans with amputations is the extension of benefits—funded in July 2019 through the Specially Adaptive Housing program—up to $98,000 to cover remodeling and retrofitting their homes for better accessibility (Copp, 2019). Overall, multiple issues and therapeutic approaches can be used by clinical military counselors to assist veterans with amputations in achieving optimal psychosocial adjustment.

TREATMENT, MANAGEMENT, AND PREVENTION OF CHRONIC PAIN

Best practices for managing chronic pain conditions with service members and veterans have been a challenge in military health care for quite some time. The opioid epidemic combined with the military mental health crisis has resulted in a high incidence of PTSD, depression, anxiety, and substance use disorders. Military suicides also occur at significantly higher rates because of medical and physical conditions. There appears to be bipartisan interest in the U.S. Congress, the U.S. Department of Defense (DoD), and the VA health care system to form partnerships confronting the critical physical and mental health conditions of military service members and veterans.

One example of advancing military health care and the comorbidity of chronic pain and co-occurring mental health conditions is the U.S. Army Surgeon General's formation of the Pain Management Task Force in 2009 (Pain Management Task Force, 2010). This task force was composed of medical and subject matter experts from the U.S. Army, U.S. Navy, and U.S. Air Force. They provided recommendations to Congress and the DoD for comprehensive treatment planning for a pain management strategy in the U.S. Armed Forces. The mission of this task force was to provide integrative approaches in an optimal quality-of-care environment, particularly for those service members who have acquired combat-related polytrauma. This multidisciplinary approach uses holistic treatment strategies that combine medical technology with CIH treatments. It also acknowledges military families and other natural supports that can assist in a healing partnership.

Historically, treating chronic pain in the VA's system of health care was done through the regular and consistent use of high doses of opioids (Evans et al., 2018). Despite the use of nonpharmacological therapies for many patients with pain, support for alternative or integrative treatments was not well endorsed. A major shift in pain management practice in the DoD and VA system advocates for CIH therapies. For example, the Pain Management Task Force's (2010) final report endorses the pursuit of CIH modalities such as Reiki—a Japanese medicine body energy approach to healing chronic illnesses and rebalancing the body's system of chakras (Gantt & Orina, 2020). The Center for Reiki Research (https://www.centerforreikiresearch.org/) is the primary clearinghouse for evidence-based Reiki research. There are more than 60 research hospitals and clinics throughout the United States that offer Reiki as a healing modality for persons with chronic pain as well as a variety of other health conditions.

Another CIH modality that has its origins in Eastern traditions is MBSR programs (Kabat-Zinn, 1990). The MBSR program is one of the most extensively researched CIH modalities and is now adapted for use with the military (Brintz et al., 2020). MBSR uses mindfulness meditation approaches to self-regulate mood, affect, and attention to bring awareness of the mind, body, and spirit with the intention of achieving a pure relaxed state of being. MBSR is particularly useful in treating chronic pain, anger management issues, substance use disorders, anxiety, and depression experienced by many active-duty service personnel and veterans across the life span.

Also, a departure from the traditional opioid pharmacological approaches is the growth of yoga for use with military service members and veterans. In fact, yoga has been integrated into the military's evolving pain management model because of its mind-body benefits that help individuals with back pain, headaches and migraines, fibromyalgia, as well as other medical conditions (Miller et al., 2017). Yoga has also been endorsed in the Pain Management Task Force's (2010) final report. Yoga classes are now seen at military installations, military treatment facilities, and Wounded Warrior transition units.

Another nonpharmacological pain intervention that has demonstrated efficacy in decreasing chronic pain symptoms has been traditional Chinese acupuncture. Acupuncture has been extensively researched for its use with military patients. In one study, Peacock et al. (2019) compared the treatments of (a) acupuncture; (b) the Tennant Biomodulator, which was a commercially produced, hand-held type of self-administered transcutaneous electrical nerve stimulation (TENS) device; and (c) the traditional TENS unit. Peacock et al. found a 16% reduction in the service member's report of pain using traditional Chinese acupuncture and the TENS unit. The Tennant Biomodulator also reportedly performed as well as the two other treatments.

A promising future for CIH modalities is expanding treatment options for service members and veterans with chronic pain conditions. Military women tend to utilize CIH treatments more than men (36% vs. 26%; Evans et al., 2018). Therapeutic interventions are enhanced when CIH treatment options are offered to service members and veterans. Decreasing dependence on opioids to treat chronic pain conditions is essential for optimal healing of the mind, body, and spirit.

CONCLUDING REMARKS

This chapter addressed the medical and psychosocial aspects of chronic pain and other types of medical conditions (e.g., SCI, traumatic amputation) that present unique opportunities for healing the mind, body, and spirit of veterans. Guidelines for the screening, treatment, management, and prevention of chronic pain conditions have been offered. Training in this area is essential because pain is one of the most frequently reported physical complaints in the military medical treatment setting. Traditional approaches to pain management within the VA and DoD have not provided a model for premier health care because of the opioid and mental health crisis. Current research has shown considerable improvement in the military's pain management, treatment, and prevention programs using CIH approaches. Current models and programs in the military advocate for the responsible partnering of medical, allied health, and mental health providers to achieve the best quality of care and outcome for service members, veterans, and their families.

REFERENCES

Blakey, S. H., Wagner, H. R., Naylor, J., Brancu, M., Lane, L., Sallee, M., Kimbrel, N. A., VA Mid-Atlantic MIRECC Workgroup, & Elbogen, E. B. (2018). Chronic pain, TBI, and PTSD in military veterans: A link to suicidal ideation and violent impulses? *The Journal of Pain, 19*(7), 797–806. https://doi.org/10.1016/j.jpain.2018.02.012

Brintz, C. E., Miller, S., Olmsted, K. R., Bartoszek, M., Cartwright, J., Kizakevich, P. N., Butler, M., Asefnia, N., Buben, A., & Gaylord, S. A. (2020). Adapting mindfulness training for military service members with chronic pain. *Military Medicine, 185*(3–4), 385–393. https://doi.org/10.1093/milmed/usz312

Brown, R. E., & Wu, T. Y. (2003). Use of "spare parts" in mutilated upper extremity injuries. *Hand Clinics, 19*(1), 73–87. https://doi.org/10.1016/s0749-0712(02)00143-9

Brundage, J. F., & Rubertone, M. V. (2014). Absolute and relative morbidity burdens attributable to various illnesses and injuries, U.S. Armed Forces. *Medical Surveillance Monthly Report, 22*(4), 5–10.

Calati, R., Bakhiyi, C. L., Artero, S., Ilgen, M., & Courtet, P. (2015). The impact of physical pain on suicidal thoughts and behaviors: Meta-analyses. *Journal of Psychiatric Research, 71,* 16–32. https://doi.org/10.1016/j.jpsychires.2015.09.004

Center for Deployment Psychology. (n.d.). *Chronic pain.* https://deploymentpsych.org/disorders/chronic-pain

Cohen, M., Quintner, J., & van Rysewyk, S. (2018). Reconsidering the International Association for the Study of Pain definition of pain. *Pain Reports, 3*(2), Article e634. https://doi.org/10.1097/PR9.0000000000000634

Cohen, S. P., & Raja, S. N. (2016). Pain. In L. Goldman & A. I. Schafer (Eds.), *Goldman-Cecil Medicine* (25th ed., pp. 133–143). Elsevier Saunders.

Copp, T. (2019, July 10). *As amputee veterans age and move, will government cover special housing needs?* https://www.mcclatchydc.com/news/nation-world/national/national-security/article232502822.html

Curthoys, K. (2018, February 4). Army working on more ways to manage soldiers' pain in fighting against opioid use. *Army Times.* https://www.armytimes.com/news/your-army/2018/02/02/army-working-on-more-ways-to-manage-soldiers-pain-in-fight-against-opioid-abuse/

Defense & Veterans Center for Integrative Pain Management. (n.d.). *Pain Assessment Screening Tool and Outcomes Registry (PASTOR).* https://www.dvcipm.org/clinical-resources/pain-assessment-screening-tool-and-outcomes-registry-pastor/

Evans, E. A., Herman, P. M., Washington, D. L., Lorenz, K. A., Yuan, A., Upchurch, D. M., Marshall, N., Hamilton, A. B., & Taylor, S. L. (2018). Gender differences in use of complementary and integrative health by U.S. military veterans with chronic musculoskeletal pain. *Women's Health, 28*(5), 379–386. https://doi.org/10.1016/j.whi.2018.07.003

Falvo, D. R., & Holland, B. E. (2018). *Medical and psychosocial aspects of chronic illness and disability* (6th ed.). Bartlett & Jones.

Fordyce, W. E. (1982). Foreword. In J. Barber (Ed.), *Psychological approaches to the management of pain* (pp. v–x). Brunner/Mazel.

Furlan, J. C., Gulasingam, S., & Craven, B. C. (2019). Epidemiology-related spinal cord injury among war combatants: A systematic review. *Global Spine Journal, 9*(5), 545–558. https://doi.org/10.1177/2192568218776914

Gantt, M., & Orina, J. A. T. (2020). Educate, try, and share: A feasibility study to assess the acceptance and use of Reiki as an adjunct therapy for chronic pain in military health care facilities. *Military Medicine, 185*(3–4), 394–400. https://doi.org/10.1093/milmed/usz271

Garfield, C. A. (1979). *Stress and survival: The emotional realities of life-threatening illness.* Mosby.

Gatchel, R. J., McGeary, D. D., Peterson, A., Moore, M., LeRoy, K., Isler, W. C., Hryshko-Mullen, A. S., & Edell, T. (2009). Preliminary findings of a randomized controlled trial of an interdisciplinary military pain program. *Military Medicine, 174*(3), 270–277. https://doi.org/10.7205/milmed-d-03-1607

Goodwin, L. R., Jr. (2016). Treatment for substance use disorders. In I. Marini & M. A. Stebnicki (Eds.), *The professional counselor's desk reference* (2nd ed., pp. 457–468). Springer.

Ilgen, M. A., Zivin, K., Austin, K. L., Bohnert, A. S., Czyz, E. K., Valenstein, M., & Kilbourne, A. M. (2010). Severe pain predicts greater likelihood of subsequent suicide. *Suicide and Lifethreatening Behavior, 40*(6), 597–608. https://doi.org/10.1521/suli.2010.40.6.597

Institute of Medicine. (2011). *Relieving pain in American: A blueprint for transforming prevention, care, education, and research.* Washington Academies Press.

International Association for the Study of Pain. (2011). *Classification of chronic pain* (2nd ed.). https://www.iasp-pain.org/PublicationsNews/Content.aspx?ItemNumber=1673

Kabat-Zinn, J. (1990). *Full catastrophic living: Using the wisdom of your body and mind to face stress, pain, and illness.* Dell.

Kearns, R. D., & Heapy, A. (2016). Advances for pain management in veterans: Current status of research and future directions. *Journal of Rehabilitation Research and Development, 53*(1), vii–x. https://doi.org/10.1682/JRRD.2015.10.0196

Knotkova, H., Crucian, R. A., Tronnier, V. M., & Rasche, D. (2012). Current and future options for the management of phantom limb pain. *Journal of Pain Research, 5,* 39–49. https://doi.org/10.2147/JPR.S16733

Lazarus, R. S. (1999). *Stress and emotion: A new synthesis.* Springer.

LeShan, L. (1979). The world of the patient in severe pain of long duration. In C. A. Garfield (Ed.), *Stress and survival: The emotional realities of life-threatening illness* (pp. 273–279). Mosby.

Marini, I. (2016). Counseling caregivers. In I. Marini & M. A. Stebnicki (Eds.), *The professional counselor's desk reference* (2nd ed., pp. 513–517). Springer.

Marini, I., & Brown, A. D. (2016). Family care and spinal cord injury. In M. J. Millington & I. Marini (Eds.), *Families in rehabilitation counseling: A community-based approach* (pp. 193–212). Springer.

McCarberg, B. H., Stanos, S., & Williams, D. A. (2012). Comprehensive pain management: Improving physical and psychological functioning (CME multimedia activity). *American Journal of Medicine, 125*(6), Article S1. https://doi.org/10.1016/j.amjmed.2011.10.004

McFarland, L. V., Choppa, A. J., Betz, K., Pruden, J. D., & Reiber, G. E. (2010). Resources for wounded warriors with traumatic limb loss. *Journal of Rehabilitation Research and Development, 47*(4), 1–13. https://doi.org/10.1682/JRRD.2009.02.0017

Milks, J. W. (2012). Pain. In E. T. Bope & R. D. Kellerman (Eds.), *Conn's current therapy* (pp. 24–31). Elsevier Saunders.

Miller, S., Gaylord, S., Buben, A., Brintz, C., Olmsted, K. R., Asefnia, N., & Bartoszek, M. (2017). Literature review of research on chronic pain and yoga in military populations. *Medicines, 4*(3), Article 64. https://doi.org/10.3390/medicines4030064

Mitchell, S. L., Hayda, R., Chen, A. T., Carlini, A. R., Fike, J. R., & MacKenzie, E. J. (2019). The Military Extremity Trauma Amputation/Limb Salvage (METALS) study. *The Journal of Joint and Bone Surgery, 101*(16), 1470–1478. https://doi.org/10.2106/JBJS.18.00970

Moodley, R., & West, W. (2005). *Integrating traditional healing practices into counseling and psychotherapy.* Sage.

Myers, J. E., & Sweeney, T. J. (2005). *Counseling for wellness: Theory, research, and practice.* American Counseling Association.

Nahin, R. L. (2017). Severe pain in veterans: The impact of age and sex, and comparisons to the general population. *Journal of Pain, 18*(3), 247–254. https://doi.org/10.1016/j.jpain.2016.10.021

National Defense Authorization Act for Fiscal Year 2010, Pub. L. 111–84 (2009, October 28). https://www.govinfo.gov/content/pkg/PLAW-111publ84/pdf/PLAW-111publ84.pdf

National Spinal Cord Injury Statistical Center. (2017, June). *Spinal cord injury facts and figures at a glance.* https://msktc.org/lib/docs/Data_Sheets_/SCIMS_Facts_and_Figures_2017_August_FINAL.pdf

Pain Management Task Force. (2010, May). *Providing a standardized DoD and VHA vision and approach to pain management to optimize the care for warriors and their families.* https://www.dvcipm.org/site/assets/files/1070/pain-task-force-final-report-may-2010.pdf

Peacock, K. S., Stoerkel, E., Libretto, S., Zhang, W., Inman, A., Schlicher, M., Cowsar, J. D., Jr., Eddie, D., & Walter, J. (2019). A randomized trail comparing the Tennant Biomodulator to transcutaneous electrical nerve stimulation and traditional Chinese acupuncture for the treatment of chronic pain in military service members. *Military Medical Research, 6*(1), Article 37. https://doi.org/10.1186/s40779-019-0227-4

Reisman, M. (2016). PTSD treatment for veterans: What's working, what's new, and what's next. *Pharmacy and Therapeutics, 41*(10), 632–634.

Ruff, R. L., Ruff, S. S., & Wang, X. F. (2009). Improving sleep: Initial headache treatment in OIF/OEF veterans with blast-induced mild traumatic brain injury. *Journal of Rehabilitation Research and Development, 46*(9), 1071–1084. https://doi.org/10.1682/jrrd.2009.05.0062

Runnals, J. J., Van Voorhees, E., Robbins, A. T., Brancu, M., Straits-Troster, K., Beckham, J. C., & Calhoun, P. S. (2013). Self-reported pain complaints among Afghanistan/Iraq era men and women veterans with comorbid posttraumatic stress disorder and major depressive disorder. *Pain Medicine, 14*(10), 1529–1533. https://doi.org/10.1111/pme.12208

Sapolsky, R. M. (1998). *Why zebras don't get ulcers: An updated guide to stress, stress-related diseases, and coping*. Freeman.

Schlitz, M., Amorok, T., & Micozzi, M. S. (2005). *Consciousness and healing: Integral approaches to mind-body medicine*. Elsevier.

Sheng, J., Lui, S., Wang, Y., Cui, R., & Zhang, X. (2017). The link between depression and chronic pain: Neural mechanisms in the brain. *Neural Plasticity, 2017*, Article 9724371. https://doi.org/10.1155/2017/9724371

Stebnicki, M. A. (2017). *Disaster mental health counseling: Responding to trauma in a multicultural context*. Springer.

Stiller, R. (1975). *Pain: Why it hurts, where it hurts, when it hurts*. Thomas Nelson.

Tick, E. (2014). *Warrior's return: Restoring the soul after war*. Sounds True.

U.S. Department of Veterans Affairs. (2019, February 6). *VA research on spinal cord injury*. https://www.research.va.gov/topics/sci.cfm

Van Der Kolk, B. (2014). *The body keeps the score: Brain, mind, and body in the healing of trauma*. Penguin Books.

Wallace, D. (2012). Trends in traumatic limb amputation in allied forces in Iraq and Afghanistan. *Journal of Military and Veteran Health, 20*(2), 31–35.

Weil, A. (2000). *Spontaneous healing: How to discover and embrace your body's natural ability to maintain and heal itself*. Ballantine Books.

Williams, L. S., Jones, W. J., Shen, J., Robinson, R. L., Weinberger, M., & Kroenke, K. (2003). Prevalence and impact of depression and pain in neurology outpatients. *Journal of Neurology, Neurosurgery, and Psychiatry, 74*(11), 1587–1589. https://doi.org/10.1136/jnnp.74.11.1587

Winterowd, C., & Sims, W. F. (2016). Counseling persons with chronic pain. In I. Marini & M. A. Stebnicki (Eds.), *The professional counselor's desk reference* (2nd ed., pp. 565–570). Springer.

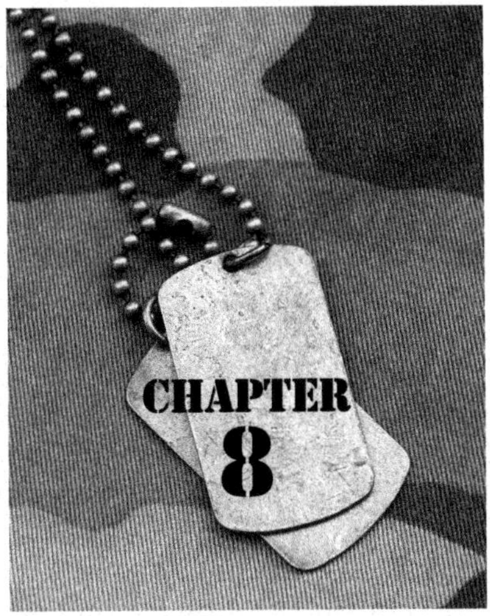

BLAST INJURIES AND TRAUMATIC BRAIN INJURY IN THE MILITARY

I've been blown up at least 3 or 4 times
during my last deployment . . .
Oorah!

—Statement from one of my
military clients, 2012

★ ★ ★

Traumatic brain injury (TBI) and blast injuries have been a frequent source of severe and catastrophic injury that can have life-threatening consequences in the U.S. military. TBI has been coined "the signature injury" of Operation Iraqi Freedom (OIF) and Operation Enduring Freedom (OEF). TBI or blast wounds sustained during military exercises or during combat operations have long-term physical and psychological effects on service members and veterans. Some aspects of blast injuries mimic postconcussive syndrome or mild TBI (MTBI). Other aspects are critical and require immediate medical attention in a military trauma facility. In this chapter, I discuss some of the distinct differences between blast injuries and TBI. I also explore improved (a) battlefield neurological assessments, (b) postdeployment medical evaluations, as well as (c) veteran mental health and neurocognitive care in outpatient services and postacute TBI rehabilitation hospitals.

Because of the increased incidence and prevalence of survival of severe blast wounds or TBI, military medical researchers and practitioners have taken an increased active role to understand specialized assessments, treatments, and preventive measures to achieve optimal physical and mental health. Combining research from various disciplines in battlefield technology, trauma medicine, psychology, and rehabilitation, the U.S. Department of Defense (DoD) has implemented a system of various strategic goals to monitor the progress of interventions and quality of care received.

The relevance of this chapter for mental health providers is to highlight the clinical symptoms (e.g., posttraumatic stress disorder [PTSD], major depressive disorder, substance use disorders, suicidality) that need to be addressed to treat complex trauma. One of the most critical aspects of complex TBIs and blast injuries is the significantly higher rates of suicide among military personnel. Thus, having a combination of physical and psychological conditions places service members and veterans in a significantly higher risk category.

BLAST INJURIES IN THE MILITARY

In my earlier years of working with active-duty Marines and veterans across all branches of the military, I would hear my clients say, "I got blown up three or four times" (just like in the movies). I would observe my client's metacommunication and think to myself, "Wow, you look pretty good for getting blown up 3–4 times; you look nothing like the patients on the acute care TBI rehabilitation unit where I used to work 60 hours per week." After session, I would review my client's brief medical records to find that they typically had a minimal U.S. Department of Veterans Affairs (VA) disability rating for an MTBI but slightly higher ratings for other physical and mental health conditions (e.g., low back, high neck, or knee injury; chronic pain; PTSD). Interestingly, there was minimal documentation of symptoms related to MTBI or blast injuries. Did it not exist? Was my client not being honest with me? Perhaps my client had repressed memories or was in denial?

The reality was that my client was being totally honest with me. My comprehensive clinical assessment revealed symptoms related to the daily or weekly presence of migraine headaches, some vertigo, and decreased memory and concentration, which are all clinically significant symptoms of TBI and blast injuries. The common theme I found out later is that the blast injuries were never recorded in after-action reports, in the combat theater trauma registry, or in the medical records of a military trauma facility (e.g., no Purple Hearts were awarded in the battle because the "O-6" said so, or it was an off-the-books mission). The principle remains true that "if it wasn't documented, it didn't happen." However, clear documentation is a critical component of good physical and mental health care.

This narrative reflects some of the battlefield medical documentation reported in the literature that took place during OIF and OEF. The typical scenario is that if the combat operator did not sustain a more severe acute injury (e.g., TBIs, traumatic amputations, muscular skeletal and soft tissue injuries, burns) or did not require immediate emergency medical attention, then they likely sustained a primary blast injury or concussion and were able to return to duty. If the symptoms were not immediately present in the heat of the battle, then the service member and medical professionals may have not detected their condition until a postdeployment medical evaluation.

Blast injuries are physically and psychologically devastating to military service personnel and family members. Consequently, blast injuries or TBIs, whether sustained during military exercises or combat operations, have the potential to be life threatening. Thus, early detection is critical. Medical professionals must have good documentation of the patient's history so that appropriate medical evaluation and treatment can be delivered. As for clinical military counselors, having a good medical record that accurately communicates the person's medical conditions and residual functional capacity (e.g., neuropsychological, physical therapy, and duty restrictions) will assist in developing and implementing an appropriate mental health and rehabilitation counseling plan to maximize physical and mental health improvement.

Good documentation has been problematic in battlefield medicine regarding blast injuries and MTBIs. This deficiency was recognized by an Army Dismounted Complex Blast Injury Task Force (2011) report that identified the medical documentation challenges for trauma physicians. This documentation applies to all phases, including when soldiers are wounded in action, treated at a military trauma facility, and returned to duty. Solutions have been slow in development.

To correct problems in the medical documentation protocols, the U.S. Congress directed the DoD in December 2019 to document service members' blast exposure in combat and training exercises. The mandate is to include these critical incidents within the service member's medical records. Moving forward, blast injuries are now identified as a "covered incident" and will be eligible for disability benefits (Sisk, 2019). There are significant advantages in knowing the etiology of physical and psychological symptoms and conditions acquired during one's military service. Appropriate medical and psychological evaluation can assist health care providers in managing treatment options. Veterans are deserving of medical and monetary benefits to compensate them for the sacrifice they have made.

Military medical researchers have referred to a plethora of data and statistics that document the seriousness of acquired blast injuries (Bryan & Clemans, 2013; Centers for Disease Control and Prevention [CDC], n.d.; Chase et al., 2016; Kirkman et al., 2011; Warden, 2006; Wightman & Gladish, 2001; Wolf et al., 2009). The following data highlight current issues and problems in military blast injuries:

- Approximately 22% of all combat casualties from OIF and OEF involve TBIs, compared with 12% during the Vietnam War.
- Military blast injuries rose fourfold (conservatively) between 1999 and 2006 and eightfold worldwide.
- Suicide is currently the second leading cause of death among military personnel. Repetitive blast injuries develop into more severe TBIs. TBI and co-occurring mental health conditions place service members and veterans in a significantly higher risk category for suicide completion.
- The combination of blast injuries and PTSD complicates the individual's physical, neurocognitive, neurobehavioral, and neuropsychological healing. The critical statistic is the negative long-term physical and mental health implications of having both TBI and PTSD.
- Cumulative and repetitive blast injuries that are unrecognized, untreated, undertreated, and undocumented have negative long-term health effects and life-threatening implications for service members, veterans, and their families.
- Blast injuries and TBIs predispose service members and veterans to significantly higher rates of PTSD, depression, anxiety, and substance use disorders.
- Most blast injuries occur during military combat operations or exercises. However, terrorist attacks by homemade improvised explosive devices have risen dramatically in the United States (e.g., Times Square and Port Authority bombings in 2017, Boston Marathon bombing in 2013, Oklahoma City federal building bombing in 1995, University of Illinois at Chicago bombing in 1978). Thus, civilian medical and mental health providers require training for the triage, evaluation, and treatment of these catastrophic injuries because of the unique and complex patterns of injury that are seldom seen outside combat operations. Thus, treating blast injuries with the highest level of skill and competence is required by both civilian and military medical professionals.

Blast injuries or wounds are slightly different than open- or closed-head TBI injuries even though the medical and physical conditions can be the same. For example, many service members who have sustained blast injuries also have the neurocognitive and neuropsychological characteristics of an MTBI. These characteristics include, but may not be limited to, migraine headaches; vertigo; tinnitus; wake-sleep disorders; PTSD; major depressive disorder; irritability; as well as memory, concentration, and attention deficits. In the physics of explosions, the blast results in an instantaneous conversion from solid or liquid material to a toxic gas after detonation. This toxic gas—depending on the magnitude, distance, and other variables—accelerates rapidly (may exceed 831 mph) outward from the point of the high-intensity detonation and causes (a) an immediate rise in air pressure creating a supersonic blast wave or blast wind; (b) an immediate blast of propellants that may contain shrapnel (e.g., rocks, nails, ball bearings, scrap metal, and other solid objects to maximize the lethality); (c) toxic inhalants of dust, fumes, particles, smoke, carbon monoxide, and other chemicals that burn from hot gases; and (d) secondary fires. Almost half of blast injury victims die because of a severe TBI or significant lung or pulmonary injuries.

Service members who are blast injury survivors may sustain other catastrophic injuries if they are thrown toward an immovable object (e.g., a building, the ground) or if shrapnel penetrates soft tissue or the muscular skeletal system. Moreover, the consequence of crushing injuries and structural collapse of internal organs (e.g., lungs, pulmonary, cardiovascular) creates multiple medical complications requiring long-term healing.

Blast injuries are categorized into the following four separate categories:

1. *Primary.* This category results from the blast overpressure that is transmitted to the individual that can cause tissue damage. The most common types of injuries during a primary blast are pulmonary barotrauma of the lungs, middle ear tears and ruptures, abdominal hemorrhage and perforation, eye rupture, and concussion without physical signs of a closed- or open-head TBI.
2. *Secondary.* This category results from the blast overpressure or blast wind hurling debris that can cause penetrating or blunt trauma injuries. These objects are accelerated by the energy of the explosion, simulating injuries comparable in appearance with stab wounds, physical assault, and ocular injuries.
3. *Tertiary.* This category occurs when the person is physically displaced by the force of the overpressure and blast wind, resulting in closed-head injuries, blunt abdominal trauma, tissue contusions, and fractures.
4. *Quaternary and quinary (miscellaneous blast).* This category was developed independently of the other blast injury categories because of the unique medical characteristics documented in medical case studies. In this category, the blast injuries are like the other categories and may cause burns and toxic substance exposure, such as radiation, carbon monoxide, and cyanide poisoning that may cause asphyxia. Most notable types of injuries in this category are burns, crushing injuries, open and closed brain trauma, development of acute and chronic obstructive pulmonary diseases, angina, hyperglycemia, and hypertension.

Over the last 5 years, military medical researchers and clinicians have investigated the unique clinical characteristics of blast injuries as they relate to triage, assessment, and treatment. For instance, in primary blast injuries, clinical symptoms are often subtle and delayed. Yet, the problem remains that service members are at higher risk for chronic long-term and life-threatening illnesses and disabilities. Medical management of pulmonary diseases is critical because of the toxic inhalants consumed in the blast energy. Thus, the military medical community advocates for early diagnosis and aggressive treatment of blast injuries to prevent future complications.

The medical, mental health, and psychosocial implications of blast injuries—which are offered to mental health clinicians to assist them in treatment planning for therapeutic resources that deal with this complex type of trauma—include the following:

- Repetitive blast injuries increase the number of physical and mental health risk factors. Mental health providers should anticipate that clients may report migraine headaches; vertigo; tinnitus; wake-sleep disorders; PTSD; major depressive disorder; irritability; as well as memory, concentration, and attention deficits. Thus, therapeutic goals will require partnering with multiple other resources and medical providers to achieve optimal health care.
- Mental health providers should familiarize themselves with the Rancho Los Amigos Levels of Cognitive Functioning Scale (Hagan et al., 1972), the Glasgow Coma Scale (GCS; Jennet et al., 1981), as well as other concussion protocols used for pre- and postdeployment. Refer to the TBI section for a more in-depth explanation. Scales of cognitive functioning will provide mental health providers with information on their client's neurocognitive functioning at the time of acute injury. These data may assist providers with the rehabilitation process and help them to anticipate future deficits, strengths, neurocognitive functioning, and residual functional capacity.
- Mental health providers need to take their clients seriously when they report being "blown up multiple times." Mental health providers should consider interventions beginning with the date of onset of the blast injury. Blast injuries are treated differently during the first 24, 36, or 48 hours than 1 or 2 years postinjury.
- Blast injuries are physically and psychologically traumatic to individuals. Mental health professionals will want to complete a comprehensive clinical assessment of service members and veterans to evaluate the degree of trauma exposure. Blast injuries create issues related to complex trauma because of the co-occurring physical and psychological conditions present.

- Competent mental health counselors understand the complex nature of trauma involving client issues related to anniversary dates of injuries, persistent and complex bereavement disorders, the person's perception toward the traumatic event, losses sustained, and current level of coping and resiliency.

TBI

TBI is the major cause of death and disability in the United States and increased by 53% in the civilian population between 2006 and 2014 (CDC, 2019). In 2014, it was estimated that 155 civilians per day die of TBI, with the major causes including falls, motor vehicle accidents, work-related accidents, physical assaults, violence, gunshots to the head, and blast injuries (Falvo & Holland, 2018; Loane et al., 2015). TBI is the leading cause of death among children and adolescents, primarily because of motor vehicle accidents. Males (15–24 years of age) are 4 times more likely than females to acquire a TBI because of the high-risk behaviors of younger males.

In the military, TBI is known as the signature injury of OEF and OIF. In fact, between 2000 and 2018, more than 38,300 service members acquired a TBI (Defense and Veterans Brain Injury Center [DVBIC], 2020). According to military researchers, between 12% and 23% of veterans acquire a TBI during their military service (Cooper et al., 2018; Elder et al., 2019; McKee & Robinson, 2014). Most TBIs (85%) are considered mild (MTBIs). However, the long-term consequences to one's mental, neurocognitive, and physical health have the potential to be both life threatening and catastrophic.

One of the most striking aspects of TBI statistics is the incidence of co-occurring mental health disorders that follow TBI, such as posttraumatic stress, major depression, anxiety, and substance use disorders. Additionally, there is a significantly higher risk for suicidal ideation, lethal attempts, and completions after acquired TBI. Moreover, researchers have demonstrated a relationship between TBI and dementias as well as military chronic traumatic encephalopathy (CTE; Chapman & Diaz-Arrastia, 2014; Elder et al., 2019; McKee & Robinson, 2014). Overall, TBI, PTSD, and other co-occurring disorders make this injury a priority for the military culture because of the complex physical, neurocognitive, neuropsychological, and mental health conditions that affect service members, veterans, and military families throughout the life span.

CATEGORIZATION OF TBI

Brain injuries are classified as mild, moderate, and severe. There are two types of brain injuries: *closed head* (i.e., internal injury due to blunt trauma, blow, or jolt to head and neck) and *open head* (i.e., visible skull fracture typically due to penetrating injury). The most reliable predictors of brain injury during the rehabilitation process include the (a) severity of injury and co-occurring physical and mental impairments (e.g., mild, moderate, or severe TBI; impairment in physical, cognitive, and independent functioning), (b) area of brain injured (e.g., right-left side, ocular, motor, communication), (c) residual functional capacity (e.g., motor skills, neurocognitive deficits, expressive-receptive communication abilities, personality, behavioral changes), and (d) predisability characteristics (e.g., previous physical and psychological conditions, other TBIs, educational level, age). Potential consequences of brain injury vary considerably depending on the aforementioned factors. The following categories of brain injury are offered to mental health professionals with the intent of assisting you, your client, and their family members to prepare for the physical limitations that are anticipated to affect psychological functioning (Beers et al., 2003; CDC, 2019; DVBIC, 2020; Falvo & Holland, 2018).

MTBI

Most TBIs (85%) fall into this category. Approximately 3 months postinjury, 78% of service members have persistent headaches, 59% have memory problems, and 34% are unable to return to duty. Characteristics and symptoms associated with this level of injury include the following:

- Loss of consciousness for approximately 3–30 minutes;
- GCS score of 13 or higher;
- Limitations in concentration, focus, attention, memory, and learning new tasks;
- Clinically significant symptoms of migraine headaches, vertigo, tinnitus, wake-sleep disorders, depression, irritability; and
- Concussion (also referred to as *postconcussion syndrome*, which is considered an MTBI and has similar deficits in residual functioning; many concussions in the military go unrecognized until key clinical symptoms appear, such as those listed earlier).

Moderate TBI

Characteristics and symptoms associated with this level of injury include the following:

- Loss of consciousness for a few minutes or hours;
- GCS rating of 9–12;
- Lethargy, confusion, and disorientation and more moderate deficits in concentration, focus, attention, memory, learning new tasks, ability to complete independent living tasks, and motor skills; and

- Physical, neurocognitive, and motor skill deficits that are quite apparent and that last for months and years (the majority of individuals do not return to duty).

Severe TBI

Characteristics and symptoms associated with this level of injury include the following:

- Prolonged state of unconsciousness for days, weeks, or months; individual does not react to any stimuli and basically remains comatose;
- GCS rating of 8 or less;
- Disorientation to person, place, and time;
- In a vegetative state of consciousness (note that no interventions currently are available to reverse long-standing vegetative states);
- No purposeful and meaningful voluntary movements; and
- Persistent state of agitation with no purposeful voluntary responses.

BRAIN INJURIES REQUIRING CRITICAL CARE

Brain injuries in the military occur while engaging in multiple situations and activities. These activities include, but are not limited to, military readiness training exercises, engaging enemy combatants, Humvee rollovers, falls, parachute injuries, improvised explosive device attacks, penetrating wounds, and other physical activities. During initial or primary impact, the head goes through a coup-contrecoup motion in which the head and brain rock violently forward and backward, ripping and shearing motor and sensory neurons at the basal ganglia.

Although the brain is bathed in cerebral spinal fluid that helps cushion it from everyday bumps and mishaps, when TBI occurs, the brain tissue begins to swell. This edema causes bleeding or intracranial hemorrhaging that creates the formation of a hematoma (sac filled with blood). Thus, at this point, the brain injury—even an MTBI—becomes a critical event because the skull cannot accommodate the expansion of tissue and fluid, depriving the brain of blood supply and oxygen. If pressure builds up and the intracranial fluid cannot be released, death can occur. Edema in the brain may also cause seizure activity. Other serious injuries (e.g., traumatic amputation, muscular skeletal disabilities) of course complicate one's ability to maximize their physical and psychological abilities.

TBI ASSESSMENTS AND CONCUSSION SCREENINGS

Recent attention has focused on blast wounds and combat-related injuries. However, it should be noted that MTBIs can be acquired in military life in many ways, such as through combat readiness exercises (e.g., falls, blows to the head, parachute accidents). Thus, many service members who acquired a concussion or an MTBI did not receive proper neurological, neurocognitive, and neuropsychological examinations. Starting in 2008, service members have been required to take baseline computerized neurocognitive evaluations using the Automated Neuropsychological Assessment Metric before they deploy (DVBIC, 2020). DVBIC has been designated by the DoD with responsibilities to implement a system-wide program referred to as the Neurocognitive Assessment Tool. The goal of this tool is to ensure that all service personnel are neurocognitively tested predeployment. DVBIC has also been charged with implementing any follow-up testing using concussion protocols as well as clinical practice guidelines set forth by military medical providers for neurocognitive and neuropsychological diagnosis and treatment. The following TBI assessments and concussion screening instruments are currently implemented by military medical practitioners.

Military Acute Concussion Evaluation–2 (MACE-2)

In 2018, the MACE-2 screening instrument (DVBIC, 2020) was implemented as a multimodal assessment tool to assist medical providers at various military treatment facilities in the assessment and diagnosis of concussion injuries. The MACE-2 is a standardized test that incorporates 17 different areas in which to test neurological and physical symptoms, orientation, memory, concentration, history of other injuries, as well as vestibular and ocular-motor abilities.

DVBIC 3 Question TBI Screen/ Brief Traumatic Brain Injury Screen

The DVBIC 3 Question TBI Screen (DVBIC, 2020), also referred to as the Brief Traumatic Brain Injury Screen (Schwab et al., 2006), is a basic three-item screening instrument to evaluate military personnel who may require additional neurological and neurocognitive testing for an MTBI. The three items evaluate (a) any injuries sustained while deployed (e.g., vehicle accidents, bullet fragments, falls), (b) any injuries sustained that resulted in various neurocognitive symptoms (e.g., dazed, confused, dizzy, loss of consciousness), and (c) any current symptoms as a result of possible head injury (e.g., headaches, tinnitus, vertigo, memory problems). This brief instrument, typically completed postdeployment by military medical personnel, provides a rapid assessment of other mandated TBI follow-up evaluations and treatments required for all new deployments.

GCS

The GCS (Jennet et al., 1981) is a widely used standardized tool that was constructed to assess the patient's degree of consciousness. It is typically used in early phases postinjury within the emergency and critical care unit. The GCS provides a baseline of subsequent changes in neurological and neurocognitive functioning and measures three distinct areas of functioning: eye open, verbal response, and motor response. Repeated observation and measurement provide a general measure of neurological and neurocognitive functioning. The scale itself assesses the level of consciousness along a continuum ranging from being comatose to being alert. Scores range from 3 to 15, with lower scores indicating a deeper level of unconsciousness.

Rancho Los Amigos Levels of Cognitive Functioning Scale

The Rancho Los Amigos Levels of Cognitive Functioning Scale (Hagan et al., 1972) is used to establish a baseline with repeated observation and measurement of neurological and neurocognitive functioning. The scale ranges from 1 (*no response*; person does not respond to visual, auditory, or tactile stimuli) to 8 (*purposeful/appropriate*; oriented to person and place, typically overestimates functional ability, difficulty relating in social interactions, needs assistance with activities of daily living) and up to 10 (*postacute/stable*; person is independently able to complete tasks at home, work, or leisure; may need extra time for tasks). Higher scores indicate higher levels of functioning.

FUNCTION AND STRUCTURE OF THE BRAIN AND RESIDUAL FUNCTIONAL CAPACITY

The brain and spinal cord make up the joint forces and command center of the human body. The brain and spinal cord regulate various neurochemical reactions in the body. Besides regulating all neurochemical reactions, the brain regulates body temperature, blood pressure, respiration, cardiovascular health, immune system functioning, cognitive abilities, motor skills, expressive and receptive communication, sensory mechanisms (such as vision, hearing, tactile), as well as many more elements that make people more intelligent than other species.

The brain is an elegant organ that gathers, analyzes, stores, integrates, coordinates, and interprets all information required to function and control the body systems described earlier. The prognosis and residual functional capacity of brain injury depend on the severity of the individual's injury and what parts of the brain are most affected. The consequence of brain injuries has a profound impact on the individual's physical, neurological, neurocognitive, neuropsychological, and overall ability to function. People's personality; behaviors; social, emotional, and mental health; and overall well-being depend on the brain to properly function.

Although the right and left sides of the brain have different functions and are responsible for different skills, the two sides must work in coordination to complete various tasks. For instance, the architect designing a magnificent bridge must have good analytical skills (left brain) while possessing some artistic and three-dimensional abilities (right brain). The same is true of playing a musical instrument, which requires some ability to do math (left brain) yet the talent to create music (right brain).

The following information is a brief overview and description of the right and left hemispheres of the brain. The intention is for readers to possess a beginning understanding of the motor, sensory, communication, processing, and other aspects of the brain that may have been impaired during a blast injury; concussion; or mild, moderate, or severe TBI. Injuries to specific parts of the brain inform medical and allied health providers of the prognosis, treatments, and goals for therapy, which can assist clinical military counselors in future therapeutic interventions with the TBI survivor and their family members.

Right Brain

Damage to the right hemisphere affects the person's ability to utilize expressive communication. This hemisphere is responsible for (a) artistic awareness and imagination, such as in expressive arts and music; (b) intuition; (c) the ability to see three-dimensional objects and figures; and (d) personality traits that may include how people project their quirkiness, eccentric behaviors, and emotions that define them as a person. Right brain injury impairs the individual's ability to communicate expressively to others, which is also referred to as *Broca's aphasia*. The individual typically can comprehend spoken words but has difficulty expressing or communicating their thoughts. Broca's aphasia is typically marked by articulation errors as well as speech that is hesitant and laborious with reduced vocabulary. The individual's reading ability is typically much better than their writing ability. The right hemisphere controls left brain motor and physical functioning. Likewise, the left hemisphere controls right brain motor and physical functioning. If the individual has injury to the right brain, it will impair motor skills on the left side of the body, which may be apparent by some degree of paralysis or weakness. Conversely, if the individual has injury to the left brain, it will impair motor skills on the right side of the body.

Left Brain

Damage to the left hemisphere affects the person's receptive language skills. This hemisphere is responsible for (a) spoken and written language, (b) technical and scientific skills, (c) number skills, and (d) analytical thinking. Left-side impairments create receptive aphasia, also referred to as *Wernicke's aphasia*. This type of aphasia creates impairment with one's ability to understand and process information.

Speech and grammar typically function normally. However, one's ability to comprehend even basic information is impaired. Overall, individuals with left-side damage typically have poor reading and auditory comprehension abilities.

TBI Implications

Consequently, TBI has multiple functional deficits and long-term implications for the individual. The following summary represents deficits in physical, neurocognitive, behavioral, personality, and mental health functioning. The frequency, degree, and intensity of these deficits depend on the location and severity of the service member's or veteran's brain injury:

- Difficulties with comprehending and processing information that is communicated to them (caused by receptive aphasia);
- Difficulties with communicating or articulating using speech as well as putting words and sentences together (caused by expressive aphasia);
- Motor coordination and balance problems;
- Problems with depth perception, ability to judge distances, and interpreting visual stimuli;
- Difficulties with activities of daily living, such as eating, swallowing, bowel and bladder function, cooking, cleaning, and bathing safely;
- Cognitive problems of memory, concentration, and attention deficits;
- Difficulties with concept formation, judgment, reasoning, and insight;
- Proneness to irritability, anger outbursts, labile emotions, and depression;
- Exhibition of socially and interpersonally inappropriate behaviors; and
- Problems with wake-sleep disturbance, depression, irritability, and anger.

CTE

CTE is now being recognized in the military as a serious condition that can affect the service member's neurocognitive functioning long after separation from military service. CTE results from repeated blows to the head, much like what is seen in the National Football League, in the National Hockey League, and among professional boxers.

Repetitive blast wounds, concussions, and MTBI all contribute to possible neurocognitive and neuropsychiatric deficits among older veterans. Statistically, a decline in neurocognitive functioning occurs after age 55 in the civilian population. However, previous head injury predisposes veterans to greater vulnerability to acquiring CTE. The prevalence and incidence of veteran CTE are currently unknown because this specialty area in neuroscience research is in the early stages of development (McKee et al., 2013).

CTE appears as a distinct pathology from other neurodegenerative diseases such as dementias and Alzheimer's disease, although they may co-occur with CTE (McKee et al., 2013). Neurocognitive researchers have shown significant neurodegenerative changes within certain structures of the brain where abnormal tissue develops (Chapman & Diaz-Arrastia, 2014; Elder et al., 2019; McKee et al., 2015). These neurodegenerative changes can occur months, years, or even decades after the person's last concussion. Consequently, a combination of reduced cognitive functioning occurs, including memory loss, confusion, impaired judgment, poor concentration and focus, paranoia, low impulse control, major depression, aggression, dementias, and the early presentation of Parkinson's disease.

Blast injuries, concussions, and MTBIs are taken seriously in the military. Current treatment protocols in the U.S. Armed Forces require more detailed and mandatory neurological and neuropsychological screenings both before and after deployment. This specialty area of military research has revealed the short- and long-term neurocognitive and neuropsychological deficits present among active-duty personnel and veterans. Multiple considerations are under way regarding military technology, improved battlefield protection (e.g., body armor, helmets), and other preventive measures to reduce serious head injuries.

PSYCHOSOCIAL ASPECTS OF BLAST INJURIES AND TBI

Besides the physical, neurocognitive, and neuropsychological changes that occur with blast injuries and TBIs, the person and their family experience several psychosocial issues, which are the focus of this section.

The therapeutic goals for medical providers, allied health specialists (e.g., physical, occupational, speech therapists), and mental health counselors depend on the patient's specific phase of brain injury rehabilitation treatment. Neurorehabilitation efforts in the military typically follow the course of (a) trauma stabilization in a treatment facility overseas; (b) neurorehabilitation in an acute or postacute facility either overseas or in the United States, depending on the level of injury and medical stability; and (c) admission to a long-term neurorehabilitation center in the United States for patients who are more medically impaired. The VA health system has significantly increased its capacity for state-of-the-art research, innovative educational programs, and rehabilitative care for the 4,300 veterans identified in 2018 with a TBI who separated from military service with polytrauma conditions (DVBIC, 2020). The VA has created a model for long-term care that operates in five polytrauma rehabilitation centers throughout the United States (Minneapolis, MN; Palo Alto, CA; Richmond, VA; San Antonio, TX; and Tampa, FL). Statistics from the VA polytrauma rehabilitation centers show that after 5 years of long-term care rehabilitation, 56%–85% of veterans reach independent functioning (Whyte et al., 2013). Besides the 12 military base rehabilitation hospitals located throughout the United States and the one in Germany, many additional private for-profit brain injury rehabilitation centers around the United States specialize in veteran TBI and other polytrauma conditions. For example, U.S. News and World Report has ranked the top 50 neurorehabilitation centers in the United States (https://health.usnews.com/best-hospitals/rankings/neurology-and-neurosurgery).

Psychosocial adjustment and adaptation to blast injuries and TBIs involve co-occurring physical, neurocognitive, and neuropsychological challenges that affect the individual's mood, emotion, behaviors, personality, thoughts, and overall mental health functioning. The following guidelines are offered to clinical practitioners for consideration during comprehensive clinical assessments and the development of mental and behavioral health treatment strategies for service members and veterans with blast injuries and TBIs:

- The present chapter serves as a primer or introduction to blast injuries and TBIs. Competent and ethical clinical providers engage in training activities and clinical supervision when working with a specific cultural or disability group. Mental health practitioners are encouraged to enroll in continuing education courses and seminars that address the neurocognitive and neuropsychological aspects of treating blast injuries and TBIs. Because of the complex clinical characteristics and skills required to work competently with military personnel who have sustained blast injuries and TBIs, it is important to understand the unique approaches to assessments, resources, allied health specialists, and co-occurring mental health conditions (e.g., PTSD, depression, anxiety, substance use disorders) associated with these injuries.
- Consider elements of the psychosocial adjustment and adaptation to disability presented in Chapter 6 to anticipate and plan appropriate strategies within the rehabilitation process. Stage models can provide practitioners with a general impression of the person's expected psychosocial functioning and clinical interventions to facilitate the rehabilitation treatment process. Psychosocial adjustment to brain injury rehabilitation follows specific patterns of physical, neurocognitive, neuropsychological, and mental health functioning that can assist providers with developing goals and treatment strategies.

- Review the characteristics and residual functional capacity deficits of the person's blast injuries or TBI presented in this chapter (e.g., deficits in memory, attention, concentration, motor skills, and level of independent functioning). Examine the person's medical and allied health providers' records that address specific information related to residual functional capacity. Medical records provide clinicians with valuable information related to the development of appropriate therapeutic goals to address the individual's interpersonal, social, emotional, sexual, education and career, and overall independent functioning.
- Some clinical manifestations of blast injuries and TBIs are associated with other symptoms related to PTSD, major depressive disorder, anxiety, and substance use disorders. Given the complex and poly-traumatic nature of blast injuries and TBIs, competent mental health providers partner with medical specialists, allied health providers, and other resources to coordinate the person's care and treatment.
- Mental health practitioners should consider the traumatic nature of repetitive blast injuries and TBIs as it relates to the clinically significant symptoms of persistent complex bereavement disorders. An interplay of TBI and complex bereavement may contribute to the person's feelings of grief, loss, and mourning. For example, bereavement becomes clinically significant for service members or veterans who experienced the death of other unit members. Competent clinicians also consider anniversary dates of their client's injury as well as injuries or deaths of other unit members.
- Multiple losses experienced by the person require processing and normalizing, including the loss of career, personal identity as a member of an elite unit, one's independence, and neurocognitive functions.
- Recognize the person as a "survivor" rather than a victim. Viewing the person as a survivor increases their ability to cope and adapt to adversity, empowering them with coping and resiliency strategies.
- Depending on the severity of the person's blast injury or TBI, there will be neurocognitive deficits that require adaptation and accommodation for independence. Partnering with allied health providers (e.g., speech, occupational, and physical therapists) supports a direction for behavioral and mental health treatment. Facilitate goals that reinforce, generalize, and incorporate global strategies to optimize maximum functioning.
- Neurocognitive deficits—such as impaired memory, concentration, and focus—affect all areas of the person's life. Behavioral and mental health therapists may want to reinforce the idea of making lists and keeping charts, notebooks, and calendars as memory aids, particularly for provider visits and other life activities. Incorporate natural cues, prompts, or reminders in the natural environment to accommodate neurocognitive deficits.

- Wake-sleep disorders are a common clinical feature of blast injuries and TBIs. This area should be evident from the mental health provider's comprehensive clinical assessment. Addressing good sleep hygiene is another important therapeutic goal.

CONCLUDING REMARKS

Blast injuries and TBIs—the signature injuries of OIF and OEF—produce complex sequelae of physical, psychosocial, neurocognitive, neuropsychological, and mental health conditions for service members, veterans, and their families. Military neuroscience researchers have demonstrated the unique similarities and differences between blast injuries and MTBI. Because of the increased incidence of blast injuries and TBIs, military neuroscience researchers have taken an active role in developing improved diagnostic and treatment protocols. The primary objectives are to reduce physical, neurocognitive, neuropsychological, and mental health risk factors in service members and veterans.

In this chapter, I also explored advancements in improved battlefield neurocognitive and neuropsychological assessments administered before and after deployment. Military personnel who have sustained blast injuries and TBIs are at significant risk for military suicidality. Strategic goals implemented by the DoD mandate a system to monitor the neurocognitive and neuropsychological health of service members and veterans. One of the most critical aspects of blast injuries and TBIs involves dealing with the mental health challenges of complex PTSD and its co-occurring conditions (e.g., major depressive disorder, substance use disorders, suicidality). Veteran health care for the future remains a priority in treating the neurocognitive, neuropsychological, and mental health conditions of those who have survived repetitive blast injuries and TBIs.

REFERENCES

Army Dismounted Complex Blast Injury Task Force. (2011, June 18). *Dismounted complex blast injury.* https://www.jsomonline.org/TCCC/06%20TCCC%20Reference%20Documents/DCBI%20Task%20Force%20Report%20Final%20(Redacted)%20110921.pdf

Beers, M. H., Fletcher, A. J., Jones, T. V., Porter, R., Berkwits, M., & Kaplan, J. L. (2003). *The Merck manual of medical information* (2nd ed.). Merck Research Laboratories.

Bryan, C. J., & Clemans, T. A. (2013). Repetitive traumatic brain injury, psychological symptoms, and suicide risk in a clinical sample of deployed military personnel. *JAMA Psychiatry, 70*(7), 686–691. https://doi.org/10.1001/jamapsychiatry.2013.1093

Centers for Disease Control and Prevention. (n.d.). *Explosions and blast injuries: A primer for clinicians.* https://www.cdc.gov/masstrauma/preparedness/primer.pdf

Centers for Disease Control and Prevention. (2019, March 11). *TBI: Get the facts.* https://www.cdc.gov/traumaticbraininjury/get_the_facts.html

Chapman, J. C., & Diaz-Arrastia, R. (2014). Military traumatic brain injury: A review. *Alzheimer's & Dementia, 10*(Suppl. 3), S97–S104. https://doi.org/10.1016/j.jalz.2014.04.012

Chase, R. P., McMahon, S. A., & Winch, P. J. (2016). "Tell me what you don't remember": Care-seeking facilitators and barriers in the decade following repetitive blast exposure among Army combat veterans. *Military Medicine, 181*(2), 116–122. https://doi.org/10.7205/MILMED-D-14-00471

Cooper, L. N., Holliday, R. P., Holder, N. D., Jackson, J., North, C. S., & Suris, A. M. (2018). Working with trauma-related mental health problems among combat veterans of the Afghanistan and Iraq conflicts. In I. Marini & M. A. Stebnicki (Eds.), *The psychological and social impact of illness and disability* (7th ed., pp. 311–343). Springer.

Defense and Veterans Brain Injury Center. (2020, May 15). *DoD worldwide numbers for TBI.* http://dvbic.dcoe.mil/dod-worldwide-numbers-tbi

Elder, G. A., Ehrlich, M. A., & Gandy, S. (2019). Relationship of traumatic brain injury to chronic mental health problems and dementia in military veterans. *Neuroscience Letters, 707,* Article 134294. https://doi.org/10.1016/j.neulet.2019.134294

Falvo, D. R., & Holland, B. E. (2018). *Medical and psychosocial aspects of chronic illness and disability* (6th ed.). Jones & Bartlett Learning.

Hagan, C., Malkmus, D., & Durham, P. (1972). *Rancho Los Amigos Levels of Cognitive Functioning Scale.* Rancho Los Amigos Hospital.

Jennet, B., Snoek, J., Bond, M. R., & Brooks, N. (1981). Disability after severe head injury: Observations on the use of the Glasgow Outcome Scale. *Journal of Neurology and Neurosurgical Psychiatry, 44*(4), 285–293. https://doi.org/10.1136/jnnp.44.4.285

Kirkman, E., Watts, S., & Cooper, G. (2011). Blast injuries research model. *Philosophical Transactions of the Royal Society B: Biological Sciences, 366*(1562), 144–159. https://doi.org/10.1098/rstb.2010.0240

Loane, D. J., Stoica, B. A., & Faden, I. A. (2015). Neuroprotection for traumatic brain injury. In M. Aminoff, F. Boller, & D. F. Swaab (Eds.), *Handbook of clinical neurology* (Vol. 127, pp. 343–366). Elsevier.

McKee, A. C., & Robinson, M. E. (2014). Military-related traumatic brain injury and neurodegeneration. *Alzheimer's & Dementia, 10*(Suppl. 3), S242–S253. https://doi.org/10.1016/j.jalz.2014.04.003

McKee, A. C., Stein, T. D., Kieman, P. T., & Alvarez, V. E. (2015). The neuropathology of chronic traumatic encephalopathy. *Brain Pathology, 25*(3), 350–364. https://doi.org/10.1111/bpa.12248

McKee, A. C., Stern, R. A., Nowinski, C. J., Stein, T. D., Alvarez, V. E., Daneshvar, D. H., Lee, H.-S., Wojtowicz, S. M., Hall, G., Baugh, C. M., Riley, D. O., Kubilus, C. A., Cormier, K. A., Jacobs, M. A., Martin, B. R., Abraham, C. R., Ikezu, T., Reichard, R. R., Wolozin, B. L., . . . Cantu, R. C. (2013). The spectrum of disease in chronic traumatic encephalopathy. *Brain, 136*(1), 43–64. https://doi.org/10.1093/brain/aws307

Schwab, K. A., Baker, G., Ivins, B., Sluss-Tiller, M., Lux, W., & Warden, D. (2006). The Brief Traumatic Brain Injury Screen (BTBIS): Investigating the validity of a self-report instrument for detecting traumatic brain injury (TBI) in troops returning from deployment in Afghanistan and Iraq. *Neurology, 66*(5), Article A235.

Sisk, R. (2019, December 26). *Pentagon ordered to add blast exposure to troops' medical histories.* Military.com. https://www.military.com/daily-news/2019/12/26/pentagon-ordered-add-blast-exposure-troops-medical-histories.html?utm_source=Sailthru&utm_medium=email&utm_campaign=EBB%2012.26.19&utm_term=Editorial%20-%20Military%20-%20Early%20Bird%20Brief

Warden, D. (2006). Military TBI during the Iraq and Afghanistan wars. *Journal of Head Trauma Rehabilitation, 21*(5), 398–402. https://doi.org/10.1097/00001199-200609000-00004

Whyte, J., Nakase-Richardson, R., Hammond, F., McNamee, S., Giacino, J. T., Kalmar, K., Greenwald, B. D., Yablon, S. A., & Horn, L. J. (2013). Functional outcomes in traumatic disorders of consciousness: 5-year outcomes from the National Institute on Disability and Rehabilitation Research Traumatic Brain Injury Model Systems. *Archives of Physical Medicine and Rehabilitation, 94*(10), 1855–1860. https://doi.org/10.1016/j.apmr.2012.10.041

Wightman, J. M., & Gladish, S. L. (2001). Explosions and blast injuries. *Annals of Emergency Medicine, 37*(6), 664–678. https://doi.org/10.1067/mem.2001.114906

Wolf, S. J., Bebarta, V. S., Bonnett, C. J., Pons, P. T., & Cantrill, S. V. (2009). Blast injuries. *Lancet, 374*(9687), 405–415. https://doi.org/10.1016/S0140-6736(09)60257-9

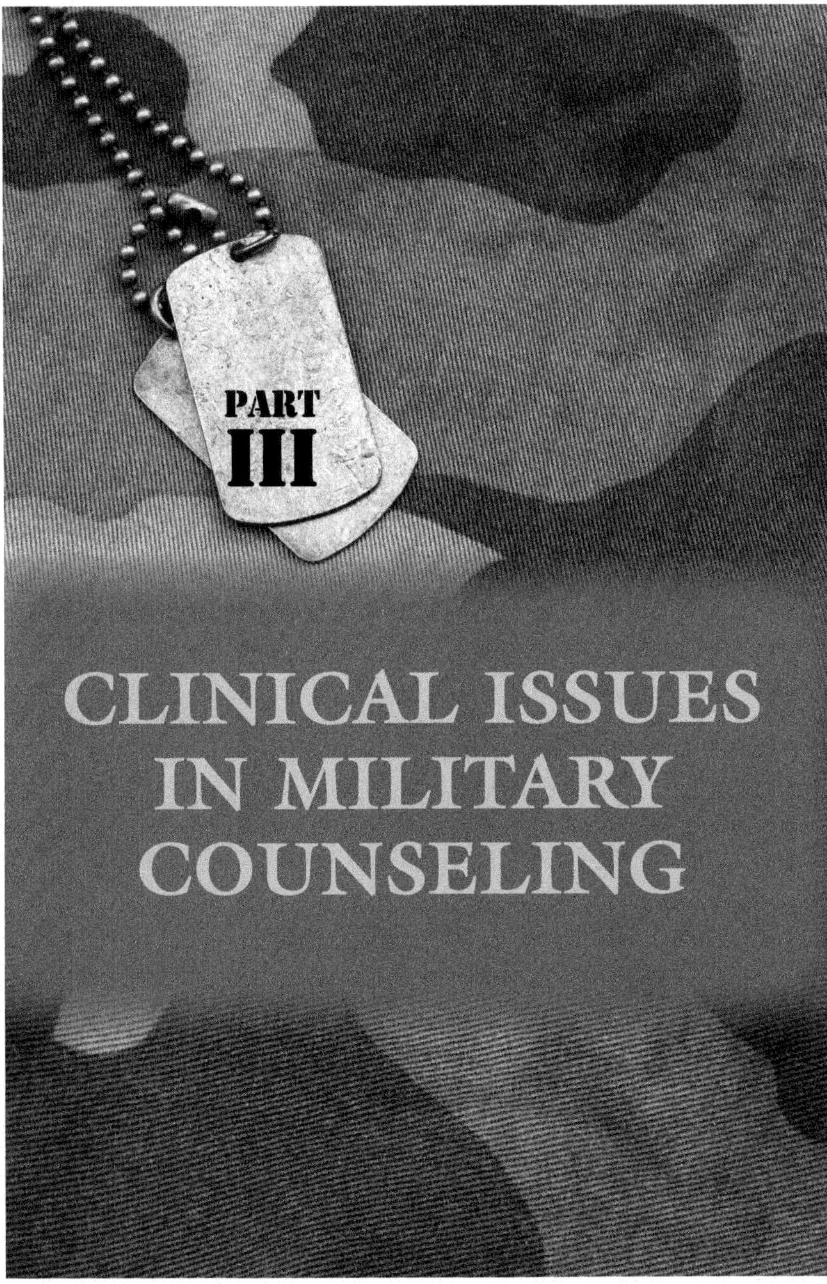

PART III

CLINICAL ISSUES IN MILITARY COUNSELING

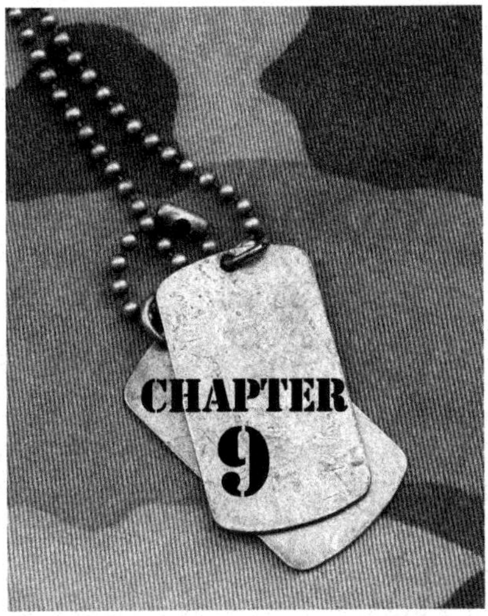

SPIRITUALITY, MORAL INJURY, AND TRAUMA IN MILITARY LIFE

If soul loss is a spiritual illness that
causes emotional and physical disease,
then we better get boots on the ground
to go find it.

—Mark A. Stebnicki, 2020

★ ★ ★

There is a growing body of literature regarding military psychology, moral injury, and trauma that suggests a strong association between having good spiritual well-being and military resiliency and readiness (Doehring, 2019; Smith-MacDonald et al., 2017). Extraordinary stressful and traumatic events in military life have long-term implications for service members' and veterans' mental, physical, and spiritual well-being. Many experiences in warfighting will never be disclosed by service members and veterans to others outside their units or as reflected in after-action reports. Exposure to frequent killing of enemy combatants; the threat of being attacked, killed, or captured; witnessing death and injury; and handling injured and dead bodies of unit members, civilians, and enemy combatants change the military service member in a profound way. Consequently, service members and veterans are challenged spiritually, ethically, and morally by these warfighting experiences (Knobloch et al., 2019; Smith-MacDonald et al., 2017; Tick, 2014; Wortmann et al., 2017).

Healing the mind, body, and spirit of service members and veterans is enhanced by integrating their spiritual and religious belief systems into the therapeutic process. The use of psychospiritual approaches in therapy enhances the service member's ability to cope with military life stressors, depression, and suicidality; these approaches also help with engagement in spiritual care activities and increase one's awareness for good emotional, social, and psychological health and resiliency (Sterner & Jackson-Cherry, 2015; Thomas et al., 2018).

When using spiritual care to treat military moral injury, one must consider the service member's and veteran's unique religious and spiritual worldview. Competent and ethical practitioners utilize their training and out-of-session resources to provide multiple opportunities for healing trauma of the mind, body, and spirit. Relying solely on psychotherapy approaches—without understanding the resources that chaplains, pastoral counselors, and religious leaders can bring to the service member's and veteran's life—risks "medicalizing" the individual's moral injury as a mental health condition (Graham, 2017).

The beneficial effects of increased spiritual well-being help bring meaning to one's military career, particularly during the loss and grief associated with combat-related death and warfighting (Doehring, 2019; Ramsay, 2019; Tick, 2014). Accordingly, integrating spirituality within military mental health counseling practice has emerged as one of the most powerful approaches for healing trauma and moral injury. In this chapter, I explore the implications of integrating psychospiritual practices with the intention of healing moral injury and military trauma. Guidelines are also offered for practitioners who are open to exploring other healing resources with their military clients.

CONCEPTUALIZING SPIRITUALITY IN CLINICAL PRACTICE

Integrating spirituality and religiosity in mental health counseling is one of the most misunderstood areas in therapeutic practice. Many clinicians believe that issues related to spirituality should be addressed primarily by those trained in theology (e.g., pastors, rabbis, priests) or military chaplains. Although military chaplains certainly do play an important role in dealing with issues of spirituality, clarifying religious beliefs and values, performing rituals, and dealing with matters related to moral injury and trauma, it becomes problematic when coordination of therapeutic effort is not maximized across the various disciplines. It is akin to clinicians not discussing client medications prescribed by a psychiatrist or family medical practitioner during their session (e.g., list of medications, dosage, side effects, benefits). Accordingly, addressing spirituality and religiosity brings meaning to traumatic experiences and moral injury in military life.

Cashwell and Young (2020), as well as their contributing colleagues, have discussed integrating spirituality and religion into the therapeutic setting. Research and practice in this area have developed into core competencies and skills that are delineated by the Association for Spiritual, Ethical, and Religious Values in Counseling (ASERVIC), which is a division of the American Counseling Association. The core competencies are listed in the following domains: (a) Culture and Worldview, (b) Counselor Self-Awareness, (c) Human and Spiritual Development, (d) Communication, (e) Assessment, and (f) Diagnosis and Treatment. The intention is that each of these domains translates into therapeutic skills facilitated in conjunction with evidence-based practices in counseling and psychology. ASERVIC (n.d.) has published a white paper to assist in clarifying the definition, meaning, and construct of spirituality for clinical mental health practitioners. Delineated in ASERVIC's definition and construct are principles related to (a) a life force that expands beyond individual consciousness; (b) the integration of naturally occurring events within one's environment; (c) individual and cultural meaning of spiritual events; (d) one's personal growth and development nurtured by love, transcendence, connectedness, compassion, wellness, wholeness, and creativity; and (e) integrating a specific system of beliefs, values, and practices.

Many clients with a religious or spiritual orientation bring the following types of existential questions to session: "Why am I being punished?" "Why has God abandoned me?" "What kind of God would allow this to happen to me?" (Young & Cashwell, 2020). Particularly in times of crisis or trauma, competent clinical military counselors facilitate therapeutic strategies that address such concerns to assist military clients in contemplating, clarifying, bringing meaning and significance, and taking actions related to their life.

Coordination of care can be enhanced by multiple disciplines, viewpoints, and therapeutic approaches when healing trauma and moral injury of the mind, body, and spirit.

Spirituality is a subjective experience and exists in the hearts and minds of all cultures (Stebnicki, 2016b; Vaughan, 1991). In contrast to religion, spirituality describes the relationship between the person and a transcendent being or higher power. There is no universal language or way to communicate one's spirituality like in religious practices (e.g., religious texts, references, rituals performed). Thus, many individuals have an emotional connection or experience as they describe their spiritual belief system (Csordas, 1990).

Early researchers and psychotherapists contended that spirituality is a natural part of being human (Assagioli, 1965, 1971; Jung, 1937/1973; Worthington, 1988). It is interwoven within the individual's physical, mental, cognitive, and emotional psyche (Ellison & Smith, 1991; Myers et al., 2000). Spirituality is a way to construct personal meaning and purpose regarding one's life and culture (Frankl,

1959; Myers et al., 2000; Stebnicki, 2016a, 2016b; Tillich, 1952). It oftentimes becomes paradoxical for the individual because it is difficult for the therapist to observe their client's spirituality (Hayes, 1984). Spirituality is the courage to look within oneself; to trust a transcendent spiritual being; or to have a deep sense of belonging, wholeness, connectedness, and openness to the infinite (Shafranske & Gorsuch, 1984).

Religiosity has a more direct meaning because it involves ascribing to a set of religious beliefs, doctrines, and rituals. It can be observed by others and most often is institutionally based in a church, temple, mosque, or faith-based organization (Shafranske & Malony, 1990, 1996; Vaughan, 1991). Religion is recognized as being a part of the individual's spiritual belief system and is the expression of one's spirituality (Myers et al., 2000).

The psychology and counseling literature indicates that clients who have religious and spiritual concerns oftentimes bring these issues into therapeutic settings (Francis, 2016). Yet, few therapists address spiritual concerns with their clients. The search for personal meaning in one's chronic illness, disability, or traumatic experience is an existential and spiritual pursuit (Stebnicki, 2016b). Thus, possessing the awareness, knowledge, and skills of how to integrate spiritual practices within the therapeutic environment is essential for working optimally within a multicultural counseling perspective (ASERVIC, n.d.; Corey & Corey, 2021; Miller, 2003; Moodley & West, 2005; Myers & Sweeney, 2008; Shannonhouse et al., 2016; Stebnicki, 2008, 2016b; Stebnicki & Cubero, 2008).

INTEGRATING SPIRITUALITY IN CLINICAL MILITARY COUNSELING

Spirituality and faith-based practices have emerged as a unique topic of interest within military psychology, mental health counseling, and its related disciplines (e.g., pastoral and chaplaincy psychology, military medicine and psychiatry, veteran health care). More recently, integrating psychospiritual practices within the therapeutic environment has been deemed worthy of empirical study by the U.S. Department of Defense (DoD). The clinical application of psychospiritual practices can be found in current evidence-based treatment programs, and these practices are also part of multiple military wellness and resiliency programs (Knobloch et al., 2019; Smith-MacDonald et al., 2017; Thomas et al., 2018).

The resurgence of religious and spiritual values represents a growing trend in psychology and counseling for service members and veterans. Complementary and integrative health approaches that incorporate spiritually based strategies provide opportunities outside traditional psychotherapy and include such healing arts as yoga, meditation, mindfulness-based stress reduction, acupuncture, expressive arts, and animal-assisted therapy. Spiritual health is an especially important issue for service members and veterans who are challenged by extraordinary stressful and traumatic events that create distress and moral injury. Making sense and meaning of military service for many is a spiritual journey given the existential nature of war.

Integrating psychospiritual approaches in military psychology and counseling practice has been slow in its development. Several explanations have been offered for this delay. First, as with any specific counseling theory or strategy, the integration of psychospiritual approaches may depend on the mental health practitioner's level of interest, motivation for its use, and advanced training that they may or may not have acquired. Second, some agencies, organizations, and clinical programs may perceive psychospiritual approaches as being overly religious or too faith based for their secular mental health practices. Lastly, it is recognized that there are few resources outside of pastoral, chaplain, and theological education where mental health practitioners have training opportunities for integrating psychospiritual practices within the therapeutic environment. Interestingly, spiritually based outpatient and residential treatment programs (e.g., Alcoholics Anonymous, Narcotics Anonymous, Celebrate Recovery, 28-day rehabilitation treatment programs) have been offered by clinical mental health and addiction counselors to nonmilitary clients for decades (Benshoff & Janikowski, 1999; Goodwin, 2002; Juhnke et al., 2009; Robertson, 2016).

In military life, multiple extraordinary stressful and traumatic events can be life altering, causing serious psychological problems and leading to spiritual and moral injury (Bremault-Phillips et al., 2019; Ramsay, 2019). Consequently, trauma and moral injury negatively affect the individual's spiritual well-being. One instrument developed by early researchers to measure spiritual well-being is the Spiritual Well-Being Scale (SWBS; Paloutzian & Ellison, 1982). The SWBS is considered the most extensively researched subjective measure of spiritual well-being (Ellison & Smith, 1991; Ledbetter et al., 1991; Watson et al., 1990). It consists of 20 items evenly divided into two subscales of religious well-being and existential well-being. This self-report instrument has been used in a variety of settings, including colleges, universities, seminaries, hospitals, recreational therapy practices, mental health clinics, and prisons. Several studies have shown a positive correlation between the SWBS and increased psychological health among persons with chronic medical illnesses and life-threatening disabilities (Baldwin, 1995; Campbell, 1988; Carson, 1990; Carson et al., 1990; Granstrom, 1987; Heintzman, 1999; Kaczorowski, 1989; Kohlbry, 1986; Richter, 2002; Riley et al., 1998).

More recently, a shortened version of the SWBS was used to evaluate psychometric properties with seven key items of this original

20-item scale (Malinakova et al., 2017). On the basis of the data, these researchers concluded that the shortened version supports a two-factor model of the SWBS and has satisfactory internal consistency, suggesting it is suitable for measuring spiritual well-being in secular environments.

In one of the few studies available, Johnson et al. (2015)—using a small sample of veterans diagnosed with posttraumatic stress disorder (PTSD) receiving services from the U.S. Department of Veterans Affairs (VA)—utilized two versions of the Functional Assessment Chronic Illness Therapy–Spiritual Well-Being Scale, which is a 12-item scale, to measure spiritual well-being in the veteran population. The interested reader will want to consult this study for greater detail. This complex design utilized a three-factor model (Peace, Meaning, and Faith) and two-factor model (Peace combined with Meaning and Faith) and then compared the results with a four-factor model (Peace, Meaning, Faith, and Spirituality) and the three-factor model. Results indicated that the three-factor model (Peace, Meaning, and Faith) had the best fit to measure veteran spiritual well-being. The results and conclusion of this study suggest that treatment of veterans with PTSD should include an evaluation of the person's spiritual well-being. This evaluation could potentially be integrated with veteran medical and mental health services because of the influence that spiritual well-being has on treating veteran complex trauma.

Fundamentally, integrating psychospiritual approaches in military counseling settings is relevant and should be a high priority for healing the wounds of trauma and moral injury. For psychospiritual research, theory, and practice to advance in clinical military counseling settings, it is essential that researchers and practitioners learn how to evaluate and integrate relevant psychospiritual intervention with military cultural concerns.

For the last 30 years—from a human growth and development perspective—research in psychology and counseling has defined, evaluated, measured, and clinically described developmental characteristics of one's spirituality, faith, and religious and moral beliefs (Myers et al., 2000; Worthington, 1989). This body of research has resulted in other paradigms that have led to the development of wellness theories and their application for mental health practice. Wellness theories have the intention to cultivate optimal functioning for the individual and human potential for everyday life. The shift in utilizing one's religious beliefs, values, and practices in therapy is culturally sensitive and is pivotal in the psychospiritual wellness movement in clinical mental health counseling. Wellness theories have also provided a means to communicate the principles of integrative healing approaches, tapping into the unused potentials of the mind, body, and spirit. The unique wisdom offered in clinical practice suggests that wellness practices can be utilized in everyday life for everyday people—not just for those with chronic and persistent medical and mental health conditions (American Counseling Association, 2006; Shannonhouse et al., 2016).

The shift to current models of wellness began with Myers et al.'s (2000) foundational work on the wheel of wellness (WoW). The WoW is a theoretical model that combines empirical research from 17 specific areas of health, longevity, and quality of life. This model suggests that there are five life tasks central to healthy human functioning: (a) work, (b) friendship, (c) love, (d) self, and (e) spirituality. Although there are 17 categories of wellness in the WoW model, spirituality is hypothesized to be the most essential aspect of wellness and healthy human functioning (Myers et al., 2000).

Wellness programs in the military culture offer opportunities for health prevention related to one's physical, mental, cognitive, behavioral, psychological, social, emotional, occupational, and spiritual health. The DoD and VA have devoted time and money to the development of wellness programs for more than 20 years because of their success in preventing physical and mental health conditions. The positive results in wellness research suggest that prevention and treatment on the front end of therapy serve as a cost-saving measure on the back end after the service member or veteran has a physical or mental health crisis (Carrola & Corbin-Burdick, 2015; Parker et al., 2001).

The U.S. Army's Comprehensive Soldier and Family Fitness program (https://readyandresilient.army.mil/CSF2/index.html), based on the U.S. Army's (2014) Regulation 350–53, is one example of a wellness model approach that serves as a key component of the U.S. Army's readiness and resiliency objectives to promote optimal resiliency in the service member's physical and mental well-being. The U.S. Army's Master Resiliency Training Course, part of the Comprehensive Soldier and Family Fitness program, focuses on five core areas (i.e., physical, emotional, social, family, spiritual) of leadership training to assist in building mental toughness, character, strength, and strong relationships that are modeled to others in the unit and the military community. These core areas are aligned with other wellness models and particularly advocate for spiritual and religious practices as a pathway to optimal functioning of mind, body, and spirit.

Other programs based on this DoD directorate—known as U.S. Army Sharp, Ready, & Resilient—implement wellness strategies for enhancing soldier personal readiness through building connections with mental and physical health providers (e.g., military crisis hotline, safe helpline for sexual assault support, programs for psychological health and traumatic brain injury). These programs have six core components: (a) health assessment utilizing a wellness questionnaire, (b) physical fitness, (c) healthy nutrition, (d) stress management utilizing stress education and biofeedback, (e) general wellness education, and (f) tobacco education. The focus of these programs is on military life and the impact of combat operational stress, which can lead to co-occurring physical and mental health conditions such as PTSD, depression, suicidality, and traumatic brain injury.

Overall, a coordinated effort by military medical and mental health practitioners is required to achieve successful coping, adaptation, and adjustment to physical, mental, psychological, emotional, social, spiritual, and moral injuries. Service members and veterans have multiple resources with which they can reach out and take responsibility for their personal wellness.

SPIRITUALITY AND MORAL INJURY

In this section, I explore the relationship between spirituality and moral injury from a biopsychosocial and spiritual perspective. Given the complex nature of moral injury, researchers and practitioners alike have little guidance for the assessment, yet alone treatment, of an ambiguous collection of clinically significant symptoms that mirror multiple diagnostic categories such as PTSD, depression, and anxiety disorders. Presently, there is a lack of agreement within the mental health profession about the specific symptoms associated with moral injury and its development after extraordinary stressful and traumatic events (Currier et al., 2020). One thing that most researchers and practitioners would agree on is that moral injury appears to have clinically significant symptoms of an unhealthy physical, social, emotional, and spiritual nature. It is an invisible wound of war, unlike physical disabilities sustained during combat operations.

A plethora of research demonstrates how religiosity and spirituality enhance military and nonmilitary mental, physical, and spiritual well-being after acquired trauma. As for warfighters, religion and spirituality may help mediate the relationship between morally injurious experiences that increase the symptoms associated with PTSD, depression, and other co-occurring mental health conditions that reach a level of clinical crisis.

Trauma exposure from warfighting creates a type of soul wound or morally injurious trauma. A deep inner psychospiritual wound is thought to occur as the result of one's battlefield experiences (Tick, 2014). The excruciating struggle in the search for meaning in this soul wounding experience has led contemporary researchers to try and identify the unique set of clinically significant symptoms that differentiates moral injury from other trauma experiences.

To my knowledge, the term *moral injury* was first used in print by Shay (1991). It is described as "a betrayal of what's right by someone who holds legitimate authority (in the military—a leader) in a high stakes situation" (Shay, 2012, p. 59; Shay, 2014). Litz et al. (2009) has offered another definition that includes perpetrating, failing to prevent, witnessing, or learning about acts of humanity that violate deeply held moral beliefs. Implied in most definitions of moral injury is the invisible wound that often becomes visible by the service member's behaviors and actions. This wound may be exhibited by service members who become disloyal to the Uniform Code of Military Justice, lack dedication to the mission, exhibit loss of confidence by dishonoring unit leadership and command, perpetrate crimes against humanity, and question one's religious-spiritual beliefs. Thus, moral injury is contextualized within the warrior ethos of the military culture.

The impact of trauma and war has been described by Tick (2014) as the reshaping of one's essential self and soul. War is humanity at its worst. The outcome is expressed by the warfighter's anger; rage; and isolation from family, friends, and society and has the overall risk of suicidality. However, if moral injury does not defeat the individual, then it can provide the impetus for posttraumatic growth. The impact of trauma and war on the soul has the potential to transform the warfighter's identity through the attunement of their feelings, emotions, and experiences. A journey into healing moral injury increases one's compassion for all humanity. It is manifested by the warfighter's level of social and emotional intelligence.

The construct of the soul and soul wounding has deep theological, psychospiritual, and cultural indigenous meaning and significance. For many spiritual leaders, shamans, sages, and mystics, the soul is the seat of emotional and moral consciousness (Stebnicki, 2016b). Among indigenous North American Indian cultures, soul loss results from multiple traumas experienced both individually and by tribal members. Modern psychology and counseling have elucidated the clinical identification, assessment, diagnosis, and treatment of traumas. However, the historical traumas experienced by indigenous tribes and other racial and ethnic minority groups are difficult to describe within a clinical diagnostic framework. Hence, moral injury as prompted by one's traumatic experiences is also difficult to assess and treat. Primarily, moral injury is not a diagnostic category with clinical symptomatology to be reported as a diagnosable condition.

From a classical and traditional spiritual-religious perspective, the traumatized person's soul has disappeared into nonordinary states of consciousness and has been lost to the dark side of an unseen spirit world. Therefore, a shaman would be appointed to perform a soul retrieval because of soul wounding or loss. Shamans navigate the multidimensional spirit world to find healing spirits that assist in patient healing and retrieving one's soul that has been lost to extraordinary stressful and traumatic events (Ingerman, 1991). In many indigenous cultures, religious-spiritual rituals are performed with both the tribe and individual to heal the mind, body, spirit, and soul.

The military unit is a modern-day version of an indigenous tribe that fights and heals together. Except today, military service members and veterans attend the rituals of psychotherapy and are prescribed psychiatric medications to treat their trauma and soul loss. The competent and skilled psychotherapist partners with other resources (e.g., chaplains, spiritual leaders) to assist their clients in mending the fragmented self. Interestingly, many North American Indian tribes use sweat lodge ceremonies within the veteran Indian culture to heal traumas. Traditional healing approaches are utilized alongside evidence-based treatment received through the VA system of health care. Currently, service members and veterans are utilizing complementary and integrative spiritually based health approaches (e.g., mindfulness-based stress reduction, meditation, yoga) at more frequent rates than any other military generation.

So how do modern-day medicine healers evaluate and treat soul loss that results from morally injurious behaviors that mirror PTSD? Inquiring into these issues is critical for healing moral injury among the military community. The human spirit and soul are at stake for service members who might be involved in disaster relief or combat operations. The serious psychological conditions associated with moral injury that are clinically significant and are debilitating for the individual include intrusive thoughts that are negative and disturbing, impulsivity that turns to rage and anger, suicidal ideation, sleep disturbances, substance misuse, avoiding and socially isolating oneself because of specific internal and external triggers, as well as self-harming and demoralizing behaviors (Bremault-Phillips et al., 2019; Frankfurt & Frazier, 2016; Koening et al., 2018; Ramsay, 2019; Tick, 2014).

From a qualitative perspective, interviews with combat veterans who identify with the experience of moral injury reveal that they have an identifiable loss, question the meaning of the mission, are disillusioned by their faith, and question the presence and acceptance of a higher power or God (Doehring, 2015). Consequently, many veterans lack an understanding of their experience of moral injury. Most veterans experience a significant shift in their spiritual-religious values, beliefs, practices, and behaviors. Given the complex traumas associated with warfighting, it is critical to measure the veteran's experience of moral injury to prevent further development of clinically distressing symptoms and to treat this unique and complex mental health condition.

More recently, current tools to measure the experience and expression of moral injury among the military culture have shown promise. One example is the 17-item Expressions of Moral Injury Scale–Military Version (EMIS-M; Currier et al., 2018) screening tool. This measure has been constructed on the basis of the theoretical, empirical, and qualitative literature related to moral injury. The interested reader will want to consult the references for an in-depth review of the EMIS-M. Currier et al. (2018) have noted that the EMIS-M can be utilized as a brief initial assessment of military moral injury. The EMIS-M can be offered alongside other functional measures (e.g., PTSD, anxiety) to complete a comprehensive clinical assessment of military clients.

Another example of a recent tool for measuring moral injury is the short form of the 45-item Moral Injury Symptom Scale–Military Version (MISS-M; Koenig et al., 2018). The MISS-M is a brief screening tool to assist clinicians in measuring the service member's and veteran's feelings and experiences of moral injury. The MISS-M consists of 10 subscales that comprehensively assess the clinical symptoms reported by the veteran. These subscales all relate to the veteran's betrayal, guilt, shame, moral concerns, loss of trust, loss of meaning, difficulty in forgiving, feelings of failure, religious struggles, and loss of religious faith. The short form version is reported to be strongly correlated with symptoms related to PTSD, depression, and anxiety disorders. The interested reader will want to consult the references for a complete review.

Specific themes from qualitative researchers, factors in scale development studies, and the literature conceptualizing the constructs of moral injury all have reported areas to help the therapist screen clients for morally injurious experiences acquired during military life. The following abbreviated list is offered to show the common themes and clinically relevant symptoms that merit follow-up evaluation of your service member's or veteran's experience of moral injury:

- Feelings and experiences of shame, guilt, and anger toward self and others in witnessing or perpetrating injury or death related to civilian children, adults, and conscripted enemy combatants;
- Nondisclosure (because of operational security issues) to others outside the special operations unit of critical events related to injuring and killing enemy and non-enemy combatants, torture, rape, and other traumas witnessed or perpetrated by the individual;
- Disassociation, rejection, repression, or denial of traumatic events witnessed or perpetrated during combat operations or humanitarian missions;
- Loss of meaning of self, with the increased experiences of guilt, shame, and failure as a human being;
- Decreased ability to forgive self and others for engaging in or completing a mission that resulted in injury, death, and other horrors of war;
- Loss of meaning or feelings of disgust with one's military career, occupational specialty, mission purpose, and overall life;
- Questioning of combat-related orders and the mission as well as distrust of unit and command leadership;
- Feelings of personal and operational failure that manifest as guilt, shame, and moral concerns;
- Struggles with and loss of religious faith and spiritual practices that lead to a soul wounding experience; and
- Manifestation of clinically significant symptoms related to the diagnostic categories of PTSD, anxiety, depression, substance use disorders, and suicidality.

Healing the mind, body, spirit, and soul from war requires a transformative experience by the service member and veteran. For some, it may require a soul retrieval to heal the invisible wounds of war. For others, it may require reaching out to a competent mental health practitioner who can guide them in their personal journey from a dark night of the soul to a pathway into the light. The dehumanizing aspects of war, the grief and loss of human life, and the suffering of one's soul are all part of the ambiguous experience of moral injury. Integrating psychospiritual approaches in therapeutic interactions is another channel for a healing journey.

INTEGRATING PSYCHOSPIRITUAL ISSUES IN THERAPY

One of the most intriguing areas of scientific inquiry relates to the long-term medical and mental health impact that extraordinary stressful and traumatic events have on service members and veterans. Quantitative analysis works well with biophysiological and psychological measures of one's physical and mental health. However, mapping the pathways for the psychospiritual healing of moral injury and traumas requires qualitative approaches (e.g., phenomenological, ethnographic, case studies, historical, narrative models) to unravel the psychological, social, emotional, cognitive, behavioral, and persistent stressors that ensue during and after military life.

Indeed, spirituality plays a prominent role in the lives of individuals from most world cultures and is integrated within the identity of the culture itself (Stebnicki, 2016b). Therefore, to work effectively with the individual's spiritual identity and worldview, many experts in psychology and counseling have advocated for quite some time that mental health practitioners need to intentionally inquire about the client's spiritual health during session (Bishop et al., 2003; Cashwell & Young, 2020; Myers et al., 2000; Myers & Williard, 2003; Pargament & Zinnbauer, 2000; Polanski, 2003; Richards & Bergin, 1997; Shafranske & Gorsuch, 1984; Shannonhouse et al., 2016; Stebnicki, 2006). Many times, spiritual health circles back to one's mental and physical health and well-being. From a military life perspective, integrating the service member's and veteran's religious and spiritual beliefs is foundational for healing physical and psychological injury (Bremault-Phillips et al., 2019; Doehring, 2019; Knobloch et al., 2019; Sterner & Jackson-Cherry, 2015).

The therapeutic relationship itself and earning the circle of trust with military clients are pivotal in developing a strong working alliance. Paramount to this relationship are the communication dynamics that emerge consciously and unconsciously as the therapist examines their own attitudes, perceptions, values, and beliefs about military life. Consequently, practitioners must be aware of the meta-transference and countertransference that take place within the therapeutic relationship because of the potential conflict that may arise in the client-counselor working alliance. The following guidelines are offered for consideration in the exploration and integration of your military client's religious-spiritual beliefs:

- Earn the circle of trust first, before integrating any religious-spiritual approaches.
- Invite clients to explore any religious-spiritual beliefs, values, and practices. Often opening this door gives permission for clients to discuss deeply held religious-spiritual beliefs, values, and concerns.
- Be open and honest with clients regarding your own religious-spiritual beliefs, values, and practices.
- Explore the positive and negative impacts that your own religious-spiritual values and beliefs may have on the therapeutic relationship.
- Disclose to clients any formal or informal professional training you received related to the integration of psychospiritual practices (e.g., professional credentials, spiritually based assessments, therapy practices in faith-based settings and programs).
- Explore personal and professional growth opportunities for continuing education and training for the purpose of increasing cultural competence with religious-spiritual treatment issues.
- Organize and manage resources that provide clients with ample referrals outside of therapy, which may include a list of local churches to attend, faith-based counseling services available in the area, or contacts for spiritual leaders and chaplains.
- Seek consultation from religious-spiritual teachers, leaders, clergy, or chaplains that could assist in the integration of psychospiritual issues in session.

The following religious-spiritual questions can be integrated into the military client's initial intake interview to explore religious-spiritual values, beliefs, and practices in future therapy sessions:

- How would you describe or characterize your religious-spiritual beliefs and values?
- Do you practice any rituals, observe any religious holidays, or find any other types of religious-spiritual practices comforting?
- What role, meaning, or purpose do your religious-spiritual beliefs play in your life?
- Are there any religious-spiritual beliefs that cause you anxiety or confusion?
- What do you believe your God (Higher Power) has to teach you in life?

- Are there particular religious-spiritual texts and practices that speak to you or bring deep meaning?
- What kind of religious-spiritual growth do you see yourself making in your future?
- What are some of your earliest memories of religious-spiritual practices?
- Have you ever had any transpersonal or transformational experiences that were extraordinary (e.g., prayers answered; peak experiences bringing about resolve, comfort, or a deeper knowledge than ever before; contacts with positive spirit entities such as angels)?
- What challenges exist for you connecting with religious-spiritual resources?
- Where are you at now on your spiritual journey?

CONCLUDING REMARKS

The search for personal meaning in one's traumatic experiences is an existential or spiritual pursuit. The experiences of warfighting place military clients at risk for moral injury, which is an invisible wound that has a profound sense of soul loss or wounding. Openness to integrating religious-spiritual practices in psychotherapy session is vital to practice within a multicultural counseling framework. Exploration of the client's religious-spiritual beliefs, values, and practices opens the door to healing opportunities. Overall, integrating psychospiritual practices assists practitioners in increasing client coping and resiliency skills. Advancing complementary and integrative spiritually based practices inside and outside the therapeutic environment provides other channels for healing complex trauma.

REFERENCES

American Counseling Association. (2006, February 22). *ACA's Taskforce on Counselor Wellness and Impairment*. https://www.counseling.org/news/updates/2006/02/23/aca's-taskforce-on-counselor-wellness-and-impairment

Assagioli, R. (1965). *Psychosynthesis: A manual of principles and techniques*. Viking Press.

Assagioli, R. (1971). *Psychosynthesis*. Viking Press.

Association for Spiritual, Ethical, and Religious Values in Counseling. (n.d.). *ASERVIC white paper*. http://www.aservic.org/resources/aservic-white-paper-2/

Baldwin, L. C. (1995). Spirituality, health, and occupational therapy. In *Conference abstracts and resources* (pp. 165–166). American Occupational Therapy Association.

Benshoff, J. J., & Janikowski, T. P. (1999). *The rehabilitation model of substance abuse counseling*. Brooks-Cole.

Bishop, D. R., Avila-Juarbe, E., & Thumme, B. (2003). Recognizing spirituality as an important factor in counselor supervision. *Counseling and Values, 48*(1), 34–46. https://doi.org/10.1002/j.2161-007X.2003.tb00273.x

Bremault-Phillips, S., Pike, A., Scarcella, F., & Cherwick, T. (2019). Spirituality and moral injury among military personnel: A mini-review. *Frontiers in Psychiatry, 10,* Article 276. https://doi.org/10.3389/fpsyt.2019.00276

Campbell, C. D. (1988). *Coping with hemodialysis: Cognitive appraisals, coping behaviors, spiritual well-being, assertiveness, and family adaptability and cohesion as correlates of adjustment* [Doctoral dissertation, Western Conservative Baptist Seminary]. *Dissertation Abstracts International, 49,* 538B.

Carrola, P., & Corbin-Burdick, M. F. (2015). Counseling military veterans: Advocating for culturally competent and holistic interventions. *Journal of Mental Health Counseling, 37*(1), 1–14. https://doi.org/10.17744/mehc.37.1.v74514163rv73274

Carson, V. B. (1990). *The relationships of spiritual well-being, selected demographic variables, health indicators, and AIDS related activities to hardiness in persons who were serum positive for the human immune deficient virus or were diagnosed with acquired immune deficient syndrome* [Unpublished doctoral dissertation]. University of Maryland, School of Nursing.

Carson, V. B., Soeken, K. L., Shanty, J., & Toms, L. (1990). Hope and spiritual well-being: Essentials for living with AIDS. *Perspectives in Psychiatric Care, 26*(2), 28–34. https://doi.org/10.1111/j.1744-6163.1990.tb00306.x

Cashwell, C. S., & Young, J. S. (2020). *Integrating spirituality and religion into counseling: A guide to competent practice* (3rd ed.). American Counseling Association.

Corey, M. S., & Corey, G. (2021). *Becoming a helper* (8th ed.). Cengage Learning.

Csordas, T. J. (1990). The psychotherapy analogy and charismatic healing. *Psychotherapy: Theory, Research, Practice, Training, 27*(1), 79–90. https://doi.org/10.1037/0033-3204.27.1.79

Currier, J. M., Farnsworth, J. K., Drescher, K. D., McDermott, R. C., Sims, B. M., & Albright, D. L. (2018). Development and evaluation of the Expressions of Moral Injury Scale–Military Version. *Clinical Psychology & Psychotherapy, 25*(3), 474–488. https://doi.org/10.1002/cpp.2170

Currier, J. M., Isaak, S. L., & McDermott, R. C. (2020). Validation of the Expressions of Moral Injury Scale–Military Version–Short Form. *Clinical Psychology & Psychotherapy, 27*(1), 61–68. https://doi.org/10.1002/cpp.2407

Doehring, C. (2015). Resilience as the relational ability to spiritually integrate moral stress. *Pastoral Psychology, 64*(5), 635–649. https://doi.org/10.1007/s11089-015-0643-7

Doehring, C. (2019). Military moral injury: An evidence-based and intercultural approach to spiritual care. *Pastoral Psychology, 68*, 15–30. https://doi.org/10.1007/s11089-018-0813-5

Ellison, C. W., & Smith, J. (1991). Toward an integrative measure of health and well-being. *Journal of Psychology and Theology, 19*(1), 35–48. https://doi.org/10.1177/009164719101900104

Francis, P. C. (2016). Religion and spirituality in counseling. In I. Marini & M. A. Stebnicki (Eds.), *The professional counselor's desk reference* (2nd ed., pp. 559–570). Springer.

Frankfurt, S., & Frazier, P. (2016). A review of research on moral injury in combat veterans. *Military Psychology, 28*(5), 318–330. https://doi.org/10.1037/mil0000132

Frankl, V. (1959). *Man's search for meaning*. Pocket Books.

Goodwin, L. B. (2002). *The button therapy book: A practical psychological self-help book and holistic cognitive counseling manual for mental health professionals*. Trafford.

Graham, K. L. (2017). *Moral injury: Restoring wounded souls*. Abingdon.

Granstrom, S. L. (1987, November). *A comparative study of loneliness, Buberian religiosity, and spiritual well-being in cancer patients* [Paper presentation]. Conference of the National Hospice Organization.

Hayes, S. C. (1984). Making sense of spirituality. *Behaviorism, 12*(2), 99–110.

Heintzman, P. (1999). Spiritual wellness: Theoretical links with leisure. *Journal of Leisurability, 26*(2). http://benefitshub.ca/entry/spiritual-wellness-theoretical-links-with-leisure/

Ingerman, S. (1991). *Soul retrieval: Mending the fragmented self*. HarperSanFrancisco.

Johnson, B. D., Bormann, J. E., & Glaser, D. (2015). Validation of the Functional Assessment Chronic Illness Therapy–Spiritual Well-Being Scale in veterans with PTSD. *Spirituality in Clinical Practice, 2*(1), 35–45. https://doi.org/10.1037/scp0000052

Juhnke, G. A., Watts, R. E., Guerra, N. S., & Hsieh, P. (2009). Using prayer as an intervention with clients who are substance abusing and addicted and who self-identify personal faith in God and prayer as recovery resources. *Journal of Addictions and Offender Counseling, 30*(1), 16–23.

Jung, C. G. (1973). Psychology and religion: East and West. In W. McGuire (Ed. & Trans.) & R. F. C. Hull (Ed. & Trans.), *The collected works of C. G. Jung* (Vol. 11, pp. 5–105). Princeton University Press. (Original work published 1937)

Kaczorowski, J. M. (1989). Spiritual well-being and anxiety in adults diagnosed with cancer. *The Hospice Journal, 5*(3–4), 105–116. https://doi.org/10.1080/0742-969x.1989.11882658

Knobloch, L. K., Owens, J. L., Matheson, L. N., & Dodson, M. B. (2019). Evaluating the effectiveness of REBOOT Combat Recovery: A faith-based combat trauma resiliency program. *Military Psychology, 31*(4), 306–314. https://doi.org/10.1080/08995605.2019.1630228

Koening, H., Ames, D., Youssef, N. A., Oliver, J. P., Volk, F., Teng, E. J., Haynes, K., Erickson, Z. D., Arnold, I., O'Garo, K., & Pearce, M. (2018). Screening for moral injury: The Moral Injury Symptom Scale–Military Version Short Form. *Military Medicine, 183*(11–12), e659–e665. https://doi.org/10.1093/milmed/usy017

Kohlbry, P. W. (1986). *The relationship between spiritual well-being and hope/hopelessness in chronically ill clients* [Unpublished master's thesis]. Marquette University, College of Nursing.

Ledbetter, M. F., Smith, L. A., Vosler-Hunter, W. L., & Fischer, J. D. (1991). An evaluation of the research and clinical usefulness of the Spiritual Well-Being Scale. *Journal of Psychology and Theology, 19*(1), 49–55. https://doi.org/10.1177/009164719101900105

Litz, B. T., Stein, N., Delaney, E., Lebowitz, L., Nash, W. P., Silva, C., & Maguen, S. (2009). Moral injury and moral repair of war veterans: A preliminary model and intervention strategy. *Clinical Psychology Review, 29*(8), 695–706. https://doi.org/10.1016/j.cpr.2009.07.003

Malinakova, K., Kopcakova, J., Kolarcik, P., Geckova, A. M., Solcova, I. P., Husek, V., Kracmarova, L. K., Dubovska, E., Kalman, M., Puzova, Z., van Dijk, J. P., & Tavel, P. (2017). The Spiritual Well-Being Scale: Psychometric evaluation of the shortened version in Czech adolescents. *Journal of Religious Health, 56*(2), 697–705. https://doi.org/10.1007/s10943-016-0318-4

Miller, G. (2003). *Incorporating spirituality in counseling and psychotherapy: Theory and technique.* Wiley.

Moodley, R., & West, W. (2005). *Integrating traditional healing practices into counseling and psychotherapy.* Sage.

Myers, J. E., & Sweeney, T. J. (2008). Wellness counseling: The evidence base for practice. *Journal of Counseling & Development, 86*(4), 482–493. https://doi.org/10.1002/j.1556-6678.2008.tb00536.x

Myers, J. E., Sweeney, T. J., & Witmer, J. M. (2000). The Wheel of Wellness counseling for wellness: A holistic model for treatment planning. *Journal of Counseling & Development, 78*(3), 251–266. https://doi.org/10.1002/j.1556-6676.2000.tb01906.x

Myers, J. E., & Williard, K. (2003). Integrating spirituality into counselor preparation: A developmental wellness approach. *Counseling and Values, 47*(2), 142–155. https://doi.org/10.1002/j.2161-007X.2003.tb00231.x

Paloutzian, R. F., & Ellison, C. W. (1982). Loneliness, spiritual well-being, and the quality of life. In L. A. Peplau & D. Perlman (Eds.), *Loneliness: A sourcebook of current theory, research, and therapy* (pp. 224–237). Wiley.

Pargament, K. L., & Zinnbauer, B. J. (2000). Working with the sacred: Four approaches to religious and spiritual issues in counseling. *Journal of Counseling & Development, 78*(2), 162–171. https://doi.org/10.1002/j.1556-6676.2000.tb02574.x

Parker, M. W., Fuller, G. F., Koenig, H. G., Vaitkus, M. A., Bellis, J. M., Barko, W. F., Eitzen, J., & Call, V. R. (2001). Soldier and family wellness across the life course: A developmental model of successful aging, spirituality, and health promotion. *Military Medicine, 166*(6), 485–489.

Polanski, P. J. (2003). Spirituality and supervision. *Counseling and Values, 47*(2), 131–141. https://doi.org/10.1002/j.2161-007X.2003.tb00230.x

Ramsay, N. J. (2019). Moral injury as loss and grief with attention to ritual resources for care. *Pastoral Psychology, 68*(8), 107–125. https://doi.org/10.1007/s11089-018-0854-9

Richards, P. S., & Bergin, A. E. (1997). *A spiritual strategy for counseling and psychotherapy.* American Psychological Association.

Richter, R. J. (2002). Correlation of psychological well-being and Christian spiritual well-being at a small Christian liberal arts college in the urban Midwest. *CHARIS, 2*(1), 39–46.

Riley, B. B., Perna, R., Tate, D. G., Forchheimer, M., Anderson, C., & Luera, G. (1998). Types of spiritual well-being among persons with chronic illness: Their relation to various forms of quality of life. *Archives of Physical Medicine & Rehabilitation, 79*(3), 258–264. https://doi.org/10.1016/s0003-9993(98)90004-1

Robertson, H. C. (2016). Spirituality, substance use, and the military. *VISTAS Online,* Article 95. https://www.counseling.org/docs/default-source/vistas/spirituality-substance-use-and-the-military.pdf?sfvrsn=821d4a2c_4

Shafranske, E. P., & Gorsuch, R. L. (1984). Factors associated with the perception of spirituality in psychotherapy. *Journal of Transpersonal Psychology, 16*(2), 231–241.

Shafranske, E. P., & Malony, H. N. (1990). Clinical psychologists' religious and spiritual orientations and their practice of psychotherapy. *Psychotherapy, 27*(1), 72–78. https://doi.org/10.1037/0033-3204.27.1.72

Shafranske, E. P., & Malony, H. N. (1996). Religion and the clinical practice of psychology: The case for inclusion. In E. P. Shafranske (Ed.), *Religion and the clinical practice of psychology: A case for inclusion* (pp. 561–586). American Psychological Association.

Shannonhouse, L. R., Myers, J. E., & Sweeney, T. J. (2016). Counseling for wellness. In I. Marini & M. A. Stebnicki (Eds.), *The professional counselor's desk reference* (2nd ed., pp. 617–623). Springer.

Shay, J. (1991). Learning about combat stress from Homer's *Iliad. Journal of Traumatic Stress, 4*(4), 561–579. https://doi.org/10.1002/jts.2490040409

Shay, J. (2012). Moral injury. *Intertexts, 16*(1), 57–66.

Shay, J. (2014). Moral injury. *Psychoanalytic Psychology, 31*(2), 189–191.

Smith-MacDonald, L., Norris, J. M., Raffin-Bouchal, S., & Sinclair, S. (2017). Spirituality and mental well-being in combat veterans: A systematic review. *Military Medicine, 182*(11–12), e1920–e1940. https://doi.org/10.7205/MILMED-D-17-00099

Stebnicki, M. A. (2006). Integrating spirituality in rehabilitation counselor supervision. *Rehabilitation Education, 20*(2), 115–132. https://doi.org/10.1891/088970106805074494

Stebnicki, M. A. (2008). *Empathy fatigue: Healing the mind, body, and spirit of professional counselors.* Springer.

Stebnicki, M. A. (2016a). From empathy fatigue to empathy resilience. In I. Marini & M. A. Stebnicki (Eds.), *The professional counselor's desk reference* (2nd ed., pp. 533–545). Springer.

Stebnicki, M. A. (2016b). Integrative approaches in counseling and psychotherapy. In I. Marini & M. A. Stebnicki (Eds.), *The professional counselor's desk reference* (2nd ed., pp. 593–604). Springer.

Stebnicki, M. A., & Cubero, C. (2008). A content analysis of multicultural counseling syllabi from rehabilitation counseling programs. *Rehabilitation Education, 22*(2), 89–99. https://doi.org/10.1891/088970108805059444

Sterner, W. R., & Jackson-Cherry, L. R. (2015). The influence of spirituality and religion on coping for combat-deployed military personnel. *Counseling and Values, 60*(1), 48–66. https://doi.org/10.1002/j.2161-007X.2015.00060.x

Thomas, K. H., McDaniel, J. T., Albright, D. L., Fletcher, K. L., & Koenig, H. G. (2018). Spiritual fitness for military veterans: A curriculum review and impact evaluation using the Duke Religion Index (DUREL). *Journal of Religion and Health, 57*(3), 1168–1178. https://doi.org/10.1007/s10943-018-0597-z

Tick, E. (2014). *The warrior's return: Restoring the soul after war.* Sounds True.

Tillich, P. (1952). *The courage to be.* Yale University Press.

U.S. Army. (2014, June 19). *Army Regulation 350–53: Training: Comprehensive Soldier and Family Fitness.* https://readyandresilient.army.mil/CSF2/supportdocs/r350_53.pdf

Vaughan, F. (1991). Spiritual issues in psychotherapy. *Journal of Transpersonal Psychology, 23*(2), 105–119.

Watson, P. J., Morris, R. J., & Hood, R. W. (1990). Intrinsicness, self-actualization, and the ideological surround. *Journal of Psychology and Theology, 18*(1), 40–53. https://doi.org/10.1177/009164719001800104

Worthington, E. L. (1988). Understanding the values of religious clients: A model and its application to counseling. *Journal of Counseling Psychology, 35*(2), 166–174. https://doi.org/10.1037/0022-0167.35.2.166

Worthington, E. L. (1989). Religious faith across the life span: Implications for counseling and research. *The Counseling Psychologist, 17*(4), 555–612. https://doi.org/10.1177/0011000089174001

Wortmann, J. H., Eisen, E., Hundert, C., Jordan, A. H., Smith, M. W., Nash, W. P., & Litz, B. T. (2017). Spiritual features of war-related moral injury: A primer for clinicians. *Spirituality in Clinical Practice, 4*(4), 249–261. https://doi.org/10.1037/scp0000140

Young, J. S., & Cashwell, C. S. (2020). Integrating spirituality and religion into counseling: Introduction. In C. S. Caswell & J. S. Young (Eds.), *Integrating spirituality and religion into counseling: A guide to competent practice* (3rd ed., pp. 3–29). American Counseling Association.

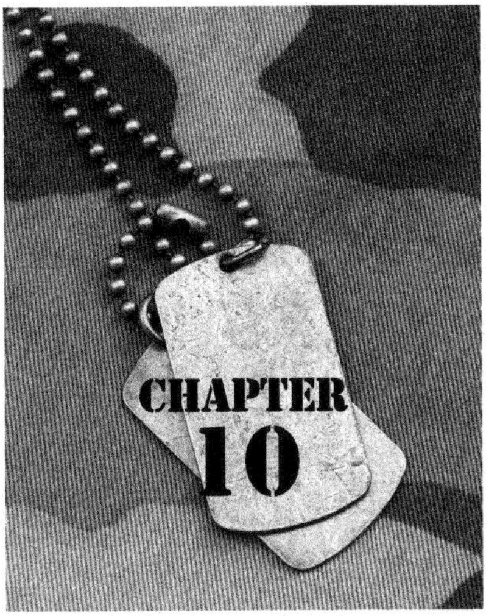

MILITARY FAMILIES AND THE DEPLOYMENT CYCLE

Grief and loss are mutually shared across all cultures and experienced by nearly all individuals over one's lifetime.

—Mark A. Stebnicki,
The Professional Counselor's Desk Reference (2nd ed.)

★ ★ ★

Since September 11, 2001, more than 2.5 million troops have been deployed in support of Operation Iraqi Freedom, Operation Enduring Freedom, Operation Inherent Resolve, and other operations around the globe to fight the war on terrorism. Many service members have successfully transitioned and reintegrated back to civilian life with their families. Yet, some service members have not because of a combination of severe physical and psychological injuries. The research and guidelines for practice in *Clinical Military Counseling* have primarily centered on the individual service member or veteran. However, in this chapter, I explore the impact that military life has on families, and I advocate for the integration of family members as a natural support system within the therapeutic process. I also discuss the unique psychosocial grief and trauma experienced by spouses, children, and parents of service members throughout the deployment cycle.

Military family members also serve but in a different capacity. This message is communicated throughout the month of November, which is considered Military Family Appreciation Month. The literature related to military families has only recently become a focus of attention. Historically, issues related to military families have been neglected. Moreover, there are deficiencies in therapeutic programs and services offered by the military, other than an occasional support group and the Family Readiness Officer on base. Building therapeutic relationships with military families is an important value of the healing process for service members and veterans. Other topics examined in this chapter relate to military families' communication, intimacy, healthy attachment, coping, and resiliency skills. Innovative programs and services are also explored, demonstrating the benefits of partnering with school systems and community-based mental health providers to assist therapeutically with military spouses as well as children and adolescents.

MILITARY FAMILIES IN THE NEW DECADE

In 2017, there were 2,103,415 military personnel enlisted in active duty and the selected reserves as well as 2,667,909 military family members, which includes spouses, children, and adult dependents (U.S. Department of Defense, 2017). During this reporting period, 44.6% of military personnel were single with no children, 33.6% were married with children, 15.8% were married without children, and 6.0% were single with children. Thus, military families are a key demographic group for whom military counselors can provide programs and services that enhance the quality of their life.

The changing demographics and focus on mental health within military families appear much different in the new decade than observed in previous wars. One example that underscores this point is the recognition of same-sex marriages among active-duty personnel. Lesbian and gay military spouses are now eligible for TRICARE health care benefits and a military spouse identification card; in addition, they can register in the Defense Enrollment Eligibility Reporting System (https://www.tricare.mil/DEERS), which enrolls military spouses in a database to qualify them for multiple military benefits. Moreover, with the use of social media and networking, several online support groups are available where military spouses can receive psychoeducation as well as social and emotional support.

PSYCHOSOCIAL STRESSORS IN THE MILITARY FAMILY SYSTEM

The psychosocial issues challenging military families are much different than civilian families. Most family system models are based on theories, research, and practices of nonmilitary families. Riggs and

Riggs (2018) have presented a family attachment network model that depicts the multiple family system issues and psychological stressors related to military families. This elegant model illustrates the role of healthy family attachment and psychological functioning throughout the deployment cycle. Because of much longer and more frequent deployments than in past wars, less time is available for healthy family attachment to take place. Viewing one's family of origin, parenting styles, and marital relationship is a beginning point that can affect healthy attachment, coping, and dealing with the multiple psychosocial stressors that ultimately affect military children and adolescents.

Historically, multiple other family system models (nonmilitary families) have depicted healthy-unhealthy family dynamics. However, military families attach, bond, communicate, and cope differently than civilian families because of the psychosocial stressors related to military life. Military families who have received couples counseling and psychotherapy services from me tend to have a close social network of other military spouses and family members. These families live in military base housing or in towns near the base. Thus, a natural support network is present when living in a military town. Many spouses feel a certain pride because they are part of an "extended family" who understands their experiences. However, within-group differences sometimes occur between enlisted and officer-rank spouses. For example, being the wife of a Marine officer carries a different level of status and responsibility within the military. There are expectations of spousal involvement in officer wives' clubs, volunteering with military organizations, planning homecoming celebrations, engaging in fundraisers, and other activities. Girlfriends, boyfriends, and partners of enlisted individuals have a much different experience than officer families and are generally not recognized by the command structure. This lack of recognition is due in part to the ambiguous, intimate, legal, and temporary nature of these relationships.

Competent clinical military counselors understand these dynamics and the within-group differences in the military community. For instance, military husbands and wives who are lesbian or gay or who have bisexual partners have a much different experience than traditional military families who are primarily composed of marriages between men and women. Within-group differences also exist between families who have children and those who do not. The social activities reflect this dynamic. Service personnel who are not married and single make up another group that may not be well connected to the traditional military family.

Single individuals in the military have postdeployment difficulties that differ from those of married military couples. This dissimilarity is particularly the case for younger enlisted personnel for whom healthy social and intimate relationships can be complicated because of developmental, social, emotional, and psychological issues. Younger personnel generally have higher risk behaviors than older service members (e.g., substance abuse, exposure to sexually transmitted diseases, risky recreational activities). There are also unresolved, untreated, or undertreated mental health conditions that are not addressed throughout the deployment cycle. Overall, individuals and families in the military can have multiple difficulties adjusting to military life. Thus, if therapeutic interventions are not pursued by military families themselves, or if the military provider system does not reach out to families, then these conflicts may be accentuated and carried through reintegration and transition from active duty to civilian life.

Families associated with the National Guard and reserve components of the military have unique psychosocial stressors that are different than those of active-duty personnel who are attached to military installations. Members of the reserve component are usually indoctrinated through an initial boot camp yet are employed with a civilian job in their hometown community. They, on average, are immersed within the military culture for 2 weeks out of the year and 1 weekend per month for training exercises, but they do not report to a duty station like active-duty service personnel. The exception to this schedule was during Operation Enduring Freedom and Operation Iraqi Freedom, in which the reserve component was called up to active duty and accounted for about 40% of personnel who deployed in support of combat operations (Tanielian & Jaycox, 2008).

For reservists and their family members, the day-to-day military operations, organizational structure, and disciplines are not part of their daily lives. However, ambiguity can occur for some reservist families when the spouse is on a long-term deployment. Oftentimes reservist and National Guard families do not live in a military community or are not attached to a military installation. These families typically immerse themselves in civilian careers, schools, and social activities. Consequently, some reservist and National Guard families may feel isolated and detached from the military culture itself (Clever & Segal, 2013; Huebner, 2019). Little social support is offered from the extended military family, and some do not have access to many of the health care benefits and natural resources that are provided in a military town.

The psychosocial aspects of families attached to the reserve and National Guard components place such families at high risk for several psychosocial problems. Generally, U.S. Army and U.S. Marine reservists have higher levels of combat deployments than active-duty personnel, which can result in a higher frequency of posttraumatic stress disorder, depression, and substance use disorders (Lane et al., 2012). Reservists generally deploy as individual augmentees in support of a combat unit that differs from their initial enlistment unit. Consequently, those reservists tend to be at high risk for substance use, posttraumatic stress disorder, and depression (Cohen et al., 2015; Ursano et al., 2018), which all increase the risk for suicidal ideation, lethal attempts, or completions. Additionally, reserve personnel typically have minimal preparation for their mission and have a higher incidence of mental health problems. Overall, the lack of training for a combat deployment affects the psychosocial health of military families attached to the reserve and National Guard components.

One psychosocial issue besides deployment that clearly creates conflict among active-duty families is when they have a permanent change of duty station (PCS) and are duty bound to another geographic location. High levels of psychosocial stress occur with families who have frequent PCSs. Significant challenges in adjusting to new situations involve new housing, schools, day care, and climates; geographic separation from family and friends as well as other support networks can also be difficult. Most military spouses have little or no input regarding geographic relocation. Changes in duty station are primarily because the service member's military occupational specialty is needed for a specific geographic location or mission inside or outside the United States. Other reasons for a PCS relate to job promotions or demotions, personal requests to be near other family members or to live in a specific climate or geographic location, or motivation for overseas travel to a foreign country. One resiliency advantage that active-duty family members have during a PCS is the natural support network of other military families that serves as a protective mechanism.

In military families, deployment of a spouse may be considered a significant loss of an intact support system, causing feelings of loneliness, isolation, and withdrawal to prevail. Financial strains, role shifts, and single-parenting overload have consequences for military children and adolescents. Anger toward the deployed spouse increases, which can precipitate significant clinical symptoms of depression, anxiety, and substance use disorders (Basham, 2013; Mailey et al., 2019; Ysasi et al., 2016). The residual impact of mental health conditions increases and becomes volatile when the deployed spouse returns home with a serious physical or psychological condition. Overall, the psychosocial stressor associated with family separation, prolonged deployment, and long-standing or preexisting family conflicts is a major concern for the military community.

One of the most significant stressors experienced by military families is when a service member is killed or is missing in action. The pain and suffering felt by military spouses and dependent children can be debilitating. A profound sense of grief and loss is also experienced by the deceased service member's parents, siblings, and significant others. The psychological nature of a combat or violent death becomes more persistent and complex in terms of how military family members grieve the loss (Stebnicki, 2018). This death event is much different than a prolonged illness in which the death is anticipated.

The U.S. Armed Forces recognize that no families have given more to their nation than those of service members who have died on the battlefield. These military families are honored and recognized by the designation of a *Gold Star family* (http://goldstarfamilies.com/), which describes a family member who has lost a loved one in military service. It is a recognition of the family's loss and implies that their loved one served with honor, commitment, and sacrifice. The United States began observing Gold Star Mother's Day in 1936, then Gold Star Wives in 1947, but it has now expanded this distinction of honor to all military family members. During a ceremony, family members are issued a Gold Star lapel pin that has a purple background surrounded by a gold wreath. These ceremonies assist in supporting and connecting spouses and family members with other Gold Star families. The Gold Star recognition serves as a good beginning on the healing journey for military families. It helps define the family's identity and brings some degree of meaning to honor their loved one's military service.

Another organization that honors and supports military families is Blue Star Families (https://bluestarfam.org/research-policy/). Founded by military spouses in 2009, this organization empowers military families with resources and support by connecting them with other civilian and military support systems. One unique goal of Blue Star Families is the mission of developing research projects; it also produces an annual comprehensive report titled "Military Family Life Survey." The results of this large-scale survey provide insights, solutions, and empirically based recommendations that affect policies and improve relations with partnering civilian organizations.

Indeed, the military family system experiences multiple psychological risk factors and stressors throughout the deployment cycle. Stressors that most frequently occur have been identified as family and marital conflict, unhealthy patterns of communication, financial problems, intimate partner violence, verbal and physical abuse toward children, and adjustment issues related to frequent geographic relocation (Institute of Medicine, 2008; Miller & Warner, 2013; Ysasi et al., 2016). At the center of this storm is the military spouse, typically a woman, who takes on most or all child care responsibilities, organizing and operating domestic tasks (e.g., finances, cleaning, meal preparation, grocery shopping, home repairs) while balancing their own educational and career goals.

Many male active-duty service members who return home from deployment and are seen in my practice do not know where they fit in with the family regarding child care duties or daily household tasks. Anecdotal evidence suggests that military spouses are independent and organized, and they may have difficulties in delegating roles and responsibilities to the active-duty service member returning home from deployment. The spouse has been operational for 9–12 months to maintain a functional household system while the service member has been deployed. This organization is typically not communicated in a healthy manner, so family and relational conflict arises.

Military family researchers and practitioners have suggested that many military spouses "walk on eggshells" in the postdeployment phase waiting to see whether behavioral, personality, or psychological changes have occurred as a result of their spouses' deployment. This behavior is another indication of an unhealthy family dynamic. In response, the service member may go out to bars and binge drink with their unit buddies, particularly after a combat deployment. They cannot talk to their spouse or children about what they experienced overseas. Thus, the real debriefing takes place with these rituals that usually commence after the homecoming. However, engaging in these types of high-risk behaviors and activities can be unhealthy and potentially has consequences for the service member's military career. Thus, unhealthy communication and the sequence of maladaptive adjustment or readjustment in military families can occur throughout various phases of deployment.

Overall, resiliency is vital in all phases of military family life. Multiple challenges are related to the deployment cycle in terms of the physical and mental health of each family member. Thus, support is essential to sustain optimal health and well-being.

MILITARY CHILDREN AND ADOLESCENTS

Much of the research on military families has focused on the chronic and unhealthy mental health patterns of service members or veterans, deficits and family system dysfunction, and other unhealthy traits. These poor outcomes have particularly been noted in research relating to military children (Easterbrooks et al., 2013). Currently, there are approximately 5,250 children of military service members killed in action, which creates a high-risk situation within the family dynamics (see the Gary Sinise Foundation Snowball Express initiative: https://www.garysinisefoundation.org/snowball-express/). This special group of children may need more intensive professional therapeutic services. The literature relating to the utilization of mental health services among military children and adolescents indicates that a much greater level of care is required (Cramm et al., 2019).

Research from a large population study of children and adolescents revealed an increase in psychiatric hospitalizations and emergency department visits among adolescents in military families (Millegan et al., 2014). All the psychosocial stressors associated with deployment (e.g., prolonged separation, family members' thoughts of injury or death of the service member, frequent geographic relocations) also affect children's and adolescents' well-being but on a different level. For instance, children of service members killed in action may be retraumatized by media reports of improvised explosive device attacks and combat casualties. Children of deployed active-duty service members may have the same emotional reaction not knowing whether their mom or dad has been injured or has died overseas. Some children and adolescents may be confused by media outlets that reflect antiwar sentiments or the politics of war and global terrorism (National Child Traumatic Stress Network, 2008).

Children and adolescents who have a parent transitioning from active duty to civilian life may feel isolated, detached, and challenged by their new neighborhood, school, and surrounding community. This transition is particularly difficult for children and adolescents who previously attended a military base school. However, some researchers have suggested that new beginnings have the potential to spark resiliency in children. Better emotional stability occurs when family members—rather than the commandant—choose a new geographic location or have a more permanent house, town, or school. Some populations of children and adolescents are also more vulnerable, such as the 220,000 active-duty and reservist family members with special physical, developmental, neurocognitive, educational, and mental health needs (Aronson et al., 2016). The U.S. Department of Defense has the Exceptional Family Member Program, which provides services to families who have children with special health and educational needs. Approximately 128,000 military family members are enrolled in this program and receive such benefits (Lester & Flake, 2013).

In a RAND Corporation study, Richardson et al. (2011) examined a large sample ($N = 44{,}000$) of U.S. Army active-duty, reservist, and National Guard soldiers and their school-age children to assess the effects and behavioral health associated with parental deployment, academic performance, and use of support systems. This study provided recommendations with the primary intention of safeguarding military children's emotional and academic needs. The following results were reported: (a) children whose parents were deployed 19 months or more since 2001 had only modestly lower achievement scores compared with those who experienced fewer or no parental deployments; (b) the number of parental deployments was not associated with academic performance accounting for the cumulative months of deployment; (c) longer cumulative parental deployments were associated with lower test scores among elementary and middle school children but were not statistically significant among high school adolescents; and (d) no statistically significant differences were found in academic performance by length of deployment, rank, seniority, gender of parent deployed, or gender of child. These researchers suggested that academic performance issues are related to 19 or more cumulative months of parent deployment. Thus, children have decreased academic and behavioral health resiliency during longer parental deployments. Indeed, many military families struggle with homework completion, test grades, motivation, as well as mood and emotional regulation when one parent is absent from the home for longer periods of time because of deployment.

TALKING WITH CHILDREN AND ADOLESCENTS ABOUT MILITARY LIFE

Regardless of the child's age, threats of war and terrorism can provoke much anxiety and stress. The impact on children and adolescents especially becomes intensified when they sense high levels of anxiety and stress among adults, such as parents, family members, and teachers. Many military children and adolescents may require some parental interventions that include calming, protection, holding, and hugging as well as an outlet to provide an open, honest expression of the child's fears and anxiety. It is important to remember that children's and adolescents' physical, cognitive, mental, and emotional reactions will differ depending on age. Adults should only discuss issues of terrorism and war at the child's or adolescent's level of understanding and comfort. Children and adolescents most affected by fears of terrorism and war will likely be those who have family members deployed to hostile areas. The dynamics within this special group will require the clinical military counselor to provide more intensive therapeutic support to help family members cope with the issues associated with marital distress, separation, divorce, and the possible loss of a parent.

Children and adolescents affected by the events of war and terrorism on a long-term basis may exhibit one or more of the following reactions:

- Recurring thoughts and emotions of incidents of their parent becoming injured or killed;
- Difficulty concentrating and maintaining focus with important daily routines such as school or extracurricular and recreational activities;
- Persistent negative feelings that may be intense or unpredictable;
- Difficulty expressing their emotions to others regarding their active-duty parent;
- Irrational fears of regular everyday routines, not wanting to leave the house, or isolation;
- Decreasing or ceasing typical or daily routines;
- Feelings of being left behind or that the parent loves their job more than family;
- Feelings of a sense of loss or chronic sadness;
- Strained interpersonal relationships and more frequent arguments with family members, such as parents or siblings;
- Changes in personality, attitudes, or behavior, such as crying, anger, frustration, externalized hostility, denial of the deployment separation, or constant negativity;

- Physical symptoms of dizziness, diarrhea, constipation, headaches, loss of appetite, restlessness, fatigue, wake-sleep disturbances, or bad dreams;
- Exacerbation of a preexisting health-related condition because of military life; and
- Increased use or abuse of tobacco, alcohol, and other addictive substances.

If these symptoms persist for more than 1 month, they may be emotional and psychological indicators that the child or adolescent should seek help from a mental health professional who specializes in military family issues.

Overall, children and adolescents have multiple mental and behavioral concerns within the military family structure. For many military families, the deployment cycle becomes the source for issues that include, but are not limited to, academic and behavioral problems at school; sleep and appetite disturbances; increased levels of stress, anxiety, and depression; increased risk behaviors related to substance misuse, physical confrontations, low impulse control, or anger management issues; and other behaviors that are potentially harmful to self and others.

THE DEPLOYMENT CYCLE

In military families, balancing family with work or career has always been a struggle. Many families live in a heightened state of stress because they understand the high-risk nature of the military as an occupation and lifestyle (Cramm et al., 2019). Deployment can create a threat to the safety and security all family members. Researchers have suggested that military spouses with a history of dependency, rejection, or enabling relationships may feel unwanted or manipulated by the spouse who leaves on deployment. This reaction is particularly the case with spouses who have had a relationship history with authoritarian or attachment figures. Deployment for some spouses is misinterpreted in an unhealthy manner by believing that their spouse "loves their job more than me." This feeling speaks clearly to the irrational fear-based and anxiety-provoking experience of deployment separations and articulates the spouse's level of adaptive-maladaptive coping and resiliency skills. These skills, as they relate to the deployment cycle, are critical because healthy adaptive coping strategies are essential for maintaining good psychological health and well-being and allowing each family member to fulfill their roles and responsibilities.

Adler and Castro (2013) have emphasized the concept of the "mission first" objective in the military culture. Implicit in this concept is an understanding that service members are expected to place themselves in harm's way, sacrifice their personal mental and physical well-being, and do whatever it takes to complete the mission. The consequences are serious for those service members who do not follow orders given by the military hierarchy of officer and non-commissioned officer ranks. In addition, within the cultural context of the military, teamwork is essential (e.g., watching your unit buddies' "6"), and failure is not an option under any circumstance. For some service members, unit buddies become closer than their biological family or spouse. Therefore, because the military is an occupation that demands so much mentally, physically, emotionally, and socially, it is not clear where the service member's family fits within the military system.

Models depicting the deployment cycle assist practitioners to predict and anticipate the physical, psychological, emotional, psychosocial, and familial reactions to deployment. Deployment is frequently a source of stress that is on a continuum of low, moderate, or high psychological and emotional difficulty. Deployment is a significant life event within the lives of military families that requires adaptation, adjustment, and multiple coping resources (Basham, 2013; Pincus et al., 2020). Deployments can occur in the continental United States or anywhere globally overseas. Some military personnel are mobilized for humanitarian missions, whereas others are deployed in support of combat operations. Service members deployed in the combat theater may be located on a joint-operations base down range, a forward operating base, or a rear base.

Models describing the deployment cycle have slight variations and interpretations. Most models describe five separate phases: predeployment, deployment, sustainment, postdeployment, and reintegration. Competent clinical military counselors understand the unique challenges for military personnel and their family members within the deployment cycle. Theoretically, successful transition through each phase requires multiple support systems as well as coping and resiliency resources that are both internal and external. Deployment cycle models apply to both the service member and their family. Overall, the deployment cycle model is beneficial for clinicians because it can assist them to (a) anticipate and predict significant mental health symptoms typically associated with each phase of deployment; (b) acknowledge, analyze, and coordinate multiple resources and psychoeducational materials beneficial for military service members and their families; and (c) coordinate community providers who have clinical expertise to assist military families with resources and therapeutic interventions (Center for Deployment Psychology, n.d.; Military One Source, n.d.; RAND Corporation, 2018; Rotter & Boveja, 1999; U.S. Department of Veterans Affairs, n.d.). The following brief description summarizes unique characteristics within the deployment cycle:

- *Predeployment:* The service member will receive a "warning order" for deployment in which they will leave their state-side base or duty station or be ordered to a PCS. Deployments can vary depending on the mission from 3 to 15 months. Unique characteristics with this stage include (a) the anticipation of family separation or denial of risks involved with jeopardizing their life, health, or safety; (b) training, becoming highly motivated for combat, and engaging in intense exercises; (c) getting all affairs in order; (d) mental or physical distancing from family, spouse or partner, and loved ones; and (e) decreased communication and intimacy with spouse or partner and emotional insulation from family members in preparation for deployment.

- *Deployment:* This stage can last up to a month, in which military spouses or partners report feelings of abandonment with a major life shift in all household and family responsibilities. Unique characteristics with this stage include (a) mixed emotions of anxiety, depression, and relief; (b) feelings of being disoriented and overwhelmed; (c) an emotional sense of loneliness, sadness, numbness, detachment, and isolation; (d) sleep disturbances; and (e) eventually feeling secure in the new environment.
- *Sustainment:* This stage can last between 2 and 5 months. It is marked by a period of establishing new resources for support with a heavy reliance on the Family Readiness Officer. This officer is typically a civilian spouse of an active-duty service member who serves in a professional capacity as a liaison and the primary coordinator of activities, events, and communications from the command on the progress of the mission. As challenges arise, spouses or partners and family members realize that they have developed some coping resources. Life is somewhat back to balance again but in a new and different way.
- *Postdeployment:* This stage is marked by the intense anticipation of a "homecoming" and the spouse's or partner's thoughts of whether the service member will be the same mentally, physically, and psychologically as before deployment. Exact return dates from deployment can vary from weeks to months, making things intense and frustrating for family members. Some military units go through 1–2 weeks of debriefing before going back to their home station or base. The psychological stress debriefings, physical examinations, and other activities are to prepare the service member to reintegrate into the mix of military-civilian life. Some postdeployment programs include spouses or partners in therapeutic, educational, and informational activities.
- *Reintegration:* Time frames for this stage are variable depending on family coping skills and resiliency traits. It is common that many military personnel desire their own space and can only handle short periods of family time and togetherness; they also may not feel any level of intimacy toward their spouse or partner. Many bases will require follow-up support services for the service member, such as mental and medical health appointments, command briefings and debriefings, family readjustment

activities, as well as other programs and services to assist with reintegration.

In the deployment cycle, military families and service members are challenged with reevaluating family roles, responsibilities, expectations, and level of parental involvement as well as dealing with any physical or psychological consequences of deployment.

BUILDING MILITARY FAMILY COPING RESILIENCY

Healthy military families within the deployment cycle demonstrate flexibility in adapting to new challenges by exhibiting an increase in the quality of respect, empathy, authentic communication, and collaboration of problem-solving strategies. These core principles from multiple studies relate to family coping and resiliency within the deployment cycle (Blue Star Families, 2013; Hammer et al., 2006; Hayden et al., 2017; Riggs & Riggs, 2018; Rotter & Boveja, 1999; U.S. Department of Veterans Affairs, 2020; Walsh, 2006; Ysasi et al., 2016). One of the first longitudinal studies designed to determine the impact of deployment on military families—the Deployment Life Study (Meadows et al., 2016)—was developed to assist U.S. Department of Defense policy makers and service providers to prepare service members and families for deployment. The Deployment Life Study evaluated outcomes related to the quality of marital and parental relationships, the psychological and physical health of family members, children's well-being, and military reintegration. This report provides a comprehensive list of recommendations that explore issues and challenges of military families. Key findings list predictive factors—such as marital separation, communication problems, parental conflicts, high-risk behaviors, and veteran homelessness—that hinder family resiliency.

The following section is not an all-inclusive guide to military family coping and resiliency. Unique issues related to each section of the deployment cycle go beyond the scope of this chapter. However, the handbooks and other materials in the reference section offer comprehensive guidelines for both families and therapists that can be facilitated as relatable kitchen-table wisdom. The following guidelines are offered for clinicians to consider and will require a deeper inquiry:

- Interpret deployment cycle characteristics for clients so that they may anticipate the expected and unexpected consequences of separation and homecoming. Providing families with psychoeducational materials at the level that they are most comfortable with can reduce clinically significant symptoms of anxiety, depression, substance misuse, or other harmful behavioral lifestyle habits.

- Apply functional assessments and screening tools for service members and families to assist in identifying any risk behaviors within the deployment cycle. Support the use of complementary and integrative therapeutic strategies to advocate for the family's unique cultural values and beliefs in healing (e.g., spiritual and religious practices, family bonding experiences such as camping or vacations, supportive social and extended family networks).
- Recognize, identify, interpret, and share (RIIS) with military families the unique patterns of adaptive-maladaptive behaviors; effective-noneffective communication; levels of intimacy-no intimacy; and other thoughts, feelings, and behaviors that can enhance good mental health and well-being.
- Teach internal and external coping and resiliency skills to service members and their families with the intention of having them RIIS healthy styles of communication while increasing protective factors that enhance good mental health functioning.
- RIIS the unique aspects and mental health needs of children and adolescents within military families. Facilitate natural supports that advocate inclusion and integration of all family members and their considerations in any therapeutic approaches (e.g., parents of service members, extended military family members).
- Coordinate care with teachers, school counselors, community providers, and other military family connections who can provide healthy synergistic support for successful integration and reintegration throughout the deployment cycle.

CONCLUDING REMARKS

Military family members also serve, just in a different capacity. This message is communicated throughout the month of November, which is considered Military Family Appreciation Month. In this chapter, I explored the considerable impact that military life has on families. The materials and resources provided advocate for the integration of all family members as a natural support system within the therapeutic process. Military families have multiple challenges within the deployment cycle to bring meaning and support of an occupation that demands a high level of commitment while balancing family needs. Clinical military counselors need to be attuned to unique psychosocial stressors that include, but are not limited to, the grief and trauma experienced by military service members while deployed; the impact that military trauma has on service members' spouses, children, and parents; and the necessary coping and resiliency skills that can be facilitated and integrated within the total family values.

REFERENCES

Adler, A. B., & Castro, C. A. (2013). An occupational mental health model for the military. *Military Behavioral Health, 1*(1), 41–51. https://doi.org/10.1080/21635781.2012.721063

Aronson, K. R., Kyler, S. J., Moeller, J. D., & Perkins, D. F. (2016). Understanding military families who have dependents with special health care and/or educational needs. *Disability and Health Journal, 9*(3), 423–430. https://doi.org/10.1016/j.dhjo.2016.03.002

Basham, K. K. (2013). Facilitators and barriers in effective clinical practice with postdeployed military couples and families. *Military Behavioral Health, 1*(1), 22–30. https://doi.org/10.1080/21635781.2012.721061

Blue Star Families. (2013). *Everyone serves: A handbook for family and friends of service members during pre-deployment, deployment, and reintegration.* https://everyoneservesbook.com/downloads/EveryoneServes.pdf

Center for Deployment Psychology. (n.d.). *Military family resources.* https://deploymentpsych.org/MilFam-Resources

Clever, M., & Segal, D. R. (2013). The demographics of military children and families. *The Future of Children, 23*(2), 13–39. https://doi.org/10.1353/foc.2013.0018

Cohen, G. H., Fink, D. S., Sampson, L., & Galea, S. (2015). Mental health among reserve component military service members and veterans. *Epidemiologic Reviews, 37*(1), 7–22. https://doi.org/10.1093/epirev/mxu007

Cramm, H., McColl, M. A., Aiken, A. B., & Williams, A. (2019). The mental health of military-connected children: A scoping review. *Journal of Child and Family Studies, 28,* 1725–1735. https://doi.org/10.1007/s10826-019-01402-y

Easterbrooks, M. A., Ginsburg, K., & Lerner, R. M. (2013). Resiliency among military youth. *The Future of Children, 23*(2), 99–120. https://www.jstor.org/stable/23595622

Hammer, L. B., Cullen, J. C., Marchand, G. C., & Dezsofi, J. A. (2006). Reducing the negative impact of work-family conflict on military personnel: Individual coping strategies and multilevel interventions. In T. W. Britt (Ed.), *Military life: The psychology of service in peace and combat: Vol. 3. The military family* (pp. 220–242). Praeger.

Hayden, S. E. W., Glosoff, H., Lopez-Baez, S., & Green, L. (2017). Addressing needs of military families during deployment: Military service providers' perception of integrating support services. *Journal of Military and Government Counseling, 5*(3), 190–212.

Huebner, C. R. (2019). Health and mental health needs of children in US military families. *Pediatrics, 143*(1), Article e20183258. https://doi.org/10.1542/peds.2018-3258

Institute of Medicine. (2008). *Gulf War and health: Physiologic, psychiatric, and psychosocial effects of deployment-related stress.* National Academies Press.

Lane, M. E., Hourani, L. L., Bray, R. M., & Williams, J. (2012). Prevalence of perceived stress and mental health indicators among reserve-component and active-duty military personnel. *American Journal of Public Health, 102*(6), 1213–1220. https://doi.org/10.2105/AJPH.2011.300280

Lester, P., & Flake, E. (2013). How wartime military service affects children and families. *The Future of Children, 23*(2), 121–141. https://doi.org/10.1353/foc.2013.0015

Mailey, E. L., Irwin, B. C., Hsu, W. W., & Joyce, J. M. (2019). InDependent but Not Alone: A web-based intervention to promote physical and mental health among military spouses. *Applied Psychology: Health and Well-Being, 11*(3), 562–583. https://doi.org/10.1111/aphw.12168

Meadows, S. O., Tanielian, T., & Karney, B. (2016). *How military families respond, before, during, and after deployment: Findings from the RAND Deployment Life Study.* https://www.rand.org/pubs/research_briefs/RB9906.html

Military One Source. (n.d.). *Deployment.* https://www.militaryonesource.mil/military-life-cycle/deployment

Millegan, J., McLay, R., & Engel, C. (2014). The effect of geographic moves on mental healthcare utilization in children. *Journal of Adolescent Health, 55*(2), 276–280. https://doi.org/10.1016/j.jadohealth.2014.01.009

Miller, P. E., & Warner, E. (2013). Postdeployment experiences of military mental health providers. *Military Medicine, 178*(12), 1316–1321. https://doi.org/10.7205/MILMED-D-13-00023

National Child Traumatic Stress Network. (2008). *Traumatic grief in military children: Information for medical providers.* https://www.nctsn.org/resources/traumatic-grief-military-children-information-medical-providers

Pincus, S. H., House, R., Christenson, J., & Adler, L. E. (2020). *The emotional cycle of deployment: Military family perspective.* Military.com. https://www.military.com/spouse/military-deployment/dealing-with-deployment/emotional-cycle-of-deployment-military-family.html

RAND Corporation. (2018). *Military force deployment.* https://www.rand.org/topics/military-force-deployment.html

Richardson, A., Chandra, A., Martin, L. T., Setodji, C. M., Hallmark, B. Y., Campbell, N. F., Hawkins, S. A., & Grady, P. (2011). *Effects of soldiers' deployment on children's academic and behavioral health.* https://www.rand.org/content/dam/rand/pubs/monographs/2011/RAND_MG1095.sum.pdf

Riggs, S. A., & Riggs, D. S. (2018). Risk and resiliency in military families experiencing deployment: The role of the family attachment network. In I. Marini & M. A. Stebnicki (Eds.), *The psychological and social impact of illness and disability* (7th ed., pp. 485–502). Springer.

Rotter, J. C., & Boveja, M. E. (1999). Counseling military families. *The Family Journal, 7*(4), 379–382. https://doi.org/10.1177/1066480799074009

Stebnicki, M. A. (2018). Psychosocial counseling aspects of grief, death, and dying. In I. Marini & M. A. Stebnicki (Eds.), *The psychological and social impact of illness and disability* (7th ed., pp. 245–256). Springer.

Tanielian, T., & Jaycox, L. H. (2008). *Invisible wounds of war: Psychological and cognitive injuries, their consequences, and service to assist recovery.* RAND Corporation.

Ursano, R. J., Wang, J., Fullerton, C. S., Ramswawh, H., Gifford, R. K., Russell, D., Cohen, G. H., Sampson, L., & Galea, S. (2018). Post-deployment mental health in reserve and National Guard service members: Deploying with or without one's unit and deployment preparedness. *Military Medicine, 183*(1–2), e51–e58. https://doi.org/10.1093/milmed/usx002

U.S. Department of Defense. (2017). *2017 demographics: Profile of the military community.* https://download.militaryonesource.mil/12038/MOS/Reports/2017-demographics-report.pdf

U.S. Department of Veterans Affairs. (n.d.). *What is deployment?* https://www.mentalhealth.va.gov/communityproviders/docs/deployment_operational_experiences.pdf

U.S. Department of Veterans Affairs. (2020, March 3). *Parenting for veterans and service members.* https://www.veterantraining.va.gov/parenting/index.asp

Walsh, F. (2006). *Strengthening family resilience* (2nd ed.). Guilford Press.

Ysasi, N. A., Silva, I., & Becton, A. D. (2016). Counseling families of active duty military and returning veterans. In I. Marini & M. A. Stebnicki (Eds.), *The psychological and social impact of illness and disability* (7th ed., pp. 409–413). Springer.

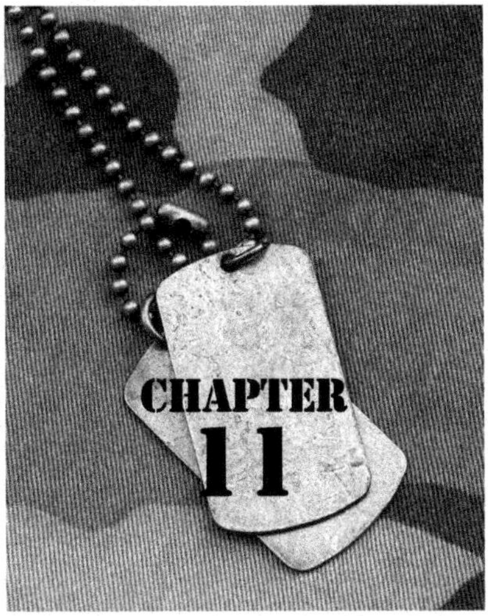

CAREER TRANSITIONS IN MILITARY LIFE: THE TRANSITION MISSION

Twenty years job experience is
simply 1-year experience—repeated over 20 times.

—Dr. T. F. Riggar,
Southern Illinois University–Carbondale, 1981

★ ★ ★

This chapter assists clinical military counselors to identify the psychosocial impact that reintegration and transition from active duty to civilian life has on veterans, veterans with disabilities, and military families. Multiple strategies can be offered by clinicians to their transitioning service members in terms of educational opportunities, career development needs, and psychosocial adjustment to any physical or mental health conditions they may carry into the life span after separation from military service. Career and vocational assessments, transferable skills analysis, career development strategies, and a model for career resiliency are offered. An extensive Military Resources to Explore (MRE) section is also available at the end of this chapter.

Recognizing and identifying psychosocial adjustment factors in veteran reintegration and transition are essential in exploring a path forward. Of paramount concern are veterans with moderate to severe physical and mental health conditions that prevent successful transition.

Veterans in transition have new rules of engagement because the new focus is on the mission of transition. Training for Operation Transition and Resiliency (OTR) requires motivation, commitment, and remaining flexible—or as Marines say, "Semper Gumby" (always flexible). The major difference in the transition mission is that the veteran is an "army of one." This designation is because career development, career choice, and job matching fall on the shoulders of the individual job seeker.

Partnering with the appropriate professionals and natural resources can assist veterans in transition to discover multiple unused opportunities. These prospects may come in the form of continued vocational or educational training, career development activities, and applying strategies that counter negative veteran perceptions that some civilian employers and organizations may have regarding the military community.

OTR

All military missions have a title that exemplifies and communicates a cultural ideology and philosophy for logistics, communication, operation tempo, troop deployment, and battlefield resupply. The theoretical mission of OTR is a metaphor I use to point out critical areas of the mission that are vital to survival in civilian life. Implied in the mission is measuring operation tempo, managing real-time resources, and building coping and resiliency skills for future career success.

Clinical military counselors understand the unique aspects of the OTR mission. One unmistakable cultural difference between military and civilian careers and occupations is the focus on how to adapt and survive, aggress—not stress, and respond to critical incidents; potential dangers of the job, such as injury or death, are also a part of military life (Adler et al., 2011). Unfortunately, some veterans after separation from service exhibit high-risk behaviors linked to their combat experiences or general difficulties that they were subjected to during military life. Veterans who reintegrate and transition successfully know how to take critical incidents and negative experiences and turn them into opportunities for new meaning. Career resiliency in the OTR mission is of paramount importance for achieving optimal mental health and well-being.

The military indeed does an excellent job in training service members for prime physical conditioning, leadership, organizational skills, problem solving, flexibility, and the ability to coordinate critical activities within the structure of a complex organizational system. The military also is successful in training personnel to work well under stress in complex and demanding situations while using a good degree of physical and mental toughness. Indeed, these worker traits and skills are excellent to promote to civilian employers and companies during job search activities, such as completing applications, cover letters, and resumes as well as job interviewing. So why is it so difficult for veterans and veterans with disabilities to prepare for, seek, and maintain employment? Why is reintegration and transition to civilian life so difficult?

Developing a career is difficult for almost everyone, regardless of whether you are a soldier or civilian. Research indicates that many veterans are relegated to unskilled or semi-skilled positions, such as retail sales, construction work, truck driving, security forces, or being a material handler working in a warehouse. One reason that veterans are drawn to these occupations is that they are plentiful and readily available in the regional and national economy. However, many veterans indicate that they prefer a *career* rather than a *job*.

The challenge for practitioners is to facilitate functional, solution-focused, reality-based counseling approaches rather than focusing all therapeutic efforts on mental health counseling. Solution-focused strategies for veterans are valuable as a career development and career counseling approach because they shift veterans' thinking patterns from a problem-oriented to a problem-solving or solution-focused approach (Green et al., 2016; Hayden & Scholl, 2017). Many veterans are challenged by new roles (e.g., stay-at-home parent or spouse), new perspectives (e.g., dealing with the stress of living life as both a civilian and a military veteran), and new meaning in their career (e.g., employment as a civilian and perhaps living with a U.S. Department of Veterans Affairs disability rating). Thus, career counselors using solution-focused approaches can assist veterans in developing optimal (a) self-identity as both a veteran and civilian, (b) ability to create new meaning from their military career and translate these strengths to civilian jobs and careers, and (c) action plans that have the potential to translate into mission objectives (e.g., career interests, job-seeking and interviewing skills).

Competent clinical military counselors know how to facilitate multiple strategies simultaneously engaging in career, mental health, and transition counseling. At some point in the therapeutic process, clinicians need to explore the client's next steps by asking, "So, what would you like to do with your life, now that you have separated from the service?" At this point, clinical military counselors can explore opportunities by brainstorming creative solutions to some challenging problems, such as unemployment, family conflicts, as well as physical and psychological health conditions requiring regular treatment. Seasoned clinical military counselors are skilled at facilitating career development strategies simultaneously with mental health therapy. The clinician's role at this point evolves into different functions, such as accomplishing career goals, facilitating next steps for educational opportunities, initiating job-seeking skills, developing resumes and cover letters, and dealing with workplace stress. Optimally, veteran motivation and job readiness coexist within the therapeutic relationship so that clinicians can help create multiple client opportunities.

PSYCHOSOCIAL ADJUSTMENTS IN THE TRANSITION MISSION

In the transition mission, no unit buddies or extended military family members support you; no unit sergeants or executive officers motivate you; and no organizational structure orders you to exercise, train, work, shower, eat, or sleep. Consequently, the transition mission comes with a significant amount of ambiguity, confusion, and psychological distress. There is a unique strain with transition and reintegration, particularly with younger veterans who may have to return home to live with their parents (Worthen et al., 2012). Military family members indeed have a substantial psychosocial adjustment to make. Many times, this adjustment parallels the veteran son, daughter, or spouse as it relates to maladaptive thoughts, feelings, and behaviors. The veterans themselves are also conscious of how family members and civilians experience or perceive them. Adjustment particularly becomes complicated when veterans have doubts about the mission, such as reflected in a Pew Research Center study reporting that 64% of veterans believed that the wars in Afghanistan and Iraq were not worth fighting given the mental and medical health consequences as well as the financial burden on the United States (Igielnik, 2019).

The lack of meaning in the mission or one's career can hinder veteran resiliency during reintegration and transition. Overall, the considerable decline in close friendships, command structure, and responsibilities can result in poor psychosocial adjustment and reintegration. This transition is also complicated by research reporting that 47% of veterans have frequent outbursts of anger; 48% have multiple family conflicts; and up to 30% have posttraumatic stress disorder, major depressive disorder, substance use disorders, or suicidal ideation (Derefinko et al., 2019; Greden et al., 2010; Porcari et al., 2017). Additional adverse factors include chronic medical conditions requiring frequent visits to health care providers (Ahern et al., 2015; Fraynt et al., 2018) and financial hardships, particularly among reservists (Griffin & Stein, 2015; Griffith, 2015)—some of which have the potential for veteran homelessness (Hayden, 2018).

Indeed, a negative shift in the veteran's identity occurs because of exposure to extraordinary stressful and traumatic events; frequent geographic relocations; separation from family, friends, and loved ones; and mandates for 24-hour availability. There are also the maladaptive behaviors of anger and alienation, a symptom of posttraumatic stress disorder (Adler et al., 2011). The social reorientation; grief and loss of camaraderie; and the feelings of alienation and estrangement from family, friends, and civilian culture all culminate in the experience of living in limbo (Danish & Antonides, 2009; Grimell, 2019; Ysasi et al., 2016).

The transition mission is hindered by multiple other factors, such as mental and physical disabilities, low or no education, lack of civilian work-related experience, and negative perceptions of veterans by some employers. Many younger student veterans find it difficult to transition into college campus life. Graf et al. (2015) reported that many combat veterans feel anxious in the classroom and are preoccupied by potential dangers in their environment. Student veterans also have difficulties forming social and intimate relationships with other college students. They feel that many of their instructors do not understand the military culture, which could assist them in classroom accommodations (Graf et al., 2015). The critical point is that postsecondary education lays the groundwork for a good career. However, if struggles occur in Phase 1 of the mission (earning a 2- or 4-year degree), then Phase 2 of the mission will have to be postponed or abandoned altogether.

WORK AND VETERANS WITH DISABILITIES

Service members do not receive enriched career transition or vocational rehabilitation services after receiving their DD-214 form. The DD-214 is a U.S. Department of Defense document that verifies one's separation from military service, authenticating such items as duty assignment at time of separation, rank, military occupational specialty, decorations, medals, badges, awards, as well as other items related to benefits and military retirement. This report helps in eligibility claims for veterans with service-connected disabilities. Depending on the severity and percentage of the U.S. Department of Veterans Affairs disability rating, some veterans may receive only a small monthly pension, making it difficult to maintain the same standard of living compared with when they were in military service. Overall, cultivating veteran resiliency in the transition process requires multiple roles and responsibilities facilitated by competent clinical military counselors.

Competent clinical military counselors understand the holistic needs of their veteran clients and how to evaluate work readiness (Stebnicki, 2017). Work readiness is basically defined by the individual's residual functional capacity and motivation to engage in work activities, which can be measured from a physical, neurocognitive, social, emotional, mental, and interpersonal perspective. It involves the assessment of physical and mental functional capacity, typically performed by medical and allied health professionals. There are also tests of vocational and neurocognitive capacities measuring the individual's abilities to perform specific job tasks, follow directions, engage and maintain work for sustained periods of time, pay attention, concentrate, make work-related decisions, and remember and carry out simple and complex instructions. Tests in other areas also provide an estimate of the accuracy, speed, and quality of work as it is typically performed in competitive employment.

Some critical areas to assess in work readiness for veterans are their ability to handle stress in the workplace as well as their emotional and mood regulation. Behaviors that would likely be perceived as maladaptive in competitive employment should also be assessed. The following sample areas may be helpful for career and clinical military counselors to functionally assess their veteran client's work readiness:

- Ability to organize, plan, and initiate work activities;
- Capacity to concentrate, stay focused, and complete work-related tasks in a timely manner;
- Display of any impulsive negative emotional and cognitive reactions of irritability, specifically directed toward supervisors, coworkers, and the public;
- Inward or outward expression of frustration and anger toward self and others in the work environment;
- Inward or outward expression of nervousness, depression, hypervigilance, as well as mental and physical stress while engaged in work activities; and
- Display of frequent or severe fatigue, low energy levels, headaches, and muscular skeletal pain.

Exposure to critical and stressful events—such as trauma, loss, grief, and death—has long-term psychosocial effects on the veteran's reintegration and return to work (Stebnicki, 2018). In terms of work readiness, consideration must be given to the (a) degree and severity of the veteran's physical and psychological health; (b) progressive nature, chronicity, and prognosis of the veteran's physical and psychological conditions; (c) veteran's level of coping and resiliency resources; and (d) veteran's level of motivation and interest to engage in vocational training, educational opportunities, and a career. Indeed, the veteran's physical and mental health are vital to building a career, maintaining a healthy self-esteem, and transcending disability to live in optimal wellness.

CAREER RESILIENCY AND THE CAREER RESILIENCY PORTFOLIO (CRP)

Career resiliency involves the individual's ability to bounce back from any physical and mental health conditions that hinder their return to work—either in the same job/same employer, different job/same employer, or different job/different employer. The greatest challenge for the individual is to be forced out of work because of disability, layoff, or business closure. In a sense, military service members who transition from active duty to civilian life are confronted with a different job/different employer situation. Thus, it is critical that career counselors and clinical military counselors assist veterans with issues related to career development, career exploration, job-seeking skills, dealing with workplace stress, and maintaining employment after a good job or career match is in place.

The CRP is one career development tool that can assist veteran clients identify career interests and aptitudes as well as increase awareness of their strengths and limitations. The CRP is useful for cultivating career resiliency traits, particularly for persons with physical and mental health conditions (Szymanski, 1999). The CRP is particularly a useful tool for veterans who have little to no vocational-technical training beyond high school. It is a valuable approach for veterans who have little (if any) civilian job experience or few specific skills and competencies that could potentially transfer into civilian occupations. Overall, the CRP can be utilized as a compass for veteran career decision-making.

Professionals can begin building resiliency with the traditional standardized career-interest inventories, aptitude tests, and intake interview questions (e.g., "Where did you work?" "How much did you earn?" "What other skills do you possess?"). However, CRPs integrate psychosocial counseling techniques that have the potential to extend beyond traditional career interventions.

CAREER COUNSELING EXPLORATION QUESTIONS FOR THE CRP

The following sample career counseling questions offer professionals an opportunity for gathering more meaningful and deeper information related to the individual's values, beliefs, philosophy, and motivation concerning jobs and careers. Skilled career and clinical military counselors understand how to listen for the emotions, cognitions, experiences, and metacommunication behind the probes.

1. What is something interesting about you as a person?
2. What is your family or home life like—what was it like when you were in the service or deployed?
3. What are some things that are unique about you—or unique regarding your cultural background?
4. Do you have any special interests, hobbies, or activities that you like to do?
5. What things in life do you feel that you are most talented or gifted at doing? What things come the easiest or natural to you?
6. What things have other people (family, friends) complimented you on in terms of what you are good at doing?
7. If you could do more of what you wanted to do in a job, occupation, or career, what would that look like for you?
8. When you think back over your life, what have been some of your greatest achievements and accomplishments?
9. What have been some of the greatest challenges or hardships that have confronted you in life?

10. What are some things that you feel would stand in the way (or would be a barrier for you) in fulfilling your employment or career goals?
11. Do you have any specific limitations that you could share with me—ones that may interfere with employment or be a barrier to your career goals?
12. Do you have any special academic, educational, or job training?
13. What jobs have you held in the past? How did you perform these jobs? What were some of the special skills or knowledge that you had to have to perform your jobs effectively?
14. What are some things in your past work that you would hope to totally avoid?
15. If you could have any job in the world, what would you want to be doing? What would be your dream job?
16. What are some short- and long-term career goals that you have at this moment?

After building a clinical picture on the basis of these sample career exploration questions, skilled counselors will want to complete a transferable skills analysis by requesting follow-up information from their veteran client by attaining (a) a complete work history detailing their military occupational specialty and any advanced training; (b) their perception regarding the role and function of their past jobs; (c) their work tasks, job duties, and tools and materials used to completely perform their job; (d) any knowledge acquired from past work, specialized training, and any other (nonconfidential) information that they can share; and (e) information about educational level obtained and vocational-technical training earned. You may also want to inquire about the veteran's favorite courses taken in high school or college; their college major; whether they had any practicum internship or mentoring experiences; as well as credentials or certifications earned before, during, or after military service.

Notice that some of the questions and information that you gather during career development and counseling interventions may be more demographic in nature. However, the open-ended sample questions offered earlier will help you to acquire functional and realistic information regarding your veteran client's (a) total life experiences; (b) values and beliefs regarding career choice, education, and work ethic; (c) physical or mental health conditions that may hinder return-to-work efforts; (d) barriers to their chosen career path; and (e) resiliency traits that will assist them while in career transition.

PERSONAL LIFE STORY OR TESTIMONIAL FOR CRP

Expressive writing is a powerful tool for military veterans that has therapeutic value. Writing a personal life story or testimonial takes on many different forms. It can be particularly useful to communicate educational, occupational, and career-related successes as well as difficulties. Writing engages a different part of the brain that allows individuals to communicate deeper thoughts and insight. This career development activity is different than having your client answering yes/no questions in a structured interview. The personal life story or testimonial should include, at a minimum, work or professional experiences, interests, aptitudes, special skills and abilities, hobbies, personal military experiences, and peak insights that evolved in military life that may have significance for choosing an educational or career path.

The intention of the life story or testimonial is for your veteran client to begin reflecting and building career and personal resiliency strategies. Make sure that you help your client understand which parts of their personal story would be appropriate to share during job interviews versus areas for therapeutic engagements (e.g., substance recovery, combat missions, getting blown up). One foundational feature of the personal life story is to assist your client in finding meaning and purpose in their new life as a military veteran. This activity will hopefully build self-awareness, insight, and reflection on their life before enlistment and help them to find meaning in their present here-and-now experience. The personal life story or testimonial is also valuable for mock job interviews or role playing with your veteran client about how to respond to challenging questions by employers.

CAREER SELF-ASSESSMENT

Career self-assessments can assist your veteran client to narrow down their worker traits, interests, and goals. There are three types of career assessments: (a) tested interests (use of standardized and nonstandardized assessments), (b) manifest (those interests that were developed throughout one's lifetime), and (c) expressed interest (verbalizing interests such as the 16 career exploration questions listed earlier). Clinical military counselors may utilize some of the career self-assessment tools and the resources located in the MRE section. One example is the U.S. Department of Labor's Career One Stop for veterans (https://www.careeronestop.org/), which assists service members in transition to explore civilian careers, find transferable skills, and determine career interests.

After delving into veteran career resources, clinical military counselors can assist their veteran clients to interpret and summarize their self-assessment and career information for self-reflection. Competent counselors understand how to elicit client verbalization and expression of wants and needs. By identifying and summarizing salient features concerning career self-assessment and self-reflection, the veteran is provided with a career compass from which to navigate. As you review your veteran's career self-assessment, assist them with identifying important themes related to (a) satisfactions/dissatisfactions with specific job tasks and careers (e.g., working with things, people, or objects); (b) likes/dislikes in terms of job tasks, work environments (e.g., indoor or outdoor work), and preferences (e.g., team work, independent projects, level of supervision and mentoring); (c) unique job skills (e.g., technical, informational, expressive or written communication); (d) talents and abilities (e.g., creative vs. concrete job tasks); and (e) other relevant career areas related to tested, manifest, and expressed interests.

APPLICATIONS, COVER LETTERS, RESUMES, AND THE JOB INTERVIEW

There are multiple resources in the MRE section that are veteran friendly because they involve career self-exploration. Competent career and clinical military counselors have a keen awareness of the veteran's job search experiences; they are also aware that many service members indicate that attending their branch's Military Transition Assistance program leaves a void in multiple areas. Thus, it is important that veteran clients understand the value of completing near-perfect applications, cover letters, and resumes. These items are the first contact that the prospective employer will have with the veteran before securing a job interview. The job interviewing process is also an essential area for which to prepare your veteran client. Farley (2010, 2013) as well as many other career experts (Buzzetta et al., 2017; Green et al., 2016; Hayden & Scholl, 2017) have identified critical tasks in transition and career development to assist career counselors who are working with veterans. The interested reader should consult these sources and the MRE section at the end of this chapter. The following important areas regarding cover letters, resumes, and the job interview process should be communicated by career and clinical military counselors to their veteran clients:

- Establish the type of jobs and careers you want on the basis of your strengths, interests, aptitudes, the occupational outlook, and labor market. You can construct one to three different resumes on the basis of your job goals and career objectives.
- Effectively communicate to employers with written and verbal communication. Accentuate your leadership capabilities, motivation, organization, time management skills, work ethic, and ability to work under stress.
- Avoid communication regarding use of jargon, deployments, combat-related experiences, and other hardships in military life. You can discuss such topics in general terms as they relate to your coping skills and resiliency strengths. If the prospective employer is a U.S. Department of Defense contractor or military-friendly business, different rules apply as to how your

military life experiences are discussed. Take cues from others in the work environment.
- Identify key marketable skills to prospective employers regarding self-management, technical, job-specific, and transferable or functional skills. Communicate verbally and in writing how these skills directly translate into specific civilian jobs or occupations.
- Communicate personal strengths and attributes rather than military stereotypes. Some employers may perceive veterans as too rigid or lacking in creativity. Emphasize how the military taught you to be flexible.
- Highlight your military career from a strengths-based perspective (mental and physical), identify with the core mission values of the organization, and describe your military life experiences that have provided optimal wellness of body and mind.

Career and clinical military counselors can be a valuable resource to support optimal veteran communication to employers of their unique set of skills, talents, and motivations for the prospective new job opportunity. Overall, as a professional, you can assist veteran job seekers to find good employment matches in the most positive and supportive work environments.

CONCLUDING REMARKS

Veteran transition and career development is a life-long process. Transitioning from active duty to civilian life requires a "GPS" to navigate this major change. Clinical military counselors can serve in multiple roles to assist simultaneously as a mental health provider as well as a facilitator and coordinator of resources; they can also engage in career development and exploration with veteran clients. Optimal career choices for veterans with severe disabilities will require more intensive psychosocial adjustment and counseling. Thus, clinical military counselors can assist veterans in job accommodation needs to achieve optimal functioning in the work environment. Initiating CRPs as a career development tool will also assist veterans in taking the necessary risks required for a healthy transition and placing one foot on the career path. Overall, the resources in the MRE section at the end of this chapter offer valuable career self-exploration tools for both professionals and veterans.

REFERENCES

Adler, A. B., Britt, T. W., Castro, C. A., McGurk, D., & Bliese, P. D. (2011). Effect of transition home from combat on risk-taking and health-related behaviors. *Journal of Traumatic Stress, 24*(4), 381–389. https://doi.org/10.1002/jts.20665

Ahern, J., Worthen, M., Masters, J., Lippman, S. A., Ozer, J., & Moos, R. (2015). The challenges of Afghanistan and Iraq veterans' transition from military to civilian life and approaches to reconnection. *PLoS One, 10*(7), Article e0128599. https://doi.org/10.1371/journal.pone.0128599

Buzzetta, M., Hayden, S. C. W., & Ledwith, K. (2017). Creating hope: Assisting veterans with job search strategies using cognitive information processing theory. *Journal of Employment Counseling, 54*(2), 63–74. https://doi.org/10.1002/joec.12054

Danish, S. J., & Antonides, B. J. (2009). What counseling psychologists can do to help returning veterans. *The Counseling Psychologist, 37*(8), 1076–1089. https://doi.org/10.1177/0011000009338303

Derefinko, K. J., Hallsell, T. A., Isaacs, M. B., Colvin, L. W., Salgado Garcia, F. I., & Bursac, Z. (2019). Perceived needs of veterans transitioning from the military to civilian life. *The Journal of Behavioral Health Services & Research, 46,* 384–398. https://doi.org/10.1007/s11414-018-9633-8

Farley, J. (2010). *Military-to-civilian career transition guide: The essential job search handbook for service members* (2nd ed.). JIST Works.

Farley, J. (2013). *Quick military transition guide: Seven steps to landing a civilian job.* JIST Works.

Fraynt, R., Cooper, D., Edwards-Stewart, A., Hoyt, T., Micheel, L., Pruitt, L., Skopp, N., & Smolenski, D. (2018). An evaluation of mobile applications designed to assist service members and veterans transitioning to civilian life. *Psychological Service, 15*(2), 208–215. https://doi.org/10.1037/ser0000205

Graf, N., Ysasi, N. A., & Marini, I. (2015). Assessment of military viewpoints regarding post-secondary education: Classroom preferences and experiences. *Rehabilitation Counseling Bulletin, 59*(1), 18–29. https://doi.org/10.1177/0034355214558937

Greden, J. F., Valenstein, M., Spinner, J., Blow, A., Gorman, L. A., Dalack, G. W., Marcus, S., & Kees, M. (2010). Buddy-to-Buddy, a citizen soldier peer support program to counteract stigma, PTSD, depression, and suicide. *Annals of the New York Academy of Sciences, 1208*(1), 90–97. https://doi.org/10.1111/j.1749-6632.2010.05719.x

Green, L. A., Dawson-Fend, L., Hayden, S. C. W., Crews, C., & Painter, A. (2016). From combat to the classroom: Understanding and addressing veteran transition. *Journal of Military and Government Counseling, 4*(2), 118–133.

Griffin, C. L., & Stein, M. A. (2015). Self-perception of disability and prospects for employment among U.S. veterans. *Work, 50*(1), 49–58. https://doi.org/10.3233/WOR-141929

Griffith, J. (2015). Homecoming of soldiers who are citizens: Re-employment and financial status of returning Army National Guard soldiers from Operations Iraqi Freedom (OIF) and Enduring Freedom (OEF). *Work, 50*(1), 85–96. https://doi.org/10.3233/WOR-131794

Grimell, J. (2019). Revisiting living in limbo to illustrate a pastoral psychological understanding of transition from military to civilian life. *Pastoral Psychology, 68*(4), 393–405. https://doi.org/10.1007/s11089-019-00881-6

Hayden, S. C. W. (2018). Supporting veterans experiencing homelessness through a theoretically based career development group. *Journal of Military and Government Counseling, 6*(4), 215–223.

Hayden, S. C. W., & Scholl, M. B. (2017). Solution-focused career counseling with a male military veteran. In L. A. Busacca & M. C. Rehfuss (Eds.), *Postmodern career counseling: A handbook of culture, context, and cases* (pp. 259–271). American Counseling Association.

Igielnik, R. (2019, November 7). *Key findings about America's military veterans.* Pew Research Center. https://www.pewresearch.org/fact-tank/2019/11/07/key-findings-about-americas-military-veterans/

Porcari, C., Koch, E. I., Rauch, S. A. M., Hoodin, F., Ellison, G., & McSweeney, L. (2017). Predictors of help-seeking intentions in Operation Enduring Freedom and Operation Iraqi Freedom veterans and service members. *Military Medicine, 182*(5–6), e1640–e1647. https://doi.org/10.7205/MILMED-D-16-00105

Stebnicki, M. A. (2017). *Disaster mental health counseling: Responding to trauma in a multicultural context.* Springer.

Stebnicki, M. A. (2018). Psychosocial counseling aspects of grief, death, and dying. In I. Marini & M. A. Stebnicki (Eds.), *The psychological and social impact of illness and disability* (7th ed., pp. 245–256). Springer.

Szymanski, E. (1999). Disability, job stress, the changing nature of careers, and the Career Resiliency Portfolio. *Rehabilitation Counselor Bulletin, 42*(4), 279–289.

Worthen, M., Moos, R., & Ahern, J. (2012). Iraq and Afghanistan veterans' experiences living with their parents after separation from the military. *Contemporary Family Therapy, 34*(3), 362–375. https://doi.org/10.1007/s10591-012-9196-4

Ysasi, N. A., Silva, I., & Becton, A. D. (2016). Counseling families of active duty military and returning veterans. In I. Marini & M. A. Stebnicki (Eds.), *The professional counselor's desk reference* (2nd ed., pp. 409–413). Springer.

MILITARY RESOURCES TO EXPLORE (MRE)

Books and Resources

Career One Stop—Veteran and Military Transition Center: https://www.careeronestop.org/Veterans/ExploreCivilianCareers/YourSkillsAndInterests/interest-assessment.aspx

Farley, J. I. (2010). *Military-to-civilian career transition guide: The essential job search handbook for service members.* JIST Works.

Farley, J. I. (2013). *Quick military transition guide: Seven steps to landing a civilian job.* JIST Works.

Other Resources

Military.com
https://www.military.com/

Military One Source—Strategies for wounded warriors to adjust and recover from serious injury
http://www.militaryonesource.mil/health-and-wellness/wounded-warrior?content_id=282472

Social Security Disability Advocates—North Carolina application and appeals help
https://www.disabilityapplicationhelp.org/Default.aspx?p=North%20Carolina&gclid=CJqXx42248oCFcYlgQodUmQJbw

U.S. Department of Veterans Affairs—Veterans Employment Toolkit
https://www.va.gov/vetsinworkplace/docs/em_fullversionResources.asp

Occupational Specialty Codes

U.S. Air Force enlisted AFSC (Air Force Specialty Code) classifications
http://www.af.mil/AboutUs/FactSheets/Display/tabid/224/Article/104609/enlisted-afsc-classifications.aspx

U.S. Air Force officer AFSC classifications
http://www.af.mil/AboutUs/FactSheets/Display/tabid/224/Article/104484/officer-afsc-classifications.aspx

U.S. Army military occupational specialty (MOS) codes search tool
http://army.com/info/mos/all

U.S. Marine Corps rank insignia, ranks, and pay grade
http://www.military-quotes.com/ranks/marine-rank-insignia.htm

U.S. Navy enlisted classifications
https://navynavadmin.files.wordpress.com/2010/03/necvol2.pdf

U.S. Navy officer billet classification codes
https://www.public.navy.mil/bupers-npc/reference/noc/NOOCSVOL1/Documents/Manual%20I%2070%20PT%20C%20(NOBC).pdf

O*NET, Military Occupational Classifications, and Career Exploration and Development

Careers in the military
https://www.careersinthemilitary.com/

GoCoastGuard.com
https://www.gocoastguard.com/active-duty-careers/officer-opportunities

My Next Move for Veterans
https://www.mynextmove.org/vets/

O*NET OnLine
https://www.onetonline.org/

U.S. Army officer careers and specialties
http://www.goarmy.com/careers-and-jobs/officer-careers-and-specialties.html

U.S. Marine Corps COOL
https://www.cool.navy.mil/usmc/

U.S. Navy COOL:
https://www.cool.navy.mil/usn/

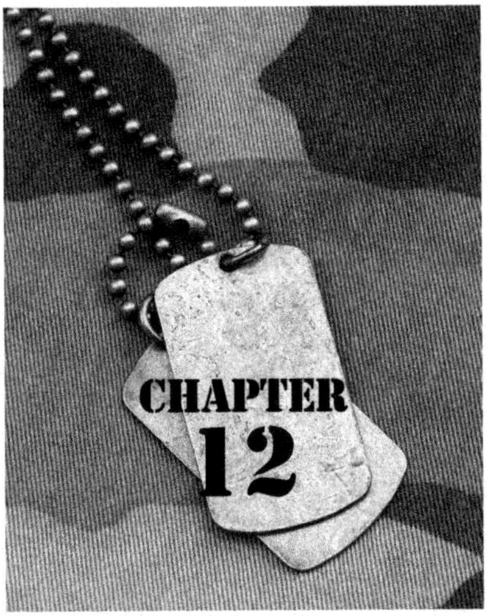

BECOMING A COMPETENT CLINICAL MILITARY PRACTITIONER: EARNING THE CIRCLE OF TRUST

Trust is the cornerstone of all relationships.

—Mark A. Stebnicki, 2020

★ ★ ★

The work presented in *Clinical Military Counseling* contributes to the literature as it relates to the medical, psychosocial, vocational, transition, family, mental health, and cultural characteristics of the military. There are indeed differences among civilian, community, and military mental health counseling. Clinicians must be attuned to working therapeutically with the unique cultural aspects of active-duty service members, veterans, veterans with disabilities, and military families. The cornerstone of any therapeutic environment is to facilitate practice in a safe and confidential setting where client self-disclosure of critical events is a natural part of the therapeutic process. Competent clinicians recognize how negative stereotypes and stigma affect the psychosocial functioning and wellness of service members and veterans seeking mental health treatment. Experienced clinicians also understand how to appraise the psychosocial impact that the deployment cycle has on military service members and their families, which is particularly important during reintegration and transition to civilian life.

Competent clinical military counselors demonstrate cultural competence when completing a comprehensive assessment with their military clients. They understand how to evaluate behavioral, psychological, and physical health concerns. Seasoned military counselors also differentiate between civilian and military social, emotional, spiritual, and interpersonal health. They also are competent in offering approaches related to career transition and cultivating strategies that best fit their client's sociocultural and family values. However, an essential prerequisite for becoming a competent clinical military counselor, before an assessment and treatment interventions are facilitated, is *earning the circle of trust*.

In this chapter, I attempt to draw similarities and differences among community, civilian, and military mental health counseling practices. Mental health and other behaviorally licensed clinicians are presented with the essential and foundational skills vital to earning the circle of trust. Ultimately, practitioners can take the knowledge and skills learned in their graduate training program and apply these theories and strategies through the cultural lens of the military.

THE ART OF CLINICAL MILITARY COUNSELING

Few training resources exist to assist mental health and other behaviorally licensed professionals to work therapeutically with military clients. Presently, it is recognized that there is a considerable cultural gap among counseling theories, models, and therapeutic strategies as they pertain to mental and behavioral health practices with military populations (Adler & Castro, 2013; Redmond et al., 2015; Stebnicki, 2016, 2017; Stebnicki et al., 2017). Thus, a multidimensional understanding is required of how counseling and psychology can inform military mental and behavioral health practice.

There are similarities and differences in building the therapeutic alliance with military and nonmilitary clients. However, translating these therapeutic approaches into clinical mental health practice presents a challenge. At the heart of *Clinical Military Counseling* are research and practice guidelines offered to assist clinicians in transcribing, translating, and replicating the foundations of counseling and psychology with considerations for a holistic practice with service members, veterans, veterans with disabilities, and military families.

Throughout the history of psychology and counseling, the essential skills of empathy have been facilitated in person-centered therapeutic environments (Corey & Corey, 2021; Egan & Reese, 2019; Hackney & Cormier, 2017; Ivey et al., 2018). Empathy is a skill that can be both developed and learned. More importantly, empathy as a way of being (Rogers, 1980) is a form of communication that involves attending, listening, observing, understanding, and responding to the concerns of others with a deep respect and genuineness. Much of what people communicate to one another is done through *meta-communication*—eye contact, body language, silence, tone of voice, gestures, facial expressions, physical space, and many other cultural characteristics. The competent therapist knows that during the comprehensive clinical assessment, less is more in terms of assessment and evaluative probes. Good attending, listening, and empathic skills present an optimal environment for accomplishing many goals within the clinical counseling process.

Corey and Corey (2021) have suggested that cultural and clinical competence is both an ethical and legal obligation of the skilled professional. Earning the circle of trust requires competent practitioners to consider the relevant cultural characteristics associated with military clients (e.g., race, ethnicity, and gender identity; enlisted or officer rank; branch of service; military occupational specialty [MOS]). Competent practitioners also understand the importance of inquiring about the military client's perception and attitude toward their career, identity within the branch of service, how they have acculturated or assimilated into the military culture as a whole, any physical and mental health challenges that hinder their ability to perform their job, and any psychosocial adjustment issues related to reintegration or transition into civilian life.

Translating the foundational counseling skills within a multicultural counseling context has been a constant challenge for researchers, counselor and psychology educators, and practitioners. This difficulty may be due, in part, to the fact that early traditional theorists generally viewed counseling and psychotherapeutic strategies as a "one size fits all" approach in the assessment, diagnosis, and treatment of mental health conditions without regard for salient cultural characteristics.

Certain aspects of community-based treatment models do not translate or differentiate well between clinical military and community-based counseling practices. This gap is sparked by disagreements on the (a) validation of assessment instruments measuring specific clinical conditions, (b) most effective evidence-based strategies and approaches to facilitate with clients, (c) lack of statistical significance between one counseling theory and another, (d) means by which clinical outcome is measured on the basis of the individual's perception and rating of "helpfulness," (e) most effective treatment settings (e.g., U.S. Department of Veterans Affairs hospitals vs. civilian residential treatment centers, military installation outpatient vs. civilian clinics), (f) specific trauma-informed treatment strategies that may focus on civilian populations and do not consider the recurring trauma exposure of frequent and lengthy combat deployments, and (g) the impact of polytrauma or complex trauma that challenges service members and veterans (e.g., complex posttraumatic stress disorder [PTSD], traumatic brain and blast injuries, grief and loss associated with combat deployments). Another prime example of why some models do not translate well culturally into military mental health treatment is the negative stigma associated with active-duty service members seeking mental health treatment and the occupational barriers that this discrimination presents to one's military career, maintaining security clearance, and overall perception of fitness for duty.

USE OF EMPATHY AS A THERAPEUTIC AND LEADERSHIP TOOL

The modern roots of empathy can be traced to its current application in research and practice as described by Carl R. Rogers (1902–1987), who published his seminal work, *Client-Centered Therapy*, in 1951. Historically, other pioneers have helped in the development of the skills and practice of empathy in therapeutic settings. The common core of knowledge and skills in empathy as well as its historical roots, cultural use, and measurement have been delineated extensively by Stebnicki (2008).

Intuitively, the use of empathy appears paradoxical for some, given the "suck it up Buttercup" culture of the military and its focus on physical toughness, not the mental and emotional qualities of communication. Yet, military leadership of the 21st century is open to multiple strategies and approaches that have been successful in civilian life. Military leadership advocates for understanding and acknowledging troop fatigue and the psychological and emotional demands of the job. Because the intention of military leadership is to improve combat readiness and postdeployment resiliency among service personnel and military families, the optimal warfighter today is trained to have the mental, cognitive, and interpersonal capacity to exhibit effective communication and leadership skills.

Empathy is a tool for building the foundation of an authentic and therapeutic relationship. It increases opportunities for earning the circle of trust. The construct and skills of empathy are much different than compassion and sympathy. It oftentimes becomes confused by pre-professional helpers and those outside the fields of psychology and counseling. Compassion has multiple definitions throughout the psychology, counseling, religious, and psychospiritual literature. It is recognized by most as a felt sense of purpose, experience, and a way of being human with the person's sense of helplessness, woundedness, pain, and suffering. Sympathy also has a felt sense of meaning for the individual but is much less proactive and is not effective in the professional helping relationship. Sympathy is in response to another person's critical life event, essentially "feeling sorry" for others' loss, grief, or pain that they may be experiencing. Sympathy and compassion are basically feeling and saying "My thoughts and prayers are with you," whereas empathy communicates to others verbally and nonverbally by affirming "My thoughts and prayers are with you . . . how can

I help?" Thus, empathy as a tool for the skilled helper is dynamic, facilitative, and the highest form of communication. Overall, the use of facilitative empathy assists therapists in earning the right to enter the private world of another person by being optimally effective in the metacommunication exchange between the client and therapist.

In military life, teamwork, leadership qualities, and working optimally under extraordinary stressful conditions are essential skills acquired through months and years of highly specialized training. Parmar (2016) posited that teamwork is the number one priority for U.S. Navy Sea, Air, and Land (SEAL) units. Given the challenging missions and environments in which SEAL teams must succeed, mental and physical toughness are required for both individual and unit survival. Having a good sense of self and others is key to mission readiness and success. It provides a level of interpersonal awareness as well as mental, emotional, and cognitive balance for warfighters and is an enduring trait to possess well after reintegration and transition to civilian life.

Kail (2011) has suggested that in military service, leadership is all about connecting with others beyond a superficial and authoritarian manner. In fact, if a unit commander relies purely on transactional leadership skills that are perceived as distant, highly structured, and impersonal, then the benefits of this style are short term at best. Some of the best military leaders understand that (a) listening to non-commissioned officers and enlisted personnel and (b) possessing flexibility as well as tolerance for a diverse range of thoughts, perceptions, and opinions regarding strategic matters all contribute to unit cohesiveness, mission readiness, and operation tempo. Allowing others to contribute to the mission exemplifies empathy and portrays ideal leadership qualities. The use of empathy in military leadership allows subordinates within the unit to find meaning in their work. It also assists the service member to take ownership and responsibility for the implementation of strategic values within the mission. The use of empathy in military leadership overall demonstrates that service members are not machines—they are to be respected for more than solely their technical skills, knowledge, and expertise in their MOS.

Card-Mina (2011) stated that there are three major factors that determine military leadership qualities in regard to dealing with mental health issues such as PTSD symptoms. These factors are values, empathy, and the Warrior Ethos. Empathy in military life allows leaders to assist peers, subordinates, and superiors by using an intense level of listening that presents opportunities to earn the person's trust and to identify their problem issues. Empathy accepts the other person's point of view. It acknowledges and understands critical issues from another person's "foxhole." Card-Mina has truly advocated for the use of empathy in military leadership because it communicates to subordinates a higher level of human caring that is essential in optimal functioning within military life. Facilitation of empathy as a leadership skill changes the focus from a "mission accomplished" perspective to valuing what the service member thinks, feels, and experiences during the deployment cycle. Overall, empathy can enhance emotional and psychological resiliency during military service.

As the military leadership literature suggests, leaders are expected to be part of the solution to help decrease the incidence of mental health conditions such as suicidality. More recently, the U.S. Department of Defense has placed a greater emphasis on mental health prevention, treatment, and resiliency. The purpose is not solely focused on troop retention but rather is to advocate for optimal mental, emotional, and psychological functioning. When military leaders openly acknowledge and discuss service members' critical mental health issues, it can serve as a type of employee assistance program for the prevention and treatment of potentially serious mental health issues such as PTSD, depression, and suicidality. The use of empathy within military leadership can be a powerful tool for change. Its use is now being explored with the intention to increase optimal levels of mental health and well-being. Overall, the identification, prevention, and mental health triage of potentially serious mental health conditions begin with both the therapist's and military leadership's use of empathy as a model.

DEALING WITH RELUCTANCE, RESISTANCE, AND DEFENSIVENESS

Clinical military counselors focus the initial therapeutic interactions on rapport building so that they can earn the circle of trust with their military clients. The intention is to cultivate a strong working alliance. However, key elements in the therapeutic process may hinder client growth and development and may dilute the therapeutic alliance, such as dealing with the reluctance, resistance, and defensiveness of the service member or veteran to engage in the therapeutic process. For many service members and veterans, attending a mental health counseling session can be quite overwhelming, especially if it is a mandated session. Military clients new to the process may have the perception that the therapist wants to enter their private and deeply personal world to see how they think, feel, act, and experience military life. Dealing with client reluctance, resistance, and defensiveness is a natural response of the process.

Competent clinical military counselors understand the therapeutic value of readiness, motivation, and timing of client self-disclosure. The intention is prevention—to decrease client reluctance, resistance, and defensiveness. Competent clinical military counselors also recognize the stigma and career cost of service members seeking mental health treatment. Accordingly, clinical military counselors may anticipate some degree of client reluctance, resistance, and defensiveness. In the following sections, I discuss how to recognize and deal with reluctance, resistance, and defensiveness in service members and veterans.

Reluctance

Reluctance is the unwillingness or disinclination to do something, and it is a natural part of seeking mental health treatment. This reaction is particularly the case for military service members and veterans for whom mental health prevention and treatment are not widely endorsed by all levels of command. Indeed, societal myths, stereotypes, and stigma are associated with being a member of the military culture. There is an occupational cost to the service member's career in terms of seeking mental health treatment and receiving a diagnosis that brings up real issues of fitness for duty and leadership. Reluctance to seek mental health treatment as a veteran is also a natural process that may have evolved before enlistment, while in active-duty service, and during transition to civilian life. Researchers have suggested that reluctance is a natural process for clients entering into mental health treatment. It is based on the individual's perception of the helpfulness and effectiveness of receiving mental health treatment. The undercurrent of reluctance is dynamic because it has multiple points in the process that can be stressful for the individual.

For instance, just thinking about and conceptualizing "change" and the experience of being in treatment, making an appointment, or the perception and stigma of what others may think may escalate the individual to the level of resistance to mental health treatment. The ambivalence for some can range from mild to moderate stress, whereas other levels of stress may be like going to the dentist for a root canal. Many researchers have suggested that reluctance—as well as the client's perception of counseling satisfaction and improvement—is directly correlated with the outcome of mental health counseling itself. This finding suggests that clinical military counselors may want to spend time with their clients discussing the benefits of receiving counseling services. Many military clients leave therapy disillusioned and with the thought that "talking to a professional" could harm their career and that their problems are way too complicated to receive any benefits at this point in their life. Just discussing the immediacy of such problems can decrease therapeutic anxiety. Although client readiness and motivation for change are important matters, if client rapport is absent and the circle of trust is not present, these issues become lost therapeutic opportunities. The following guidelines for practitioners are offered for clinical consideration:

- Before a structured or formal comprehensive clinical assessment, be mindful of good attending, listening, and empathic responding to your client with the intention of establishing optimal rapport.

- Provide the appropriate amount of information about yourself, as required by most states in terms of the professional disclosure statement, and the services you or your clinical practice have to offer.
- Address the legal and ethical obligations (and limits) to confidentiality and privacy; then, as part of an ongoing effort, reinforce the confidential nature of your sessions to strengthen the therapeutic alliance.
- Discuss reluctance with clients in an effective interpersonal manner, and describe it as a naturally occurring event. Highlight the benefits and therapeutic outcomes of receiving therapy as well as opportunities to acquire problem-solving skills and make use of available opportunities for their military life.
- Encourage clients to explore their hesitancy and ambivalence with receiving mental health treatment, with an emphasis on integrating other forms of therapy (e.g., animal-assisted therapy, expressive writing or arts, mindfulness-based stress reduction, yoga).
- Monitor your own stereotypes of the military culture, countertransference reactions, and power differential in the client-therapist role. Avoid being the "expert" by shifting some therapeutic self-care responsibilities to the client.
- Understand that your military client may be surveying your office and its surroundings by looking at windows, doors, as well as entry and exit points. This behavior is part of the military brain mapping experience in efforts to feel safe and to plan for any unpredictable or unanticipated events (e.g., fire alarm going off in building, loud voices from other surrounding therapy offices, lawn maintenance workers outside your window).
- Understand that your new military client's expressed metacommunication may be (a) part of their sympathetic-parasympathetic response, (b) a display of coping skills while being in an unknown environment, and (c) based on their military training (e.g., survival training, always knowing their surroundings). Avoid viewing these behaviors as maladaptive or unhealthy.
- Anticipate that the active-duty service member or veteran may not be able to respond to several questions that you may have for operational security reasons (e.g., geographic locations of deployments, details of their MOS). Avoid viewing these behaviors as unhealthy reluctance.

Resistance

Resistance is defined as the individual's reluctance to bring into conscious awareness any material that has been previously avoided, repressed, or denied. It can also be viewed as anything that prevents the person from dealing with painful feelings, previous trauma experiences, or personal conflicts that are primarily unconscious in nature.

The thoughts, feelings, emotions, cognitions, and behaviors related to resistance are there for a reason. At times, it can become an unhealthy response; yet, it is a natural coping mechanism. The client's way of dealing with a specific thought, feeling, emotion, cognition, or experience eventually runs its course and serves no purpose in their life. Resistance can be used as therapeutic leverage by the skilled and competent therapist who can challenge their client's thoughts, feelings, emotions, and experiences at a surface level of meaning. As the therapeutic process evolves, the client-therapist relationship may strengthen, and a deeper client awareness will ensue. However, skilled and competent clinical military counselors maintain therapeutic effectiveness because they have considered specific cultural aspects that assist in strengthening the therapeutic bond. The following guidelines for practitioners are offered for clinical consideration with the intentions of earning the circle of trust and building the therapeutic relationship:

- Recognize that resistance is a natural part of changing a behavior, thought, or feeling. By respecting your client's resistance, you will avoid having to confront or challenge your client's resistance as a perceived negative characteristic or trait. Avoid using client resistance as the focal point for therapy and artificially creating a power struggle or "pulling rank" as a requirement for change. Both client and therapist can utilize resistance as a therapeutic opportunity and examine its functional use as a coping mechanism.
- Silence does not indicate resistance. Service members were taught to respect and not challenge authority and to respond with "yes sir" or "no ma'am." Your military client may perceive that you are in a position of power. Empower your client for therapeutic partnerships that utilize you as a resource, not a gate guard.
- Many service members have a natural reluctance to attend mental health counseling because they may be perceived by others in their unit or command as weak, unable to work well under pressure, or possessing deficits in leadership qualities. Consequently, the service member may resist attending sessions because it could potentially jeopardize their career, especially if given a mental health diagnosis.
- Understand how to interpret and place into cultural context the thoughts, feelings, emotions, cognitions, and experiences of your military client. For example, anger and rage may be suppressed during therapy sessions. This suppression should not be viewed as client resistance. From the military client's perspective, this behavior could be viewed as exhibiting disrespect to someone in authority.

- Explore your client's military culture in various environments and social networks at work, on base, and at home for the purpose of understanding the mission values and expectations of their intense occupation. Skilled and competent clinical military counselors learn about the military culture by asking questions of their military clients. It is critical to remember that there is not just "one military" person. Rather, the U.S. Armed Forces of today reflect—although not proportionally—the various gender, sexual identity, racial, and ethnic groups that compose the U.S. population.
- Avoid labeling clients as resistive, hostile, noncompliant, or difficult to work with in your progress notes. Use process notes for these issues. Instead, provide a description of observable and nonjudgmental behaviors that the client exhibits within the session. Competent clinical military counselors approach all clients unconditionally and are keenly aware of issues of transference, countertransference, and other metacommunication that can diminish the therapeutic environment.

Defensiveness

Defensiveness is behavior intended to protect, and it is at the highest end of the continuum following reluctance and resistance. The display of defensive behaviors by military clients can be problematic and sometimes toxic to the therapeutic relationship. Defensiveness is exhibited by a wide range of behaviors and is different for each person. Some become physically confrontational and verbally aggressive, whereas others are passive aggressive. Multiple underlying issues are related to the client's defensiveness. Some unhealthy behaviors and clinical mental health symptoms related to defensiveness may be the unit commander's requirement for mandated treatment. Regardless of mandated treatment, defensiveness may occur because of problems in military work or home life as well as social interactions in the community (e.g., substance use disorders, anger, hostility, rage). There may also be preenlistment personality traits that clinically predispose the person to exhibit defensiveness (e.g., passive-aggressive, antisocial-personality, and borderline-personality traits).

The research suggests that defensive behaviors that go to extremes (e.g., anger and rage) indicate an underlying mood problem, such as major depressive disorder, and may be associated with behaviors of past trauma experiences (e.g., anxiety, PTSD). Some service members and veterans have a history of high-risk behaviors (e.g., suicidal ideation, going against orders of unit or post command). Additionally, defensiveness may occur as a result of psychosocial, career, or family-related issues (e.g., loss and grief within the military family, demotion in rank, less-than-honorable discharge, transition and separation from service, physical injury and disability, separation, divorce). The combination of personality, behavior, and mental health conditions requires complex treatment options facilitated by skilled and competent clinical military counselors. The following practitioner guidelines are offered for clinical consideration with the intentions of earning the circle of trust and building the therapeutic relationship:

- Monitor your reactions toward military clients who display problematic, toxic, and defensive behaviors. Clients whom you perceive as difficult or challenging to work with therapeutically can spark a range of feelings within you, such as incompetency, frustration, anger, or responding in an authoritarian manner.
- In progress (not process) notes, avoid labeling clients as defensive, resistant, hostile, noncompliant, or difficult to work with. Also, avoid clinical and diagnostic labels written into progress notes such as oppositional defiant disorder, argumentative, vindictive, and conduct disorder. Your competent and ethically derived comprehensive clinical assessment will likely document a diagnostic category (unless your client is an employee assistance program referral) that can be quite damaging to one's active-duty military career.
- In progress (not process) notes, provide a description of observable and nonjudgmental behaviors that the client exhibits within the session that may be perceived as defensiveness. Competent clinical military counselors approach all clients unconditionally and are keenly aware of issues of transference, countertransference, and other metacommunication that can diminish the therapeutic environment.
- Be mindful of who the therapist is in the room. Be proactive in deescalating unhealthy and maladaptive behaviors and leave some of your own problematic issues outside the therapeutic environment. Overall, avoid matching your behaviors and actions with your client's level of intensity.
- All feelings, thoughts, cognitions, experiences, and behaviors serve a function. For some, their defensiveness may serve as a conscious or unconscious coping mechanism. Competent clinical military counselors use client defensiveness as a personal growth opportunity. They facilitate strategies and approaches to deal therapeutically with the range of other issues that arise during one's session.

ELEMENTS OF THE MILITARY PERSON-CENTERED INTERVIEW

Because today's military demographically represents American culture in terms of gender, sexual identity, race, and ethnicity, it should be reiterated that there is not just "one" military culture. For some, the military appears primarily as a White male hypermasculine culture. The television and movie industry, as well as the electronic and print media, in part, help to form negative and positive perceptions and attitudes about individuals in uniform. As the first section of the book explains, there are societal myths and stereotypes that stigmatize service members, veterans, and families. The consequences of these myths and stereotypes have a psychological, emotional, social, vocational, educational, and family-relational cost to the individual. If the therapist directly or indirectly reinforces the military myths and stereotypes (e.g., all military members are warfighters, have PTSD, and are suicidal), then these issues can affect the therapeutic relationship. Thus, skilled practitioners have the awareness, knowledge, and skills to work competently with active-duty service members, veterans, veterans with disabilities, and military families.

Humanistic values are naturally embedded in any counseling theory and practice. Thus, therapists are not required to give up their values and personal worldview but rather anticipate and are aware of when a personal perspective may hinder the counseling process. In this section, I offer practitioners an overview of the foundational skills of the military interviewing and therapeutic process with the intention of earning the circle of trust and cultivating a strong working alliance. The following content areas of competence are offered as prerequisites for practitioners to place in their "go bag" for use within the military counseling process.

Apply the core competencies in multicultural counseling with the military culture. Everyone has a culture. Practitioners can begin by examining their cultural perceptions, beliefs, and attitudes about their military clients. Multicultural competencies require practitioners to examine their perceptions, beliefs, and attitudes toward race, gender, sexual orientation, religious and spiritual beliefs, as well as many other cultural attributes. This practice is particularly important when working with individuals in today's military, which has been described in previous chapters as more diverse than at any other time in American history. The intention for practitioners in exploring their cultural beliefs and perceptions is to ensure that their worldview does not hinder the counseling process. Even if you are a veteran mental health provider, your military life may be similar yet different than that of your clients on the basis of several cultural attributes (e.g., enlisted vs. officer rank, MOS, combat vs. noncombat operator, gender, race, ethnicity).

Differentiate among military, civilian, and community mental health core competencies in the assessment, diagnosis, and treatment of mental health disorders. Competent practitioners recognize salient aspects of military life by not imposing a generalist "one size fits all" approach to therapy. During the comprehensive clinical assessment, competent clinicians consider the cultural significance of issues related to the deployment cycle, chain of command, Uniform Code of Military Justice, and specific stressors associated with military life. Multiple other knowledge and skill areas can be acquired by practitioners through continuing education training opportunities as well as clinical experience that will inform cultural competence in military counseling.

Demonstrate an ongoing practice of attending, listening, and using cultural empathy. Attending, listening, and empathy have been the cornerstone of person-centered therapeutic interactions in Western counseling and psychology for quite some time. Competent and skilled clinical military counselors know how to adjust their attending, listening, and empathic responses for service members and veterans. If your expectations and the way in which you facilitate therapy are the same for both civilian and military mental health practice, then you have likely overlooked opportunities for facilitating therapeutic interactions within a multicultural military counseling context. For instance, level of client self-disclosure, silence during session, eye contact, body language, and metacommunication all matter in your attempts to earn the circle of trust with your military clients. Otherwise, they may feel "analyzed" or forced to disclose or retell their personal "war stories," which will likely be met with some levels of resistance or defensiveness. Ultimately, some of the most effective approaches involve the use of attending, listening deeply, cultural empathy, and communicating in a direct, honest, genuine, and unconditional manner while being mindful of all metacommunication.

Invite, encourage, and reinforce your military clients to talk at the level at which they are most comfortable. After many years of therapeutic interactions with active-duty service members, veterans, veterans with disabilities, and their families, I have found that they want to talk to a professional who has the capacity to understand their military life experience. Your military clients may communicate this desire to you both directly and indirectly. The anticipation is that many clients would like to change something about their feelings, cognitions, and experiences related to their personal and military life. Thus, you as the therapist—perhaps acting in the role of military life coach—have the opportunity now to be a part of the change that your client is inspired toward. During the rapport-building process, competent clinical military counselors avoid (a) asking multiple or closed-ended questions, (b) giving advice, and (c) performing a host of other interactions that can hinder the military client's sense of safety to disclose. In summary, competent clinical military counselors should do the following:

- Invite, encourage, and reinforce clients to talk and disclose at the level at which they feel most comfortable;
- Use good clarification, paraphrasing, and summarizing statements;

- Facilitate mostly open-ended questions to elicit client responses;
- Create a welcoming environment where clients feel safe to talk and disclose;
- Organize the office environment with appropriate lighting, low noise levels, artifacts, furniture, and décor as well as understand the therapeutic significance of creating a safe and confidential environment for military clients;
- Approach clients in a nonjudgmental and unconditional manner and communicate this acceptance both verbally and nonverbally;
- Demonstrate competence, professionalism, and ethical practices; and
- Facilitate the use of skillful observation and metacommunication while taking into consideration military mental health cultural practices.

EARNING THE CIRCLE OF TRUST THROUGH OPEN-ENDED QUESTIONS

Attending and listening are the challenging skills for clinicians to facilitate during therapeutic interactions with any type of clients. Skilled and competent clinical military counselors can acquire useful client information by asking minimal questions and facilitating the skills of attending, listening, and empathic responding through the use of clarifications, paraphrasing, and summarizing. Earning the circle of trust by using open-ended questions allows clients to elaborate and provide a clearer understanding of their problem issues. Good open-ended questioning is a strategy to gain optimal client information. The session will flow better and not be as disruptive as when the therapist asks a series of closed-ended demographic questions during the traditional intake interview or comprehensive clinical assessment. Multiple questions oftentimes can be misread by some clients as intrusive and can make them feel like they are being interrogated. This chapter focuses on rapport building and earning the circle of trust.

Of course, there are times when closed yes/no questions are useful. For example, asking the question "Did you experience these fears predeployment?" will provide you with some basic information regarding the onset and duration of such emotions. However, a follow-up, open-ended question or statement (e.g., "Help me understand how this affects you now") may provide you with information regarding frequency, duration, intensity, and the environments in which such feelings may occur with the individual. Overall, closed-ended questions provide limited information when you are trying to build rapport, particularly if you are trying to gather some basic information within a short period of time. The problems with closed-ended questioning used during the rapport-building process are described as follows:

- *What questions* most often lead to the person stating facts about a situation, a problem issue, or a significant life experience. For example, therapists who ask "What happened?" or "What are you going to do now?" can anticipate that clients will respond with basic content-related information rather than with feelings, emotions, and experiences.
- *How questions* most often lead to a discussion about processes, structure, organization, or sequences of significant life events. For example, therapists who ask "How did that happen?" or "How did you handle the situation?" can anticipate that clients will respond in a concrete manner and will "report" the event sometimes as an outside observer without acknowledging feelings, emotions, and experiences.
- *Why questions* most often lead to clients responding with a rationale or reason for why they responded or reacted to a situation. Many "why" questions are misread by the client as the therapist's projection of guilt or something that requires further justification. For example, therapists who ask "Why did you allow that to happen?" or "Why do you choose to do that?" can anticipate that their client may react defensively or feel some level of shame or remorse.
- *Could questions* are facilitative in nature and are considered open ended. This type of question allows clients to provide a range of responses that considers thoughts, cognitions, feelings, emotions, and experiences that will likely assist in bringing about awareness, understanding, and meaning to a problem issue.

Open-ended questions are the essence of effective interpersonal communication skills. These questions assist practitioners in evaluating problem issues using the most parsimonious approach. Practitioners should listen to the content, emotions, thoughts, and experiences expressed by the client, both verbally and nonverbally. During the client rapport-building process, practitioners can begin the evaluative process by asking some of the following open-ended questions:

- What brings you here to see me today?
- How did you choose to seek help at this time?
- What would you like to see get accomplished today?
- What more can you tell me about your situation?
- What else can you share to help me understand what you are trying to communicate to me?
- What current situations are happening now in your military life that make things more difficult for you (e.g., at home, while in service, as a veteran)?
- What has been your experience in talking with someone like me or another person (e.g., chaplain, unit sergeant) about these issues?

- Is our session moving in a mission-forward direction for you today?
- What do you feel would be the best tactical position right now to approach your problem issue?
- Given what you just stated, what flexibility do you have in your current plan?
- Is there anything else that comes to mind or that I may have missed that would assist me to support you?

THE MILITARY INTAKE INTERVIEW

Comprehensive clinical assessments are a vital part of ethical and competent clinical military counseling practice. This chapter emphasizes the importance of rapport building and earning the circle of trust before facilitating counseling strategies and therapeutic approaches, which requires having knowledge, awareness, and skills regarding the military culture, military families, military medical and mental health issues, stressors related to the deployment cycle, reintegration and transition, as well as other issues that are challenging in military life.

Skilled and competent clinical military counselors understand that building rapport and trust is an ongoing process. They are practiced and earned during each therapeutic encounter. Military clients, particularly those who are new to the counseling process, are prompted to share sensitive information, some of which may have never been disclosed to anyone else. The references cited at the end of this chapter contain recommendations and guidelines by counselor and psychology educators, researchers, clinicians, and other experts. Thus, becoming a skilled clinical military counselor requires an openness to the core essentials of active-duty, veteran, and military family life, recognizing the similarities and differences. Accordingly, culturally competent practitioners are sensitive and understand their military clients' verbal and nonverbal communication styles, their personal beliefs, as well as their values and philosophy about military life. Practitioners should also understand how their clients have assimilated, acculturated, and functioned overall within the culture, system, and organization of the military.

In this section, I provide sample assessment questions that relate specifically to vital areas concerning military life. The military intake interview offers structured guidelines to practitioners as a method for collecting essential material that can be utilized later during therapeutic interactions. The intention is to construct goals and interventions for optimal therapeutic outcome. The military intake interview presented in this section is not a substitute or replacement for your clinical setting's policy and guidelines for practice. Indeed, important demographic information is required during a comprehensive clinical assessment (e.g., health histories, coordination of care, professional disclosure statements). Additionally, these sample intake questions do not replace good diagnostic screening tools and standardized assessments required to make good decisions regarding client care.

Another point of distinction between military and civilian clients is that practitioners should not expect or anticipate full disclosure of information because of operational security reasons. Do not anticipate or expect your military clients to answer questions such as the following: "Where are you going to be deployed?" "What did you do on your deployment?" "Where is your next deployment?" The general categories of deployment-related questions that your military client might respond to are related in terms of (a) combat versus noncombat deployments, (b) humanitarian versus nonhumanitarian missions, or (c) military exercises inside the continental United States versus outside the continental United States. Various MOSs (e.g., counterintelligence, U.S. Marine Forces Special Operations Command, U.S. Army Special Forces) are mission sensitive, and the service member cannot disclose information because of confidentiality, operational security, or other areas that affect national security interests. Therefore, do not expect or force military clients to disclose various categories of information that may include—but are not limited to—the geographic location of their mobilization, deployment, or mission; the nature and extent of their work and what they did on their mission; and the types of tools, knowledge, machinery, weaponry, computer programs, or other materials that they dealt with while in garrison or in the combat theater of operations. Veterans may also be restricted from disclosing what they did in the military. Competent and skilled clinical military counselors understand that disclosure during the intake interview is not related to the military client's reluctance, resistance, or defensiveness.

Clinicians should also understand that female service members are more likely to experience physical and unwanted sexual advances, military sexual trauma (MST), and intimate partner violence at much higher rates than men. Thus, for military women, clinicians may want to integrate questions related to exposure to any previous interpersonal violence, particularly incidents of childhood or adult sexual abuse, harassment, or assault (either as a civilian or during training or while deployed). MST questionnaires oftentimes include questions such as the following:

- While in the military, did you receive uninvited and unwanted sexual attention, such as touching or cornering, pressure for sexual favors, or verbal remarks?
- Did someone ever use force or the threat of force to have sexual contact with you?

The service member's or veteran's perception and psychosocial response toward MST may vary. However, if the person responds in the affirmative to any of these questions, then further assessment and interpretation are warranted. Competent practitioners recognize the polytraumatic nature of these critical incidents along with the individual's coping and resiliency skills.

GENERAL INTAKE INTERVIEW SAMPLE QUESTIONS

The following sample intake interview questions are offered to practitioners as a way of gathering general information about their client's overall experiences while serving in the military:

- What is/was your MOS (U.S. Army and U.S. Marine Corps)?
- What is/was your rate (U.S. Navy pay grade) or rating (U.S. Navy occupational service)?
- What is/was your AFSC (U.S. Air Force Specialty Code)?
- What was/is your rank at the time of separation from service?
- Where did you do your basic training?
- What advanced training school have you completed?
- Do you have any academic work toward college credit, degrees, or certifications?
- Where did you earn these degrees (online vs. classroom)?
- Did you take classes while you were deployed?
- Do you use (or have you ever used) the U.S. Department of Veterans Affairs for services?
- Have you ever received mental health services before? Where (base chaplain, Military and Family Life Counseling Program)?

FAMILY-RELATED SAMPLE QUESTIONS

The following sample intake interview questions are offered to practitioners for inquiring about their client's family life experiences while serving in the military:

- Are you/were you married or dating during your time in the service (or during your deployment)?
- How did you communicate with family and friends (text, cell or satellite phone, Skype, Facebook)?
- How frequently did you communicate?
- How would you describe the quality of these interactions and communications?
- Were there any critical or stressful life events that happened while you were deployed or in the service?

DEPLOYMENT-RELATED SAMPLE QUESTIONS

The following sample intake interview questions are offered to practitioners for inquiring about their client's deployment experiences while serving in the military:

- Where were your deployments (combat, noncombat, humanitarian)?
- Do you remember any experiences that caused negative or disturbing memories?
- When you were deployed overseas, were you in a combat zone (relates to dismounted and mounted ground troops—infantry primarily), combat space (U.S. Navy and U.S. Air Force), forward operating base, or rear base?
- Did you go on combat missions and patrols or stand guard while doing your job?
- Have you ever been surrounded by the enemy? Blown up? Under fire?
- Have you witnessed the death or serious injury of anyone in your unit?
- Have you talked to anyone about these experiences?
- Are there any anniversary dates that you remember that are related to any critical or significant events while in service or things that occurred while deployed?
- Did you experience any unwanted sexual advances, intimidation, harassment, or assault?

These sample questions can assist practitioners during therapeutic engagements in several ways. The general intake questions may assist in developing MOS skills transferable to civilian occupations and educational goals based on your military client's training they received while in service. Earning a bachelor's or master's degree while in service, especially while deployed, certainly will address how well your client works under pressure or their aptitude to juggle various responsibilities. The family-related questions may assist practitioners with information regarding intimate relationships, separation, divorce, and how the service member dealt with or responded to these critical life events. The quality of communication provides practitioners with their client's interaction style but also information about how they experience and respond to interpersonal or intimate conflicts. The deployment-related questions may address the level of trauma exposure. The Combat Exposure Scale (Keane et al., 1989) may also assist as a screening instrument to determine the low, moderate, or high level of wartime stressors experienced by clients.

CONCLUDING REMARKS

The cornerstone of cultivating therapeutic relationships with the military culture is to facilitate practices in a safe and confidential setting where client self-disclosure is a natural part of the therapeutic process. Competent clinical military counselors recognize essential elements of military life and how to appraise optimal mental health functioning and wellness of service members, veterans, veterans with disabilities, and military families. Experienced clinicians also understand how to evaluate the psychosocial impact that the deployment cycle has on military service members and their families as well as other salient features of reintegration and transition to civilian life. The humanistic values embedded within the helping relationship require attunement to the foundations of attending, listening, and empathic responding with the intention of earning the circle of trust with your military clients.

REFERENCES

Adler, A. B., & Castro, C. A. (2013). An occupational mental health model for the military. *Military Behavioral Health, 1*(1), 41–51. https://doi.org/10.1080/21635781.2012.721063

Card-Mina, M. E. (2011, January–February). Leadership and post-traumatic stress symptoms. *Military Review,* 47–53. https://www.armyupress.army.mil/Portals/7/military-review/Archives/English/MilitaryReview_20110228_art009.pdf

Corey, M. S., & Corey, J. (2021). *Becoming a helper* (8th ed.). Cengage.

Egan, G., & Reese, R. J. (2019). *The skilled helper: A problem-management and opportunity-development approach to helping* (11th ed.). Cengage.

Hackney, H. L., & Cormier, S. (2017). *Professional counseling: A process guide to helping* (8th ed.). Pearson.

Ivey, A. E., Ivey, M. B., & Zalaquett, C. P. (2018). *Intentional interviewing and counseling: Facilitating client development in a multicultural society* (9th ed.). Cengage.

Kail, E. (2011, October 28). Leadership character: The role of empathy. *The Washington Post.* https://www.washingtonpost.com/blogs/guest-insights/post/leadership-character-the-role-of-empathy/2011/04/04/gIQAQXVGQM_blog.html

Keane, T. M., Fairbank, J. A., Caddell, J. M., Zimering, R. T., Taylor, K. L., & Mora, C. A. (1989). Clinical evaluation of a measure to assess combat exposure. *Psychological Assessment, 1*(1), 53–55. https://doi.org/10.1037/1040-3590.1.1.53

Parmar, B. (2016, December 13). *What to be more empathetic? Here's some advice from a Navy SEAL.* World Economic Forum. https://www.weforum.org/agenda/2016/12/what-a-navy-seal-can-teach-business-leaders-about-empathy/

Redmond, S. A., Wilcox, S. L., Campbell, S., Kim, A., Finney, K., Barr, K., & Hassan, A. M. (2015). A brief introduction to the military workplace culture. *Work, 50*(1), 9–20. https://doi.org/10.3233/WOR-141987

Rogers, C. R. (1951). *Client-centered therapy: Its current practice, implications, and theory*. Houghton Mifflin.

Rogers, C. R. (1980). *A way of being*. Houghton Mifflin.

Stebnicki, M. A. (2008). *Empathy fatigue: Healing the mind, body, and spirit of professional counselors*. Springer.

Stebnicki, M. A. (2016). Military counseling. In I. Marini & M. A. Stebnicki (Eds.), *The professional counselor's desk reference* (2nd ed., pp. 499–506). Springer.

Stebnicki, M. A. (2017). *Disaster mental health counseling: Responding to trauma in a multicultural context*. Springer.

Stebnicki, M. A., Clemmons-James, D., & Leierer, S. (2017). A survey of military counseling content and curriculum among Council on Rehabilitation Education- and Council for Accreditation of Counseling and Related Educational Programs-accredited programs. *Rehabilitation Research, Policy, and Education, 31*(1), 40–49. https://doi.org/10.1891/2168-6653.31.1.40

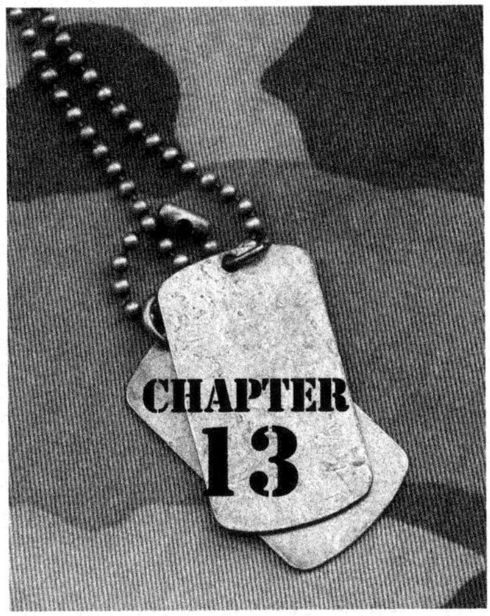

COMPLEX MILITARY PTSD AND CO-OCCURRING MENTAL HEALTH CONDITIONS

While we focus much of the research on PTSD we miss many of the equally high-risk co-occurring mental health disorders.

—Mark A. Stebnicki, 2020

★ ★ ★

Since the war on terrorism began in September 2001, more than 1.6 million U.S. troops have been deployed in support of Operation Iraqi Freedom (OIF) and Operation Enduring Freedom (OEF). These individuals have experienced more frequent and longer deployments than in any other wars overseas in U.S. history. Urban fighting takes place in an ambiguous lethal environment where the enemy combatants do not wear uniforms. Insurgents, Taliban soldiers, and other tribal fighters use unconventional warfare in a kinetic environment to inflict maximum casualties on U.S. service members through the use of improvised explosive devices, rocket-propelled grenades, snipers, and other small arms attacks. In the heat of the battle, service members are required to constantly keep their head on a swivel, stay alert on 2–4 hours of sleep per day, and maintain operation tempo in a mission-forward environment. There are no easy days.

As a result of improved body armor, cutting-edge emergency battlefield medicine, and advanced medical treatments and technology, many military service members and veterans have lived longer than in previous wars. Consequently, in more than 20 years of fighting the war on terrorism, the United States has experienced a new generation of military service members and veterans who have acquired clinically significant physical and psychological symptoms and conditions that are multidimensional in nature. The field of counseling and psychology is on the event horizon of a new complex trauma that has evolved because of surviving serious physical injuries (e.g., traumatic brain injury [TBI], blast wounds, amputation, chronic pain conditions). Additionally, the co-occurring mental health conditions of posttraumatic stress disorder (PTSD), anxiety, major depressive disorder, and substance use disorders (SUDs) are a natural fact of warfighting in the 21st century.

Historically, PTSD was rarely discussed in the early psychiatric military literature until *The Traumatic Neuroses of War* was published in 1941, authored by psychiatrist Abram Kardiner (Van Der Kolk, 2014). Kardiner's observations of World War I veterans exhibiting the clinically significant symptoms of withdrawal, detachment, depression, feelings of hopelessness, and helplessness gave way to the term "traumatic neuroses." Other terms have emerged in the literature since World War I, such as "war neurosis," "shell shock," and "battle fatigue."

The aim of this chapter is to highlight and delineate the multidimensional clinical characteristics of complex trauma. I differentiate between military and civilian trauma, and I discuss the co-occurring mental health conditions of adjustment disorder, anxiety, depression, insomnia, and SUDs. It is anticipated that most readers are licensed professionals who possess advanced skills in the diagnosis and treatment of mental health disorders. Thus, in the interest of page length and the breadth of other topics essential to articulate in *Clinical Military Counseling*, in this chapter I offer practitioner guidelines for evaluating and treating complex traumas.

PREVALENCE AND INCIDENCE OF MILITARY MENTAL HEALTH CONDITIONS

It has been estimated that between 20% and 30% of U.S. military personnel who served in OIF and OEF reported significant psychological symptoms 3–6 months after deployment (Adler et al., 2009; Liu et al., 2019). Unfortunately, according to mental health statistics, only one in three who served in OIF and one in five who served in OEF reported receiving mental health treatment (Bein et al., 2019). Approximately half of all service members in OIF and OEF who screened positive for a mental health condition ever sought mental health treatment as recommended by their postdeployment medical examination. The research in Chapter 2 related to the stigma of mental health treatment illuminates the multiple justifications why active-duty service members do not seek help (e.g., lack of trust of mental health providers, fear of losing security clearances and rank promotions, concerns that other unit members will see the person as weak or unfit for duty).

One statistic is clear in the mental health literature: Long-term physical and psychological health problems result from unrecognized, undertreated, or untreated mental health conditions. The consequence is poorer mental health outcomes, particularly for combat veterans. For instance, individuals deployed to combat operations who screened positive for posttraumatic stress symptoms (PTSSs), postdeployment, had significantly higher physical health problems than those without combat exposure. Those who were diagnosed with PTSD also had cardiovascular, dermatological, gastrointestinal, genitourinary, musculoskeletal, neurological, and pulmonary conditions requiring medical treatment (Wachen et al., 2013). Given the significant role of PTSSs and PTSD, competent military medical practitioners screen service members and veterans for several different physical, psychosocial, and mental health conditions that could potentially develop into chronic and severe health conditions.

When reporting statistics within the military medical, psychiatric, and mental health counseling literature, multiple issues do not accurately reflect the military culture. Issues of low sample size, mixing veteran data with data from active-duty personnel, and different interpretations of diagnostic criteria are just some of the methodological challenges. Accordingly, the prevalence and incidence of physical and mental health conditions are reported in ranges of low to high. The following items highlight the military medical, psychiatric, and mental health counseling concerns that hinder statistical reporting of facts among military trauma researchers:

- The literature reports that several mental health conditions have been found among active-duty personnel and veterans, which tend to cluster around positive screens for PTSD (14%–40%), major depressive disorder (5%–32%), anxiety (5%–25%), and SUDs (5%–40%; Bein et al., 2019; Buck, 2012; Cooper et al., 2018; Hitt & Massi Lindsey, 2020; J. K. Morgan et al., 2016; Rowan et al., 2020).
- Many researchers do not address adjustment disorders and do not distinguish them from other mental health conditions acquired during military service. Some researchers suggest that adjustment disorder is the most frequently diagnosed mental health condition among active-duty service members (Carta et al., 2009; P. Casey, 2009; Fielden, 2012; M. Morgan & Kelber, 2018).

- There are important statistical differences among mental health conditions, which vary by gender, sexual orientation, race, ethnicity, as well as other psychosocial factors.
- Civilian (nonmilitary) trauma oftentimes is generalized to military trauma. Although the general mind-body effects are similar, civilian and military trauma differ. Military trauma is mapped differently from a neurobiological and neurochemical perspective (see Chapter 4). Civilian and military trauma have been meshed together, in part, because of methodological design flaws, such as incorrectly mixing civilian and veteran samples as well as generalizing civilian trauma theory, constructs, and treatment to military mental health (Hitt & Massi Lindsey, 2020; Rowan et al., 2020).
- Data collected from samples of U.S. Department of Veterans Affairs (VA) patients are overrepresented in the military medical and mental health literature. VA patients tend to use physical and psychological services on a more frequent basis and represent a more chronic population. Thus, results and conclusions from some studies can be misleading.
- The U.S. Army tends to be overrepresented in sample sizes because it is the largest branch in the U.S. Armed Forces. Thus, proportionally, soldiers are seen in higher numbers at VA clinics and other military health facilities. Additionally, differences in mission, military occupational specialty (e.g., U.S. Army infantry vs. U.S. Air Force logistics), and rank (e.g., officer vs. enlisted) may account for statistical variations that cannot be generalized across all branches of service or across all active-duty service members and veterans.
- Limited research exists regarding the long-term effects of veteran mental health conditions in relation to combat exposure (e.g., low, moderate, and high ratings on the Combat Exposure Scale; Liu et al., 2019; Rowan et al., 2020). A small and emerging group of researchers are elucidating the long-term physical and psychological effects. This research is occurring, in part, because of (a) the mental health epidemic (e.g., veteran suicide, opioid use disorders), (b) private foundations and grant-based researchers who now have access to data from the U.S. Department of Defense (DoD) and the VA, and (c) the ongoing war on terrorism with more than 20 years of accumulated data.
- Most military personnel (58%) who reported physical health problems postdeployment also screened positive for a mental health condition (Britt et al., 2019).
- Researchers infrequently report mental health data in relation to the deployment cycle. Data on the intensity, frequency, and severity of mental health symptoms typically are divided into two groups: active-duty personnel and veterans. This information could be valuable for clinicians because of the considerations for multiple treatment factors, such as treatment readiness as well as adjustment to physical or mental health conditions.

Indeed, health care statistics are vital in making complex and important decisions about military physical and mental health care. Good research can assist clinicians with better standardized mental health screening and assessments, proper diagnosis, as well as prevention and treatment approaches that consider critical issues in the military community.

MILITARY ADJUSTMENT DISORDERS

Adjustment disorders are the most frequently diagnosed mental health condition among active-duty service members (Carta et al., 2009; P. Casey, 2009; Fielden, 2012; M. Morgan & Kelber, 2018). Adjustment disorders are multidimensional and multidetermined phenomena that can assist in delineating the unique clinical characteristics of complex PTSD. In the U.S. Army, adjustment disorders have been diagnosed in about 40% of active-duty service members admitted for psychiatric hospitalization and 43% attending outpatient mental and behavioral health treatment. As noted in the clinical diagnostic criteria, adjustment disorders are diagnosed within 3–6 months after the initial onset of a stressor. Thus, adjustment disorders are expected and anticipated to be resolved within 6 months of beginning treatment. Adjustment disorders can be ambiguous for many clinicians because the goals for treatment tend to focus on clinical symptoms related to anxiety and major depressive disorder. Despite the diagnostic category of a specifier (e.g., adjustment disorders with anxiety or with depression), the clinically significant symptoms of adjustment disorders typically do not resolve within 3–6 months.

Unlike posttraumatic stress (PTS) and other associated clinically significant symptoms, adjustment disorders occur when there is a presence of emotional or behavioral symptoms in response to an identifiable stressor, which can be a single incident or recurrent critical life events. Some examples are bereavement-related issues, termination of a romantic relationship, marital distress or separation, life-threatening illness, caregiver stress, being terminated from a job, or retirement. In the military culture, "retirement" may be managed as a medical separation from service. It also may be a separation from one's military career, in which transitioning from active duty to civilian life is indeed a major life adjustment. Both represent significant challenges to military personnel in transition that affect coping and resiliency skills, education and career goals, and family dynamics.

Adjustment disorders in military life are typically occupationally related and are not due to combat exposure. Combat operational stress and trauma exposure are more likely to result in positive screens for PTSD, major depressive disorder, anxiety, and SUDs. However, adjustment disorders indeed are considered a serious mental health disorder. Research in the civilian psychiatric literature has shown that 78%–96% of adults with an adjustment disorder who were admitted to inpatient psychiatric facilities reported suicidal ideation (Kryzhanovskaya & Canterbury, 2001).

The assessment, diagnosis, and treatment of adjustment disorders should be facilitated by a competent clinician. Developing the appropriate therapeutic goals and treatment strategies is important for a good therapeutic outcome. Adjustment disorders can be vague, pervasive, and nondiscrete for several reasons, including the following:

- The etiology or identification of the exact onset may mimic other mental health conditions, such as PTSD, major depressive disorder, and anxiety.
- The definition of adjustment disorders lacks clarity in the psychiatric and mental health literature. For some clinicians, adjustment disorders are not easily distinguishable from other diagnostic categories.
- Few studies exist in the behavioral health fields that delineate civilian versus military adjustment disorders and the salient characteristics that are clinically significant in the military culture.
- Longitudinal studies have indicated that service members with adjustment disorders continue to have persistent clinical symptoms 12 months after their diagnosis. In many cases, the mental health practitioner does not add a new diagnosis during the reevaluation period.
- Screening instruments to measure or evaluate adjustment disorders are lacking.
- There are multiple concerns regarding the diagnostic accuracy and inconsistency with applying the exact clinical features of adjustment disorders. This diagnostic category is now being questioned by insurers, clinicians, and administrators who are well aware of the generalized category capturing multiple other mental health conditions.
- Some clinical military counselors may avoid using other diagnostic categories (e.g., PTSD, SUD), believing that these conditions could jeopardize the service member's military career.
- Treatment protocols and interventions for adjustment disorders are not described in the clinical literature. The existing treatment for adjustment disorders mirrors that of other stress-related conditions and symptoms seen within the clinical setting.

Adjustment disorders in the military differ somewhat because of the nature of the occupation (e.g., frequent geographic relocations, multiple deployments, separation from family and friends). As a result of the identifiable stressor(s) and clinically significant symptoms, the following basic guidelines are offered to clinicians to integrate within their comprehensive clinical assessment:

- Are the symptoms and responses of the military service member or veteran a continuation of a previously diagnosed mental health condition (e.g., PTSD or major depressive disorder)?
- If the veteran has been medically separated from service because of a physical injury (e.g., back, neck, or knee injury) yet reports more substantial symptoms related to a mental health condition (e.g., PTSD, major depressive disorder, anxiety, insomnia), clinicians will want to rule out any significant mental health condition that if left untreated could lead to serious consequences (e.g., suicidality).
- If the veteran who is in transition reports clinically significant symptoms associated with other mental health conditions (e.g., depression, anxiety, insomnia), the veteran may be experiencing the normal and expected life stressors associated with transition. Thus, evaluation and therapeutic goals related to adjustment disorders may be warranted, which will enhance treatment outcomes.
- Veterans in transition (without a VA disability rating) who report chronic and persistent mental health symptoms should be reevaluated by the VA for the possibility of an undiagnosed, undertreated, or untreated mental health condition. If such a condition is not recognized by self and others, it could potentially lead to serious mental health outcomes (e.g., suicidality).
- If the veteran exhibits a normal reaction to an abnormal event (e.g., anniversary death of a unit buddy, other incidents of bereavement, intimate partner conflicts other than trauma) and an appropriate evaluation is completed, then the diagnosis and therapeutic goals of an adjustment disorder may be warranted.

Overall, multiple treatment algorithms can be consulted in various clinical references for assessment, diagnosis, and treatment of adjustment disorders. When evaluating adjustment disorders for military clients, it is important to understand the unique aspects of the military culture itself. Competent and skilled clinicians understand how to clinically evaluate and distinguish between time-limited mental health symptoms—such as those observed in adjustment disorders—and those that are chronic, persistent, and pervasive throughout one's lifetime. Ultimately, the goal is to choose appropriate treatment options for optimal healing.

MILITARY PTSD

The diagnostic category of PTSD has been reconceptualized by some military researchers as *complex PTSD*. This distinction has been made because of the serious co-occurring mental and physical health conditions associated with a range of extraordinary stressful and traumatic experiences in military life. The origins, constructs, and clinically significant criteria all relate to today's diagnostic category of PTSD in which criteria in the following domains are evaluated: (a) exposure; (b) intrusion; (c) persistent avoidance; (d) negative alterations in cognitions and mood; (e) marked alterations in arousal and reactivity; (f) duration; (g) clinically significant distress or impairment in social, occupational, or other critical areas of functioning; and (h) symptoms are not attributable to physiological effects of a substance or another medical condition.

Complex PTSD most commonly co-occurs with anxiety, major depressive disorder, sleep disorders, and SUDs. TBIs and blast injuries, known as the "signature injury" of OIF and OEF, frequently co-occur with PTSD (Elder et al., 2019). Even low-level blast exposure has been known to induce PTSD-related traits absent of any other psychological stressors (Perez-Garcia et al., 2019).

More recently in the military, there has been a focus on pre- and postdeployment screenings and assessments for PTSSs. The intention is to evaluate all significant mental health and co-occurring conditions (e.g., major depressive disorder, anxiety, and SUDs) that may require prevention or treatment approaches. The DoD has taken a strong stance on prevention approaches because of the association between PTSD—as well as other co-occurring mental health conditions—and suicidality. Unfortunately, active-duty service members who seek treatment for psychiatric problems sometimes risk notification up the chain of command, which poses significant occupational and career problems.

Many active-duty service members do not endorse the diagnostic category of PTSD because of the stigma attached to having a "disorder." Moreover, having a medical record of PTSD may hinder one's military career, such as not being promoted, losing security clearances, and not being able to carry weapons. However, according to Standard Form 86, Section 21—which asks about one's psychological and emotional health—service members or other government service workers who have had mental health counseling cannot be denied, or have revoked, their security clearance for access to a classified position handling sensitive information (Misener, 2017). Yet, there are strongly held beliefs among those employed by the DoD and the U.S. Armed Forces that such a perception exists regarding concern for security clearances and promotions.

The terms PTS and PTSSs are preferable when addressing mental health problems with active-duty service members. The term PTS normalizes the combat experience for many service members who can relate to being in a state of hypervigilance as well as having intrusive thoughts, memories of unit members being blown up, wake-sleep disturbances, feelings of depression and sadness, and the intense prolonged mind-body effects that are associated with being in the epicenter of warfighting.

It is important to note that unrecognized, untreated, or undertreated chronic and persistent PTS can escalate into a diagnosis of PTSD. Active-duty personnel who have chronic, persistent, and severe mental and behavioral health issues are typically separated from service by being forced out either voluntarily or involuntarily. Those who have mental, cognitive, and behavioral health issues are sometimes given a less-than-honorable or dishonorable discharge. Conversely, service members who are separating from military service and going through the medical board examination are encouraged to report and document all physical and psychiatric conditions that are service connected. A well-documented medical record of any service-connected disabilities assists veterans in receiving the appropriate level of earned pay and benefits associated with their military service. Thus, the DoD's disability rating and classification system exists to assist veterans with any physical and mental health conditions requiring long-term treatment.

Active-duty personnel have no incentives to report any physical or psychiatric symptoms while in military service. This finding has been corroborated by multiple studies that have shown the negative impact of mental health treatment on the service member's military career. In one particular study, Ghahramanlou-Holloway et al. (2018) examined the career effects of U.S. Marines seeking mental health treatment and found that approximately 38% of active-duty Marines held a belief that seeking mental health treatment would damage their military career. Likewise, 26% of Marines who sought mental health treatment within the past year reported that attending mental health counseling had a negative impact on their careers. Treatment-seeking Marines were also more heavily scrutinized in their jobs than non-treatment-seeking Marines. Of those Marines who received mental health treatment, many experienced legal actions because of behavioral health problems (e.g., SUDs, domestic violence, physical assault; Ghahramanlou-Holloway et al., 2018).

Despite the seriousness of chronic and persistent PTS, mental health resources are lacking for their prevention and treatment among service members deployed overseas (Ogle et al., 2012). Military installations or forward operating bases located in hostile enemy territories are not places for attending psychotherapy sessions. Thus, dealing with combat operational stress, in the short term, is generally perceived as a unit function in which behavioral health assets can provide the expertise to serve as a resource.

The unit itself may be the measuring stick for pervasive mental health problems that exist among its service members, such as those who have returned from combat patrol. Mental health assessments may be required for triaging more serious mental health symptoms (e.g., anxiety disorders, suicide threats) throughout battlefield circulation. In some combat units or platoons, PTS may be experienced as secondary PTS by service members. The clinically significant symptoms may be related to hearing stories or seeing combat casualties. PTS may also relate to unit morale issues, reduction in combat personnel, supply line and logistic problems, the length of unit personnel rotation, or other force sustainment issues.

There are some distinct differences between military and civilian PTSD and how trauma is assessed, diagnosed, and treated. For instance, many military PTSD researchers have suggested that some of the diagnostic criteria may not fit well into the military culture (Adler & Castro, 2013; Kilpatrick et al., 2013; Roitman et al., 2013). For instance, clinical protocols, algorithms, and decision trees do not consider multiple traumas acquired through military service. Thus, military and civilian PTSD differ because of the following unique aspects: (a) multiple trauma exposures on multiple combat missions during battlefield circulation; (b) several deployments that can occur within a short period of time; (c) witnessing, hearing about, or experiencing multiple loss-of-life episodes as a result of combat casualties; (d) the experience of a repeated cycle of grief, death, dying, and loss; and (e) remaining in an environment where the threat of bodily harm and witnessing physical injury and death may result in daily or weekly traumatic stressors.

THE EXPERIENCES OF COMBAT OPERATIONAL STRESS AND TRAUMA

Considerable psychosocial adjustment issues are related to military service members and veterans across the life span. These issues are due, in part, to the high-risk nature of the military as an occupation that can negatively affect the individual's physical and psychological health and well-being. Experiences of combat and operational stress are well documented in the military medical and psychological literature (France, 2018; Hoge et al., 2004; Kolbow et al., 2007; Tick, 2014). The consequences of these traumatic experiences typically exceed the service member's capacity for coping with the physical or psychological fitness standards to the point where some may be deemed "not suitable for duty." Consequently, just one of the following traumatic experiences places the service member or veteran in a higher risk category for complex PTSD:

- Experiencing the serious injury or death of a friend;
- Viewing dead or seriously injured noncombatants;
- Witnessing an accident resulting in serious injury or death;
- Smelling decomposing bodies;
- Being physically moved or knocked over by an explosion;
- Sustaining an injury not requiring hospitalization;

- Sustaining a blow to the head from any accident or injury;
- Sustaining an injury requiring hospitalization;
- Engaging in hand-to-hand combat;
- Witnessing brutality toward detainees or prisoners;
- Being responsible for the death of a civilian;
- Killing enemy combatants;
- Handling or uncovering human remains;
- Being attacked or ambushed;
- Receiving incoming artillery, rocket, or mortar fire; or
- Experiencing a close call.

Warfighters are trained to "aggress not stress" during combat operations. The life and safety of others in the unit depend on the service member's quick and decisive action to eliminate hostile actors. This responsibility is partly due to the operation tempo or pace within the mission-forward environment. When a unit buddy becomes injured or dies, there is no time to grieve the loss. For some, the delayed grief reactions and traumatic stressors may be deferred until postdeployment, reintegration, or transition. Many combat operators hold tight to their training of "suck it up," "we are the tip of the spear," or "possessing an inner warrior identity." However, trauma does not care about the messaging and motivations. From a biophysiopsychological experience, trauma becomes the persistent avoidance of distressing triggers; intrusive thoughts; dissociative reactions; flashbacks; and the symptoms associated with wake-sleep disorders, major depressive disorder, anxiety, and SUDs. In military trauma, these symptoms and conditions have a delayed reaction that follows the service member to some degree of intensity throughout civilian life.

The following items are important to consider in the overall screening, assessment, and treatment of PTS and PTSD experienced throughout the deployment cycle:

- Perceptions of extraordinary stressful and traumatic events vary across different individual factors, such as age; military experience; prior exposure to other traumatic events; frequency of deployments; critical incidents while on deployment; previous and current mental and physical health; level of coping and resiliency skills; and the overall meaning, perception, and attitude toward a variety of critical events experienced.
- A parallel experience of trauma or secondary traumatic stress exists for some within the military family or unit, particularly for those deployed to a combat theater. The mental health of the unit and its command is critical for maintaining cohesiveness, operation tempo, and sustainability. Just as in the civilian workplace culture, there are toxic and sick work environments. The major difference is that military service members cannot leave work or quit their job when things go bad.

- In traditional clinical (nonmilitary) settings, if the clinical features of one or more traumatic events last beyond 30 days, and the symptoms become chronic and persistent, then the diagnostic category of PTSD would be most appropriate. Any clinically significant symptoms before 30 days are considered acute stress disorder. Clinical military counselors will have to weigh the risks and benefits of diagnosis among active-duty service members as well as their ethical obligations in treating clients.
- Mental health practitioners must consider the clinical environment in which screening, diagnosis, and treatment are being facilitated: on a U.S. military base, on a forward operating base, or in a military treatment facility. Postdeployment screenings for PTSD and depression, such as the Post-Deployment Health Assessment (Warner et al., 2011), are typically completed immediately at the end of a deployment, before leaving the country where they have been deployed, or when the service member arrives home stateside. An important element to consider in the use of standardized screening tools is that pre- and postdeployment screening tools depend on the service member's honesty and motivations for reporting clinically significant symptoms that may be associated with PTSD.
- Several other programs are notable regarding systematic assessment of service members' expression of PTSD and other serious co-occurring mental health disorders. One example is the Battlemind training program described by Adler et al. (2009) and Foran et al. (2013). This program was designed to target service members who exhibit high-risk behaviors after deployment. The focus relates to the transition home and deals with specific issues related to safety; interpersonal, social, and intimate relationships; and the clinically relevant symptoms of combat operational stress. The interested reader should consult the reference section. However, the key point is that early intervention and prevention programs can assist service members and veterans with the intensity and frequency of symptoms acquired during warfighting.
- Approximately half of all mental and behavioral health problems among active-duty personnel go unrecognized and untreated. The issue is compounded by the negative stigma toward seeking mental health treatment. For the reserve component, untreated, undertreated, or unrecognized mental and behavioral health problems are typically much higher than for service members on military installations. Resiliency programs—such as Mental Health First Aid (Mohatt et al., 2017), the Comprehensive Solider Fitness Program (G. W. Casey, 2011), and the U.S. Army's Comprehensive Solider & Family Fitness 2 (https://readyandresilient.army.mil/CSF2/index.html)—as well as other

prevention, mental health detection, and psychoeducational approaches have significantly decreased the long-term effects associated with PTSD and co-occurring disorders. Such prevention approaches also assist in destigmatizing PTSD, particularly if they are endorsed by the chain of command. Thus, education and prevention within the military culture empowers the individual with good coping and resiliency resources.

ANXIETY DISORDERS IN THE MILITARY

The Armed Forces Health Surveillance Center (2013) indicated that between 2000 and 2012, anxiety-related medical visits by active-duty service members increased by more than 500%. Most medical visits at military treatment centers have resulted in a diagnosis of "nonspecific" anxiety disorder, which accounts for 75% of anxiety disorders. Only about one third of service members have a co-occurring diagnosis, such as major depressive disorder or adjustment disorder. Anxiety disorders are highest among service members who are female and White. Researchers have documented that anxiety disorders are associated with a variety of medical conditions, such as irritable bowel syndrome, asthma, migraines, sleep disorders, and memory dysfunction (Shelef et al., 2016). This co-occurring mind-body condition has a complex set of clinically significant symptoms that require proper medical and mental health evaluation and diagnosis to achieve the optimal treatment.

Anxiety disorders in the military overlap with some other diagnostic features of PTSD. Previously, PTSD was listed under the diagnostic category of anxiety disorders in the *Diagnostic and Statistical Manual of Mental Disorders* (4th ed.; American Psychiatric Association, 1994). Anxiety disorders, if left untreated, can escalate to the high end of the anxiety-risk continuum and morph into panic reaction, specific phobias (e.g., agoraphobia, obsessive-compulsive disorder), or a trauma and stressor-related disorder such as PTSD. Many service members and veterans who have anxiety disorders express their emotions and behaviors in maladaptive ways, such as exhibiting impulsive anger, rage, and fear. Even a generalized or nonspecific anxiety disorder can have major physical and psychological consequences for the service member or veteran.

Anxiety disorders are high among combat service members. Grossman (2009) has suggested that in his warfighting experience, there is an intense resistance to killing another person that becomes so intense that some combat infantrymen would rather die on the battlefield. There are documented reports of service members not firing their weapons (15%–20% in World War II, 45% in the Korean War, and 5%–10% in the Vietnam War). Thus, training military recruits with human-shaped targets on the firing range, and rewarding or recognizing them as expert marksmen, can reduce or desensitize combat personnel to the resistance to killing another person.

Although service members who have low levels of combat exposure may exhibit less anxious behaviors, the mind-body sensory connection still signals some level of fear or anxiety. Generalized anxiety disorders, if left untreated, can develop into more serious physical and mental health conditions in military and civilian life. Multiple situations place service members or veterans in harm's way, putting them into a higher risk category. These situations include—but are not limited to—deployment to harsh physical environments, getting only 2–4 hours of sleep each day, separation from family with little or no communication, as well as other stressors that create mood and anxiety disorders. The consequence can be disabling and can compromise good physical and mental health, particularly as the service member transitions to veteran status (Buck, 2012; Ysasi et al., 2016).

Fear is the emotional response to a real or perceived imminent threat (e.g., your jumpmaster tells you to exit the plane *now* in enemy territory), whereas anxiety is the anticipation of a future threat (e.g., flying 18 hours or floating 30 days outside of the continental United States to a rear or forward base of operations). Indeed, there is a biopsychological cost to the fear and anxiety of killing another human or being confronted with being injured or killed. The sympathetic arousal system sets into motion the fight-or-flight response, triggering a host of neurobiological responses in which substantial elevations in epinephrine, norepinephrine, cortisol, heart rate, respiration, blood pressure, and amygdala activation take place. Although the military brain is mapped for "fight not flight" and "aggress not stress," combat operational stress prompts the basic building blocks for mapping the emotions of anxiety and fear.

Predeployment psychological screenings are an important aspect of being mission ready after months of training for various special operations. However, even the best psychological screening instruments can become problematic when trying to assess personnel who are "fit for duty." This difficulty is because most service members (79%) do not report any mental health problems during predeployment psychological screenings (Wright et al., 2005). This denial is related to military stigma and career-related obstacles to seeking mental health treatment. Interestingly, on pre- and postdeployment medical screenings, most service members (58%) who seek help for a physical health condition also screen positive for a mental health condition (Britt et al., 2019). Thus, one could conclude that going to the medical versus mental health practitioner is more acceptable within the military community.

The following items are important to consider in the overall screening, assessment, and treatment of anxiety disorders experienced throughout the deployment cycle:

- Benzodiazepines have historically been used to treat anxiety disorders because of their sedative characteristics. However, clinical guidelines for military medical prescribers have multiple layers of restrictions associated with the use of any anxiolytics. These restrictions are because of the potential side effects of cognitive impairment, psychomotor incoordination, respiratory depression, as well as the risk of dependency and overdose. These issues particularly become important when assessing the service member's physical and mental fitness for deployment. Little evidence exists for the efficacy of anxiolytics for active-duty service members. Moreover, service members must be weaned off all medications, with a few exceptions, prior to deployment. The use of anxiolytics has also become a significant mental health treatment issue within the VA health care system.
- Encourage clients to seek appropriate medical evaluation for all reported symptoms that may be related to their experience of anxiety. Given the complex somatic nature of anxiety disorders, partnering with medical practitioners is vital to maintaining appropriate physical and mental health and well-being.
- Several evidence-based psychotherapy treatments, as well as complementary and alternative approaches, have been well documented to successfully treat anxiety disorders. These strategies should be adapted for the service member's personal needs within the deployment cycle. Latent anxiety disorders occur for some service members transitioning to civilian life. The traditional approaches of cognitive behavioral therapy (CBT), acceptance and commitment therapy, emotional freedom techniques, mindfulness-based stress reduction, and breathing meditation have been demonstrated to reduce the symptoms of anxiety. In addition, some behavioral health approaches—which include recreational activities and exercise (not physical therapy); good nutrition; getting connected with social supports; and eliminating or reducing smoking, drinking alcohol, or consuming large quantities of caffeine—can also lower anxiety symptoms. Finally, resiliency approaches—such as expressive arts, animal-assisted therapy, yoga, and other mind-body activities—have also successfully lessened anxiety in the military community.

MAJOR DEPRESSIVE DISORDER IN THE MILITARY

Depression in both civilian and military life is a common occurrence. It is one of the most frequently diagnosed and treated conditions in the medical and mental health settings. Depression is both a physiological and psychological condition that results in limitations of cognitive, social, independent, psychosocial, and vocational functioning (Falvo & Holland, 2018). Major depression commonly co-occurs with several other chronic illnesses and disabilities, which include—but are not limited to—TBI, spinal cord injury, chronic pain conditions, cardiovascular diseases, neurodegenerative and neuromuscular diseases (e.g., multiple sclerosis, amyotrophic lateral sclerosis, Parkinson's disease, dementia, Alzheimer's disease), diabetes, and other endocrine disorders (Falvo & Holland, 2018; Harley, 2018; Livneh & Antonak, 2018). Major depression frequently occurs among veterans age 55 years and older; in addition, patients being treated for dysthymia and depression are more likely to develop dementias than veterans not being treated (Byers et al., 2012).

Depression commonly co-occurs with TBI (Chapman & Diaz-Arrastia, 2014; Elder et al., 2019). Approximately 10%–20% of veterans deployed to Iraq and Afghanistan sustained a TBI (DePalma, 2015; Elder et al., 2010), but more than 80% went undocumented (Chase & Nevin, 2015). Major depressive disorder may be underreported because it co-occurs with and can sometimes be masked by the clinical symptoms associated with grief, loss, and bereavement (Stebnicki, 2018). Overall, the diagnostic category of major depressive disorder is likely underreported in the military and is prone to having multiple underlying conditions that co-occur with other physical health ailments.

Because of the experience of loss, grief, and bereavement sustained in military life, it may be difficult for some medical and mental health practitioners to distinguish between major depressive disorder and other psychosocial issues that pose clinical concerns (Stebnicki, 2018). Generally, a major depressive episode is a chronic, persistent, and pervasive emotion that has clinically significant symptoms present on most days. The complex symptoms associated with major depressive episodes (e.g., sadness, hopelessness, low self-concept, loss of interest or pleasure in many life areas, changes in appetite, sleep disturbance, suicidal thoughts) can develop over one's lifetime.

Diagnostically, major depression is subjective and is based on the severity index of mild, moderate, and severe with either single or recurrent episodes. Conversely, grief is typically associated with a specific event of loss but can co-occur with other positive feelings (e.g., remembering the positive traits of the individual who has died). Grief itself is a multidimensional or multidetermined phenomenon. Individual cultural traits, personality states and traits, and multiple psychosocial stressors are associated with the feelings and experience of grief. Thus, persistent and complex bereavement is expressed somewhat differently than depression. Grief experienced in military life is a normal response to abnormal events (e.g., dying as a result of enemy combatants, watching the death of a unit buddy getting blown up or burned alive).

All episodes of depression, dysthymia, and bereavement should be taken seriously by medical and mental health practitioners. The research on military suicide presents a clear picture that major depressive disorder places service members and veterans in a higher risk category for suicidal ideation, lethal attempts, and completions. The following items are important to consider in the overall screening, assessment, and treatment of major depressive disorder and persistent complex bereavement disorders experienced throughout the deployment cycle:

- Comprehensively assess and differentiate depression from traumatic bereavement disorders. Evaluate these conditions within the cultural lens of active-duty service members, veterans, and veterans with disabilities. The differential diagnoses of normal grief, major depressive disorder, PTSD, and anxiety require closer analysis, inquiry, and consultation with more seasoned clinicians.
- Consideration of the service member's or veteran's physical and psychological health is of paramount importance. Multiple medical conditions (e.g., hyperthyroidism, hypothyroidism, diabetes) mimic mental health disorders such as major depression. In today's military health care system, military treatment providers are mandated to coordinate medical and psychological services to benefit patient care. Thus, partnering and coordinating treatment goals ultimately improves the physical and mental health of service members and veterans.
- Differentiate substance use–induced mood disorders from the diagnostic criteria of major depressive disorder. A comprehensive clinical assessment can reveal the etiology, critical incidents, and history of the mental health condition(s) under consideration for treatment.
- Because of the overlapping symptoms of depression and multiple other conditions, choosing the appropriate treatment strategies is vital for optimal mental health functioning. In addition to evidence-based practices (e.g., CBT), behavioral health strategies (e.g., nutrition; exercise; reduction or elimination of caffeine, tobacco, or alcohol use) and complementary and alternative practices (e.g., yoga, meditation, animal-assisted therapy, expressive arts) can also increase overall wellness.

INSOMNIA IN THE MILITARY

The incidence of clinically diagnosed insomnia and obstructive sleep apnea in the U.S. military rose dramatically between 1997 and 2011. In fact, between 2003 and 2011, the incidence of insomnia rose 652% and sleep apnea rose 600% (Cadwell et al., 2019). There is a strong association between combat deployments and sleep-wake disorders that deserves clinical attention among military service members and veterans. Sleep-wake disorders encompass 10 separate disorders, with insomnia being the most characteristic within the military population.

The lack of quantity and quality of sleep is part of military training and is pervasive among service members for whom 2–4 hours of sleep is common during combat deployments. Insomnia can become a fixed pattern of physiological, behavioral, cognitive, emotional, and psychological functioning. The pervasiveness of insomnia among military service members should be disconcerting to unit command. The lack and quality of sleep have a cost in terms of psychomotor and neurocognitive functioning in service members. The consequences of insomnia also limit service members in other ways, such as deficits in memory, attention, focus, and concentration. The clinical features of insomnia can have life-threatening consequences for those in an occupation that demands total focus and attention.

Researchers have documented numerous long-term physical and psychological illnesses associated with sleep-wake disorders. Some of these illnesses include hypertension, diabetes, obesity, heart attack, stroke, and chronic pain conditions. Multiple mental health disorders are associated with insomnia, such as depression, anxiety, SUDs, PTSD, and suicidality. Thus, long-term sleep-wake disorders over one's lifetime have the potential to be an underlying and contributing factor to veteran mortality (Swinkels et al., 2013; Troxel et al., 2015; Wright et al., 2011).

The following items are important considerations in the overall screening, assessment, and treatment of wake-sleep disorders—particularly insomnia—experienced throughout the deployment cycle:

- Troxel et al. (2015), as well as other DoD-funded studies, have provided a wealth of research and practitioner guidelines for assessing, treating, and promoting good sleep hygiene with service members and veterans. Clinical military counselors can administer multiple self-report and screening sleep measures to clients. Readers should consult the resources found in the reference section at the end of this chapter.
- Over-the-counter antihistamines are the most used products for insomnia. The most common physician-prescribed medications to treat insomnia are traditional benzodiazepines (e.g., alprazolam, diazepam) and a newer class of benzodiazepines (e.g., zolpidem, zaleplon). Despite side effects, prescribers have found these medications effective in the frontline treatment of insomnia and other wake-sleep disorders.
- As with other mental health disorders, a comprehensive clinical assessment should evaluate any physical and co-occurring mental health disorders that present problems in the daily life of service members and veterans for optimal healing and treatment.
- It has been reported that CBT is effective in treating insomnia. In addition, some studies have reported that CBT is just as effective in treating sleep-wake disorders as pharmacological products (e.g., Troxel et al., 2015). Good sleep hygiene habits have also been effective in treating insomnia disorders (e.g., low or no light-emitting diode lights from clocks and TVs in the bedroom, proper room temperature adjusted individually, breathing meditation).

- Complementary and alternative medical and mental health treatments have been effective in treating insomnia. These approaches include—but are not limited to—mindfulness-based stress reduction, meditation, visualization, as well as a host of other behavioral health approaches (e.g., exercise, nutrition, reduction or elimination of tobacco and alcohol use).
- Medical and mental health practitioners should focus part of their comprehensive clinical assessment on substance misuse because of the overuse of alcohol as a self-prescribed method of treating insomnia during military life. SUDs often develop as an unhealthy coping strategy because of wake-sleep disorders and other stressors acquired during military life.

SUBSTANCE USE IN THE MILITARY

The relationship between trauma and SUDs is well documented in the medical, mental health, and substance use literature. Medical and mental health practitioners should not assume that trauma causes SUDs. The biopsychosocial nature of SUDs is more complex and cannot be reduced to a direct association between trauma and SUDs, in part, because SUDs are multidimensional in nature and involve one's core cultural values and beliefs regarding use of substances. The level of stress associated with one's occupation is also a contributing factor to substance use. Items such as behavioral lifestyle, personality traits, previous trauma experiences, and family members' history of use and abuse should be identifiable to clinicians. Thus, skilled and competent clinical military counselors know how to assess and predict low- and high-risk behaviors as well as client histories that predispose the individual to SUDs.

Trauma researchers have suggested that trauma exposure and SUDs are co-occurring mental health conditions that can (a) precede each other, (b) follow each other, (c) contribute to the development or course of PTSD and other disorders, and (d) be acquired independently of one another (Burke & Carruth, 2012). Exposure to trauma per se does not necessarily increase the risk of developing an SUD. Rather, SUDs are a contributing factor with other co-occurring mental health conditions (e.g., depression, anxiety, sleep-wake disorders) and psychosocial stressors (e.g., divorce, loss of a unit buddy, blast wound or TBI). Mental health and substance abuse counselors advocate for integrative treatment approaches in which each medical and mental health partner has expertise in treating primary and secondary conditions. Many state licensing boards over the last 20 years have created a separate clinical addiction specialist license. This classification is based, in part, on the rationale that addictions require specific knowledge, skills, and advance training to assess, diagnose, and treat. Ideally, all medical and mental health specialists should have a range of skills to treat clients. Overall, clients benefit from integrative behavioral health approaches in which competent practitioners can treat SUDs with other co-occurring mental health conditions that significantly affect the person's life along the developmental continuum.

SUDs are particularly relevant issues for service members and veterans who may be masking trauma, depression, anxiety, wake-sleep, or chronic pain disorders. Substance use and co-occurring disorders among service members are just one of the challenges that the military has had since the war on terrorism began in 2001. In response, the military has increased its attention and focus on improving optimal physical and mental health among service members and veterans. The following findings help present an overview of the problem and the military's response to SUDs (Butler Center for Research, 2018; National Center for PTSD, n.d.):

- Military populations experience a significantly higher rate of PTSD and SUDs than civilian populations.
- Service members who were deployed to Iraq and Afghanistan met the criteria for alcohol use disorder (58%) and PTSD (63%).
- Veterans with PTSD and alcohol use disorder had significantly elevated rates of major depression (37%), generalized anxiety disorder (44%), suicidal ideation (39%), and lethal attempts (46%).
- More than 27% of veterans receiving care from the VA are diagnosed with PTSD and SUDs.
- Because of reporting issues, approximately 10%–40% of veterans who served in Iraq and Afghanistan have an SUD.
- PTSD tends to increase opioid use disorders. These co-occurring disorders increased dramatically between 2004 and 2013.
- The most effective treatments for SUDs include relapse prevention, CBT, trauma-focused therapy programs, and treatment for specific symptoms such as chronic pain, anger, and insomnia.

Other research studies outside the DoD have provided a much different picture regarding military SUDs and co-occurring mental health conditions. For instance, the National Health Interview Survey from 2013 to 2017 compared alcohol consumption of the U.S. Armed Forces with other professions (Centers for Disease Control and Prevention [CDC], 2018). In a survey of 27,000 individuals across 25 different categories of occupations and industries (e.g., mining, construction, agriculture, utility work, manufacturing, professional, technical), using the average number of days per year alcohol was consumed by the individual, the CDC reported that the U.S. Armed Forces consumed more alcohol (130 days per year) in comparison with any other occupation. The next highest ranked occupations or industries were mining (112 days per year) and construction (106 days per year). The lowest alcohol consumption on the list was among health care and social service industry workers (68 days per year).

Alcohol use is part of the induction into the military culture, which is also marked by the initiation of heavy nicotine use, binge drinking, and prescription drug misuse (National Institute on Drug Abuse, 2019). Many researchers have suggested that veterans abuse alcohol at much higher rates than nonveterans. The Treatment Episode Data Set (Substance Abuse and Mental Health Services Administration, 2015) indicates that veterans were more likely than nonveterans to seek admission to inpatient alcohol treatment (non-VA) centers. Veteran inpatients were more likely than nonveterans to report alcohol as their primary substance of abuse (65% vs. 37% of nonveterans) and were less likely to report needing treatment for marijuana (6% vs. 13% of nonveterans) or heroin (11% vs. 21% of nonveterans).

Some researchers have shown that the rates of SUDs and co-occurring mental health problems are not unique to the military. Using samples of active-duty service members and civilians, Witkiewitz and Estrada (2011) indicated that the rates of alcohol use and binge drinking (≥5 consecutive drinks for men; ≥4 consecutive drinks for women) were similar across military and civilian populations. This study further showed that 70% of military service members who were previously deployed averaged 3 drinks per day with 3 days per week of binge drinking, compared with civilians who exhibited 4 drinks per day with 3 days per week of binge drinking. The notable difference was in regard to illicit drugs used in the military (2%) versus civilian illicit drugs use, which was significantly higher.

One major difference in military versus civilian SUDs is the cost to one's career. In fact, Article 112a in the punitive articles of the Uniform Code of Military Justice indicates that SUDs, particularly the use of illicit drugs, are punishable by court martial. If the accused service member is found "drunk while on duty" in violation of Article 112a, they may face a maximum punishment of 9 months confinement, a bad conduct discharge, and forfeiture of all allowances and pay (Joint Service Committee on Military Justice, 2019). There are some loopholes in Article 112a (e.g., persons not on duty and found to be elsewhere in a drunken state cannot be charged because they are not performing in their "official" capacity). Active-duty personnel should pursue expert legal advice to determine the extent of their violation and understand their legal options because of new case law affecting an Article 112a judgment or decision.

Besides the maximum consequence of a court martial, command has several rehabilitative efforts at their disposal for active-duty service members who test positive for any of the drugs mentioned earlier. The chain of command may refer active-duty personnel for a mandated drug and alcohol assessment completed by a qualified licensed mental health practitioner or clinical addiction specialists. At this point, a determination will be made by command according to the DoD's problematic substance abuse policy (DoD, 2014). The response from command can range anywhere from mandatory treatment to a less-than-honorable or dishonorable discharge.

The DoD requires all branches of the U.S. Armed Forces to conduct random urinalysis drug screening to detect and deter drug use among active-duty service members. As for those who would like to enlist, the U.S. Military Entrance Processing Command (https://www.mepcom.army.mil/About-Us/) has the task of determining the mental, physical, and moral fitness of every new member in the U.S. Armed Forces. Multiple disqualifying conditions restrict enlistment in military service. Thus, minimum qualifications must be met for those who would like to serve in the U.S. military, and individuals who are in active addiction or who have a record of SUD treatment are not eligible. To increase the screening mechanism of SUDs in the military, the U.S. Military Entrance Processing Command now tests for 26 different types of drugs. These drugs include a wide range of illicit and controlled substances such as amphetamines, cocaine, ecstasy or MDMA, heroin, synthetic cannabinoids, LSD (lysergic acid diethylamide), marijuana, methamphetamine, opium, street drugs such as spice and bath salts, as well as prescription medications.

Many active-duty and veteran clients whom I have treated have indicated that "my military service [name the branch] helped me refine my drinking skills," which suggests a long-term pattern of substance use and abuse preenlistment. The long-term physical and mental health effects of SUDs are no joking matter. The substantial negative consequences of SUDs among service members are a clear and present danger that escalates to the high end of the risk continuum. First, SUDs significantly affect the physical and psychological health of the service member. Second, SUDs have a major negative effect on work performance, mission readiness, and social and familial relationships within the military culture. All factors make for a combination of high-risk behaviors that have the potential to prematurely end one's military career without benefits (e.g., health care, post-9/11 educational opportunities, other benefits to family and dependents).

The screening tools commonly used by military mental health practitioners for SUDs are (a) the Alcohol Use Disorder Identification Test (Babor et al., 1989), a 10-item questionnaire that screens for hazardous and harmful alcohol use; (b) the Drug Abuse Screening Test (Skinner, 1982), a 10-item yes/no self-report that is the brief version of the longer 28-item version; (c) the Alcohol, Smoking and Substance Involvement Screening Test (World Health Organization, 2010), an eight-item questionnaire typically administered by medical professionals to screen for harmful and undetected substance use disorders in primary health care settings; and (d) the Cut-Down, Annoyed, Guilty, Eye-Opener test (Mayfield et al., 1974), a five-item yes/no tool used to screen and prompt more comprehensive SUD assessments. These assessments all have the same problems as other screening and evaluation tools because they are primarily based on self-report by the service member or veteran.

Medical and mental health clinicians have multiple challenges during the SUD screening and assessment process. These challenges particularly become relevant when self-report instruments are used. For instance, family members, spouses, and the direct unit command non-commissioned officer may or may not want to fully disclose the service member's pattern of drinking or drug use. Corroborating sources know the consequences of discussing the frequency, duration, and patterns of use and abuse. Additionally, the severity and chronicity of substance misuse may be masked by other factors on a mobilization or deployment. Thus, the pattern of use or abuse may be situational depending on the environment, unit, or billet that the service member is attached to. Moreover, cultural differences between enlisted and officer ranks affect drinking patterns. For instance, on many bases, some protections are offered to officers in the "informal drinking" network, which may endorse various drinking patterns on and off duty.

The sample intake questions offered next to practitioners can serve as a starting point for gaining a more comprehensive clinical picture of their military client's substance use. These questions should be used in conjunction with other standardized screening or assessment tools. Depending on the individual's responses, information gained from the following brief questions may be helpful in setting therapeutic goals for prevention, cutting down or eliminating the use of substances, or assisting in relapse prevention planning:

- Where do you drink or use other substances? *Consider environments such as on base, in the barracks, in the office, at home, in bars, on the street, or in natural environments such as the woods.*
- How frequently do you drink or use other substances? *Allow clinical intuition and corroborative sources to determine frequency of use. Also consider the size of the beverage (12-, 16-, or 24-oz beer, wine, or liquor) and the alcohol content (craft beers usually have a higher alcohol content [≥7%] than commercial beers [≤5%]). Generally, one standard drink is equivalent to 12 ounces of beer (5% alcohol), 5 ounces of wine (12% alcohol), and 1.5 ounces of 80-proof liquor (40% alcohol).*
- Do you smoke or chew tobacco? Do you vape? *Consider the high prevalence and incidence of nicotine addiction in the military. Practitioners may want to consider a separate nicotine use and abuse assessment if warranted. Assess the client's commitment and stage of motivation to decrease or eliminate nicotine.*
- When did you first begin drinking alcohol or using other substances? *Consider prescription and nonprescription drugs. Practitioners may have to provide examples and names of specific drugs typically abused.*

- Describe the benefits and any negative consequences of your alcohol or other substance use. *Consider medical, physical, psychological, neurocognitive, emotional, social, vocational, spiritual, and other factors.*
- How long and over what period of time do you drink? *Practitioners should evaluate the client's pattern of binge drinking (≥5 consecutive drinks typically consumed in a 2-hour period for men; ≥4 drinks in 2 hours for women).*
- What activities, situations, and events prompt you to drink or use other substances more? What prompts you to use less? *Consider work, home, social, recreational, and other situations.*
- What other things intensify your drinking and other substance use? *Consider situations and environments across different life areas.*
- What do you generally do in life to eliminate stress? *Consider healthy versus unhealthy behaviors.*
- What activities can you do without drinking or using other substances? *Consider challenging the client with the "30-day elimination" test of alcohol or other substances. Observe the client's metacommunication and listen for commitment or stage of motivation to attempt the 30-day elimination test.*
- Are there certain activities, environments, or situations you avoid when using alcohol or other substances? *Consider the degree of difficulty for the client to abstain from alcohol and other substance use. Consider whether the client is an active or passive participant in such activities, environments, or situations.*
- Does your drinking or other substance use change your behaviors in any way? *Consider all intimate, social, or recreational relationships at work and home.*
- How does your drinking or other substance use affect your relationship with others? *Consider different ways to ask the same probes to get at more refined information.*

These sample questions yield important information and content regarding your client's use of alcohol and other substances. Of course, many other assessments are administered by practitioners, which can be found in demographics questionnaires (e.g., age, education, military occupational specialty, marital status), screening devices (e.g., the Alcohol Use Disorder Identification Test and the Cut-Down, Annoyed, Guilty, Eye-Opener test), and standardized assessment tools (e.g., Addiction Severity Index [McLellan et al., 1992], Global Appraisal of Individual Needs [Dennis et al., 2008]). For a comprehensive yet brief guide to SUD assessment and treatment, refer to the reference section (see Goodwin, 2016a, 2016b) at the end of this chapter.

Ultimately, therapeutic interventions with SUDs begin with primary and secondary prevention approaches. For instance, recommendations made by various military substance abuse task force and study groups propose a four-tier substance use prevention model. The recommendations are based on the opportunity for outreach, prevention, and substance use education for all members of the U.S. Armed Forces. The model suggests that the DoD can do (a) universal prevention with all members of the U.S. Armed Forces, (b) selective prevention focusing on higher risk groups, (c) individual prevention and screening for those with combat operational stress, and (d) tertiary prevention to prevent relapse for those currently receiving treatment. This model is obviously not possible in civilian life where, for example, the school system may be the only source that has "eyes on" a high-risk student, whereas working parents, a single parent, or blended family households may not recognize the warning signs. The U.S. Armed Forces have a greater advantage than schools, families, and communities regarding substance use prevention, screening, and treatment. The total population of military service members are known by their unit, branch of service, name, rank, and serial number. Therefore, substance abuse prevention programs can be implemented system wide.

OPIOID USE DISORDERS IN THE MILITARY

Opioid use disorders, such as opioid addiction, are an epidemic in both civilian and military life. This has prompted the CDC to provide guidelines for prescribers—particularly for those patients diagnosed with chronic pain syndromes (Dowell et al., 2016)—and the VA system of health care (VA & DoD, 2017). Between 2004 and 2012, opioid use among veterans increased by 77%, with the highest use among veteran women between the ages of 18 and 34 years. Of veterans returning from Afghanistan, 44% reported a chronic pain condition, with approximately 15% prescribed opioids. Out of this group being treated for chronic pain, approximately 90% remained on their opioid medication after 90 days and 80% after 1 year. Veterans treated for PTSD within the VA health system are reported to receive much higher doses of two or more opioids during their course of treatment compared with veterans without a diagnosis of PTSD (Shiner et al., 2017). In addition to poor clinical outcomes with the use of opioids, those who have an opioid addiction also have an elevated rate of alcohol use disorder (60%).

Researchers have identified numerous variables that have significantly increased the risk of opioid use disorders, which, in turn, have created a major addiction problem in both the U.S. military and civilian populations with chronic pain syndromes. Some of these issues relate to (a) the pharmaceutical industry's lobbying access to medical providers and politicians, (b) the patient not properly taking their medications or using alternative treatments for pain, (c) providers improperly diagnosing and treating a patient with a previous history of drug addiction, and (d) multiple other psychosocial factors that go beyond the scope of this chapter.

One issue that is clear relates to the risk factors associated with opioid use. The following questions are useful in the short term for the identification, screening, and treatment of patients prescribed opioids (readers should consult the reference section for more specific medical and psychological assessment and treatment guidelines):

- Has the patient been prescribed, or is the patient prescribed, any benzodiazepines?
- Does the patient have a history of—or are they currently being treated for—an SUD?
- Does the patient have a history of—or are they currently being treated for—PTSD, major depressive disorder, anxiety, or wake-sleep disorder?
- Does the patient have a diagnosis of borderline or antisocial personality disorder?

These questions can serve as an immediate and brief functional measure to help unravel the complicated physical and psychological aspects of opioid use disorders. The increased prevalence and incidence of SUDs and co-occurring mental health conditions have peaked the interest of a variety of medical, psychological, and addiction clinical researchers. The CDC and VA-DoD guidelines on opioid use disorders emphasize that clinical mental health and substance abuse practitioners should partner with medical providers in treating SUDs. In my professional career, I have worked with internal medicine and family practice physicians in hospitals, mental health clinics, and substance abuse clinics, and I have learned the value of having medical and mental health practitioners working in a treatment team approach. Coordination of care ultimately benefits the client. Thus, clinical mental health counselors can assist physicians and other prescribers with (a) medication compliance; (b) comprehensive clinical assessments to understand the etiology of the patient's substance misuse or pattern of addiction; (c) consultation on the clinical characteristics of a mild, moderate, or severe SUD and any co-occurring mental health disorders requiring clinical attention; (d) advocating for good patient medical care and follow-up diagnostics that may lead to a better understanding of one's mental health functioning; (e) providing the appropriate mental health diagnosis that may prompt clinical attention; and (f) providing overall model patient care in a comprehensive treatment team approach.

The following items are important to consider in the overall screening, assessment, and treatment of SUDs experienced throughout the deployment cycle:

- Multiple resources and clinical treatment guidelines are available to assist clinical military counselors in the proper assessment, diagnosis, and treatment of substance use and co-occurring disorders among active-duty service members and veterans. It is acknowledged that treatment interventions will vary depending on the practitioner's treatment setting (e.g., military installation, VA system of health care, private practice TRICARE provider). Thus, some resources and brief treatment guides that serve to assist mental health practitioners in determining priorities for treatment within the deployment cycle are located in the reference section (e.g., Goodwin, 2016a, 2016b; Moore & Penk, 2019; Substance Abuse and Mental Health Services Administration, 2015; VA & DoD, 2015; Vujanovic & Back, 2019; also see https://store.samhsa.gov/substances).
- The zero-tolerance policies toward SUDs and co-occurring disorders are a disincentive for service members to seek mental health and substance abuse treatment. The lack of confidentiality with random drug screenings to detect SUDs will have career consequences.
- Despite the inconsistencies with allowing alcohol use on base during celebrations, or during deployments, medical and mental health practitioners should not view alcohol or drug use as a "rite of passage." Rather, substance use in the military should be viewed much like it is in the civilian culture—in terms of distinguishing between healthy and unhealthy use, abuse, and addiction. SUDs in the military are a serious mental health condition that can lead to life-threatening consequences (e.g., suicide).
- Appropriate screening and SUD assessments can help determine which evidence-based treatment practices are appropriate goals for service members and veterans. Treatment outcomes and goals for therapy may include (a) medically assisted withdrawal from a substance (e.g., detox treatment), (b) elimination of any substances used that have caused harm to the individual and others in their environment, (c) reduction in the consumption of substances used, (d) improvement in quality of life in terms of occupational and social functioning, (e) improvement in physical or mental functioning, (f) keeping the person engaged in treatment (e.g., harm reduction, relapse prevention), (g) improvement in co-occurring mental or physical health-related problems (e.g., depression, PTSD, chronic pain conditions), and (h) reduction in mortality (e.g., because of at-risk suicidality).
- Process or behavioral addictions have also become problematic in military life, including addictions to pornography, sex, internet use, video gaming, gambling, and shopping. Process or behavioral addictions are a new area of inquiry in the mental health and addiction literature. Currently, sufficient peer-reviewed research and evidence-based practices are not available to establish a separate diagnostic category of *behavioral addictions*.

- The development and sequelae of clinical symptoms related to process addictions, as well as tobacco use disorders, are like other SUDs. They range from mild, to moderate, to severe. Some of the diagnostic markers for process addictions relate to the following items: (a) the individual increases the amount of time spent in engaging in such activities that lead to a pattern of addictive behaviors; (b) both physiological and psychological withdrawal occur when the individual stops a behavior or quits using a substance; (c) the individual develops a loss of control or an addiction-centered (e.g., gambling-centered, pornography-centered, sex-centered) lifestyle that consumes a significant portion of their day; and (d) the unhealthy behavior or addiction has negative consequences for social, emotional, psychological, and occupational functioning as well as for other major life areas.
- Tobacco use disorders are a problematic pattern of behavior in the military. Many mental health practitioners in private practice settings underemphasize, undertreat, or do not address the client's use of tobacco during psychotherapy sessions. This oversight is particularly the case if the client does not (a) report smoking, vaping, or using electronic cigarettes (e-cigarettes) in the intake interview or during session; (b) recognize or consciously ignores the adverse impact of tobacco use with their pattern of substance misuse or addiction; and (c) see a need to change their tobacco use behaviors. Thus, during therapeutic engagements, competent and ethical clinical military counselors comprehensively assess and bring to light issues that create or have the potential to develop into adverse physical and mental health conditions.
- Tobacco use disorders follow the course of other clinically significant impairments. For instance, pairing alcohol and cigarettes (or e-cigarettes) creates a potent pattern of behavior in which one behavior reinforces the other. Thus, most clinical addiction specialists understand that clients many times replace one addiction (alcohol use disorder) for another (tobacco use disorder).
- Currently, the practice of vaping and using e-cigarettes or electronic nicotine delivery systems has become problematic. Current research is inconclusive as to the adverse health effects. However, studies in peer-reviewed journals have suggested that significant health implications have merited further research. The CDC (2020) has provided statistics, fact sheets, as well as prevention and treatment guidelines for e-cigarettes. The interested reader should consult the reference section for more comprehensive information.

CONCLUDING REMARKS

The intention of this chapter was to highlight and delineate the multidimensional clinical characteristics related to complex trauma. I discussed the co-occurring mental health conditions of adjustment, anxiety, depression, insomnia, and SUDs that are characteristic of complex PTSD. Statistically, combat exposure and the extraordinary stressful and traumatic events that occur in military life place service members, as opposed to civilians, into a significantly higher risk category for adverse physical and mental health conditions. Through a comprehensive clinical assessment, competent and ethical clinical military counselors can holistically treat the complex nature of PTSD and its co-occurring disorders. It is of paramount importance that medical and mental health practitioners partner in treatment teams to provide optimal physical and psychological benefits to military clients.

REFERENCES

Adler, A. B., Bliese, P. D., McGurk, D., Hoge, C. W., & Castro, C. A. (2009). Battlemind debriefing and Battlemind training as early interventions with soldiers returning from Iraq: Randomization by platoon. *Journal of Counseling and Clinical Psychology, 77*(5), 928–940. https://doi.org/10.1037/a0016877

Adler, A. B., & Castro, C. A. (2013). An occupational mental health model for the military. *Military Behavioral Health, 1*(1), 41–51. https://doi.org/10.1080/21635781.2012.721063

American Psychiatric Association. (1994). *Diagnostic and statistical manual of mental disorders* (4th ed.).

Armed Forces Health Surveillance Center. (2013). Anxiety disorders, active component, U.S. Armed Forces, 2000–2012. *Medical Surveillance Monthly Report, 20*(10), 2–6. https://pubmed.ncbi.nlm.nih.gov/24191766/

Babor, T. F., De La Fuente, J. R., & Saunders, J. (1989). *Alcohol Use Disorder Identification Test: Guidelines for use in primary health care*. World Health Organization.

Bein, L., Grau, P. P., Saunders, S. M., & deRoon-Cassini, T. A. (2019). Military mental health: Problem recognition, treatment-seeking, and barriers. *Military Behavioral Health, 7*(2), 228–237. https://doi.org/10.1080/21635781.2018.1526147

Britt, T. W., Sipos, M. L., Klinefelter, A., & Adler, A. B. (2019). Determinants of mental and physical health treatment-seeking among military personnel. *The British Journal of Psychiatry*. Advance online publication. https://doi.org/10.1192/bjp.2019.155

Buck, R. P. (2012). The impact of war on military veterans. In L. Lopez Levers (Ed.), *Trauma counseling: Theories and interventions* (pp. 434–453). Springer.

Burke, P. A., & Carruth, B. (2012). Addiction and psychological trauma: Implications for counseling strategies. In L. Lopez Levers (Ed.), *Trauma counseling: Theories and interventions* (pp. 214–230). Springer.

Butler Center for Research. (2018, May). *Substance use disorders among military populations.* Hazelden Betty Ford Foundation. https://www.hazeldenbettyford.org/education/bcr/addiction-research/substance-abuse-military-ru-518

Byers, A. L., Covinsky, K. E., Barnes, D. E., & Yaffe, K. (2012). Dysthymia and depression increase risk of dementia and mortality among older veterans. *American Journal of Geriatric Psychiatry, 20*(8), 664–672. https://doi.org/10.1097/JGP.0b013e31822001c1

Cadwell, J. A., Knapik, J. J., Shing, T. L., Kardouni, J. R., & Liebermann, H. R. (2019). The association of insomnia and sleep apnea with deployed and combat exposure in the entire population of the US Army soldiers from 1997–2011: A retrospective cohort investigation. *SLEEP, 42*(8), Article zsz112. https://doi.org/10.1093/sleep/zsz112

Carta, M. G., Balestrieri, M., Murru, A., & Hardoy, M. C. (2009). Adjustment disorder: Epidemiology, diagnosis, and treatment. *Clinical Practice and Epidemiological in Mental Health, 5,* Article 15. https://doi.org/10.1186/1745-0179-5-15

Casey, G. W., Jr. (2011). Comprehensive Soldier Fitness: A vision for psychological resilience in the U.S. Army. *American Psychologist, 66*(1), 1–3. https://doi.org/10.1037/a0021930

Casey, P. (2009). Adjustment disorder: Epidemiology, diagnosis, and treatment. *CNS Drugs, 23*(11), 927–938. https://doi.org/10.2165/11311000-000000000-00000

Centers for Disease Control and Prevention. (2018, August 8). *National Health Interview Survey: 2017 data release.* https://www.cdc.gov/nchs/nhis/nhis_2017_data_release.htm

Centers for Disease Control and Prevention. (2020, February 24). *Electronic cigarettes.* https://www.cdc.gov/tobacco/basic_information/e-cigarettes/index.htm

Chapman, J. C., & Diaz-Arrastia, R. (2014). Military traumatic brain injury: A review. *Alzheimer's & Dementia, 10*(Suppl. 3), S97–S104. https://doi.org/10.1016/j.jalz.2014.04.012

Chase, R. P., & Nevin, R. L. (2015). Population estimates of undocumented incident traumatic brain injuries among combat-deployed US military personnel. *Journal of Head Trauma Rehabilitation, 30*(1), E57–E64. https://doi.org/10.1097/HTR.0000000000000061

Cooper, L. N., Holliday, R. P., Holder, N. D., Jackson, J., North, C. S., & Suris, A. M. (2018). Working with trauma-related mental health problems among combat veterans of the Afghanistan and Iraq conflicts. In I. Marini & M. A. Stebnicki (Eds.), *The psychological and social impact of illness and disability* (7th ed., pp. 311–343). Springer.

Dennis, M. L., White, M., Titus, J. C., & Unsicker, J. (2008, November). *Global Appraisal of Individual Needs: Administration guide for the GAIN and related measures.* Chestnut Health Systems. https://www.researchgate.net/profile/Michael_Dennis2/publication/267224119_GAIN_Global_Appraisal_of_Individual_Needs_Administration_Guide_for_the_GAIN_and_Related_Measures/links/5d556b37a6fdccb7dc3d0dbc/GAIN-Global-Appraisal-of-Individual-Needs-Administration-Guide-for-the-GAIN-and-Related-Measures.pdf

DePalma, R. G. (2015). Combat TBI: History, epidemiology, and injury modes. In F. Kobeissy (Ed.), *Brain neurotrauma: Molecular, neuropsychological, and rehabilitation aspects* (pp. 5–14). CRC Press.

Dowell, D., Haegerich, T. M., & Chou, R. (2016, March 18). CDC guideline for prescribing opioids for chronic pain—United States, 2016. *Morbidity and Mortality Weekly Report, 65*(1), 1–49. https://www.cdc.gov/mmwr/volumes/65/rr/rr6501e1.htm

Elder, G. A., Ehrlich, M. E., & Gandy, S. (2019). Relationship of traumatic brain injury to chronic mental health problems and dementia in military veterans. *Neuroscience Letters, 707,* Article 134294. https://doi.org/10.1016/j.neulet.2019.134294

Elder, G. A., Mitsis, E. M., Ahlers, S. T., & Cristian, A. (2010). Blast-induced mild traumatic brain injury. *Psychiatric Clinics of North American, 33*(4), 757–781. https://doi.org/10.1016/j.psc.2010.08.001

Falvo, D. R., & Holland, B. E. (2018). *Medical and psychosocial aspects of chronic illness and disability* (6th ed.). Jones & Bartlett.

Fielden, J. S. (2012). Review: Management of adjustment disorder in the deployed setting. *Military Medicine, 177*(9), 1022–1027. https://doi.org/10.7205/milmed-d-12-00057

Foran, H. M., Garber, B. G., Zamorski, M. A., Wray, M., Mulligan, K., Greenberg, N., Castro, C. A., & Adler, A. B. (2013). Postdeployment military mental health training: Cross-national evaluations. *Psychological Services, 10*(2), 152–160. https://doi.org/10.1037/a0032609

France, D. K. L. (2018). *Combat vet don't mean crazy: Veteran mental health in post-military life.* NCO Historical Society.

Ghahramanlou-Holloway, M., LaCroix, J. M., Koss, K., Perera, K. U., Rowan, A., Van Sickle, M. R., Novak, L. A., & Trieu, T. H. (2018). Outpatient mental health treatment utilization and military career impact in the United States Marine Corps. *International Journal of Environmental Research and Public Health, 15*(4), Article 828. https://doi.org/10.3390/ijerph15040828

Goodwin, L. R. (2016a). Substance abuse assessment. In I. Marini & M. A. Stebnicki (Eds.), *The professional counselor's desk reference* (2nd ed., pp. 449–455). Springer.

Goodwin, L. R. (2016b). Treatment for substance use disorders. In I. Marini & M. A. Stebnicki (Eds.), *The professional counselor's desk reference* (2nd ed., pp. 457–468). Springer.

Grossman, D. (2009). *On killing: The psychological cost of learning to kill in war and society.* Back Bay Books.

Harley, D. A. (2018). Meeting the needs of rural adults with mental illness and dual diagnosis. In D. A. Harley, N. A. Ysasi, M. L. Bishop, & A. R. Fleming (Eds.), *Disability and vocational rehabilitation in rural settings* (pp. 477–503). Springer.

Hitt, R., & Massi Lindsey, L. L. (2020). Military members' perceptions of social norms about mental health for combat stress. *Military Behavioral Health, 8*(2), 181–190. https://doi.org/10.1080/21635781.2019.1630039

Hoge, C. W., Castro, C. A., Messer, S. C., McGurk, D., Cotting, D. I., & Koffman, R. L. (2004). Combat duty in Iraq and Afghanistan, mental health problems, and barriers to care. *New England Journal of Medicine, 351*(1), 13–22. https://doi.org/10.1056/NEJMoa040603

Joint Service Committee on Military Justice. (2019). *Manual for courts-marital United States.* https://jsc.defense.gov/Portals/99/Documents/2019%20MCM%20(Final)%20(20190108).pdf?ver=2019-01-11-115724-610

Kilpatrick, D. G., Resnick, H. S., Milanak, M. E., Miller, M. W., Keyes, K. M., & Friedman, M. J. (2013). National estimates of exposure to traumatic events and PTSD prevalence using *DSM-IV* and *DSM-5* criteria. *Journal of Traumatic Stress, 26*(5), 537–547. https://doi.org/10.1002/jts.21848

Kolbow, T. T., Spira, J. L., Morse, J. S., & Grieger, T. A. (2007). Post-traumatic stress disorder and depression in health care providers returning from deployment to Iraq and Afghanistan. *Military Medicine, 172*(5), 451–455. https://doi.org/10.7205/milmed.172.5.451

Kryzhanovskaya, L., & Canterbury, R. (2001). Suicidal behavior in patients with adjustment disorders. *Crisis, 22*(3), 125–131. https://doi.org/10.1027//0227-5910.22.3.125

Liu, X., Evatt, D. P., & Belsher, B. E. (2019). Development of longitudinal data analysis in mental health research for military service members. *Military Medicine, 184*(5–6), e227–e232. https://doi.org/10.1093/milmed/usy370

Livneh, H., & Antonak, R. F. (2018). Psychological adaptation to chronic illness and disability: A primer for counselors. In I. Marini & M. A. Stebnicki (Eds.), *The psychological and social impact of illness and disability* (7th ed., pp. 77–90). Springer.

Mayfield, D., McLeod, G., & Hall, P. (1974). The CAGE questionnaire: Validation of a new alcoholism screening instrument. *American Journal of Psychiatry, 131*(10), 1121–1123.

McLellan, A. T., Kushner, H., Metzger, D., Peters, R., Smith, I., Grissom, G., Pettinati, H., & Argeriou, M. (1992). The fifth edition of the Addiction Severity Index. *Journal of Substance Abuse Treatment, 9*(3), 199–213. https://doi.org/10.1016/0740-5472(92)90062-s

Misener, C. (2017, May 10). *It's okay to answer Question 21.* Defense Logistics Agency. https://www.dla.mil/AboutDLA/News/News-ArticleView/Article/1178178/its-okay-to-answer-question-21/

Mohatt, N. V., Boeckmann, R., Winkel, N., Mohatt, D. F., & Shore, J. (2017) Military Mental Health First Aid: Development and preliminary efficacy of a community training for improving knowledge, attitudes, and helping behaviors. *Military Medicine, 182*(1–2), e1576–e1583. https://doi.org/10.7205/MILMED-D-16-00033

Moore, B. A., & Penk, W. E. (2019). *Treating PTSD in military personnel: A clinical handbook* (2nd ed.). Guilford Press.

Morgan, J. K., Hourani, L., Lane, M. E., & Tueller, S. (2016). Help-seeking behaviors among active-duty military personnel: Utilization of chaplains and other mental health service providers. *Journal of Health Care Chaplaincy, 22*(3), 102–117. https://doi.org/10.1080/08854726.2016.1171598

Morgan, M., & Kelber, M. (2018, October 29). *Adjustment disorders: How are they relevant to military mental health?* Psychological Health Center of Excellence. https://pdhealth.mil/news/blog/adjustment-disorders-how-are-they-relevant-military-mental-health

National Center for PTSD. (n.d.). *For veterans and families: Understanding PTSD and substance use.* https://www.ptsd.va.gov/publications/print/sudptsdflyer.pdf

National Institute on Drug Abuse. (2019, October). *Substance use and military life: General risk of substance use disorders.* https://www.drugabuse.gov/publications/drugfacts/substance-use-military-life

Ogle, A. D., Bradley, D., Santiago, P., & Reynolds, D. (2012). Description of combat and operational stress control in Regional Command East, Afghanistan. *Military Medicine, 177*(11), 1279–1286. https://doi.org/10.7205/milmed-d-11-00454

Perez-Garcia, G., Gama Sosa, M. A., De Gasperi, R., Tschiffely, A. E., Mc Carron, R. M., Hof, P. R., Gandy, S., Ahlers, S. T., & Elder, G. A. (2019). Blast-induced "PTSD": Evidence from an animal model. *Neuropharmacology, 145*(Part B), 220–229. https://doi.org/10.1016/j.neuropharm.2018.09.023

Roitman, P., Gilad, M., Ankri, Y. L. E., & Shalev, A. (2013). Head injury and loss of consciousness raise the likelihood of developing and maintaining PTSD symptoms. *Journal of Traumatic Stress, 26*(6), 727–734. https://doi.org/10.1002/jts.21862

Rowan, A. B., Travis, W. J., Richardson, C. B., & Adams, T. R. (2020). Military mental health personnel deployment survey: A secondary analysis. *Military Medicine, 185*(3–4), e340–e346. https://doi.org/10.1093/milmed/usz275

Shelef, L., Dotan, S., Kaminsky, D., Kedem, R., & Margulis, A. (2016). Relationship between anxiety and medical disorders among compulsory military service candidates between the years 1998–2013. *Psychiatry Research, 244,* 339–344. https://doi.org/10.1016/j.psychres.2016.07.042

Shiner, B., Westgate, C. L., Bernardy, N. C., Schnurr, P. P., & Watts, B. V. (2017). Trends in opioid use disorder diagnoses and medication treatment among veterans with posttraumatic stress disorder. *Journal of Dual Diagnosis, 13*(3), 201–212. https://doi.org/10.1080/15504263.2017.1325033

Skinner, H. A. (1982). The Drug Abuse Screening Test. *Addictive Behavior, 7*(4), 363–371. https://doi.org/10.1016/0306-4603(82)90005-3

Stebnicki, M. A. (2018). Psychosocial counseling aspects of grief, death, and dying. In I. Marini & M. A. Stebnicki (Eds.), *The psychological and social impact of illness and disability* (7th ed., pp. 245–256). Springer.

Substance Abuse and Mental Health Services Administration. (2015, November 10). Veterans' primary substance of abuse is alcohol in treatment admissions. *The CBHSQ Report.* http://www.samhsa.gov/data/sites/default/files/report_2111/Spotlight-2111.pdf

Swinkels, C. M., Ulmer, C. S., Beckham, J. C., Buse, N., & Calhoun, P. S. (2013). The associate of sleep duration, mental health, and health risk behaviors among U.S. Afghanistan/Iraq era veterans. *SLEEP, 36*(7), 1019–1025. https://doi.org/10.5665/sleep.2800

Tick, E. (2014). *Warrior's return: Restoring the soul after war.* Sounds True.

Troxel, W. M., Shih, R. A., Petersen, E., Geyer, L., Fischer, M. P., Griffin, B. A., Haas, A. C., Kurz, J. R., & Steinberg, P. S. (2015). *Sleep in the military: Promoting healthy sleep among U.S. service members.* RAND Corporation. https://www.rand.org/content/dam/rand/pubs/research_reports/RR700/RR739/RAND_RR739.pdf

U.S. Department of Defense. (2014, February 20). *Department of Defense instruction.* https://www.esd.whs.mil/Portals/54/Documents/DD/issuances/dodi/101004p.pdf

U.S. Department of Veterans Affairs & U.S. Department of Defense. (2015, December). *VA/DoD clinical practice guidelines: Management of substance use disorders.* https://www.healthquality.va.gov/guidelines/mh/sud/index.asp

U.S. Department of Veterans Affairs & U.S. Department of Defense. (2017, February). *VA/DoD clinical practice guideline for opioid therapy for chronic pain.* https://www.healthquality.va.gov/guidelines/Pain/cot/VADoDOTCPG022717.pdf

Van Der Kolk, B. (2014). *The body keeps the score: Brain, mind, and body in the healing of trauma.* Penguin Books.

Vujanovic, A. A., & Back, S. E. (2019). *PTSD and substance use disorders: A clinical overview.* Routledge.

Wachen, J. S., Shipherd, J. C., Suvak, M., Vogt, D., King, L. A., & King, D. W. (2013). Posttraumatic stress symptomatology as a mediator of the relationship between warzone exposure and physical health symptoms in men and women. *Journal of Traumatic Stress, 26*(3), 319–328. https://doi.org/10.1002/jts.21818

Warner, C. H., Appenzeller, G. N., Grieger, T., Belenkiy, S., Breitbach, J., Warner, C. M., & Hoge, C. (2011). Importance of anonymity to encourage honest reporting in mental health screening after combat deployment. *Archives of General Psychiatry, 68*(10), 1065–1071. https://doi.org/10.1001/archgenpsychiatry.2011.112

Witkiewitz, K., & Estrada, A. X. (2011). Substance abuse and mental health treatment in the military: Lessons learned and a way forward. *Military Psychology, 23*(1), 112–123. https://doi.org/10.1080/08995605.2011.548651

World Health Organization. (2010, January). *The Alcohol, Smoking and Substance Involvement Screening Test (ASSIST): Manual for use in primary care.* https://www.who.int/publications/i/item/978924159938-2

Wright, K. M., Britt, T. W., Bliese, P. D., Adler, A. D., Picchioni, D., & Moore, D. (2011). Insomnia as predictor versus outcome of PTSD and depression among Iraq combat veterans. *Journal of Clinical Psychology, 67*(12), 1240–1258. https://doi.org/10.1002/jclp.20845

Wright, K. M., Thomas, J. L., Adler, A. B., Ness, J. W., Hoge, C. W., & Castro, C. A. (2005). Psychological screening procedures for deploying U.S. forces. *Military Medicine, 170*(7), 555–562. https://doi.org/10.7205/milmed.170.7.555

Ysasi, N. A., Silva, I., & Becton, A. D. (2016). Counseling families of active duty military and returning veterans. In I. Marini & M. A. Stebnicki (Eds.), *The professional counselor's desk reference* (2nd ed., pp. 409–413). Springer.

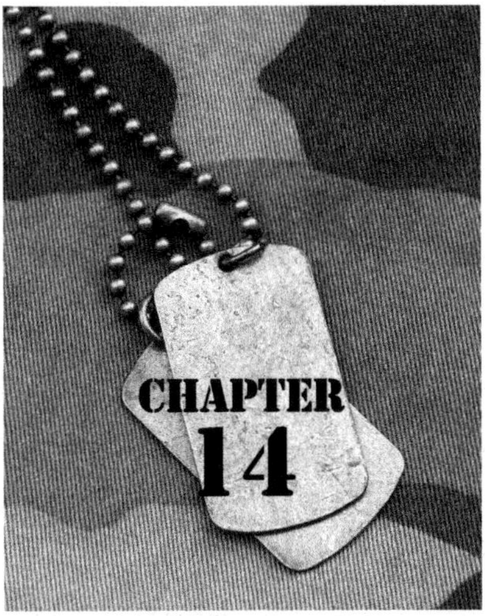

MILITARY RESILIENCY AND INTEGRATIVE TREATMENT STRATEGIES IN OPERATION MILITARY COUNSELING

New understanding and awareness springs forth
a renewed purpose for one's life.
This attitudinal and perceptual shift transforms
a sense of peaceful resolve, mending the mind,
body, and spirit.

—Mark A. Stebnicki, 2020

★ ★ ★

The impact of stress and trauma on military service members and veterans has been discussed and supported by clinical research and practice guidelines throughout *Clinical Military Counseling*. Military service places the individual at risk for complex posttraumatic stress disorder (PTSD) and co-occurring mental health (e.g., major depressive disorder, anxiety, substance use disorders, suicidality) and physical health (e.g., musculoskeletal injuries, chronic pain, traumatic brain injury [TBI], blast injuries, amputation, spinal cord injury) conditions. Research on maintaining optimal levels of mental, physical, and spiritual health is at the heart of the military wellness and resiliency initiatives (Bauer et al., 2018; France, 2018; Ysasi et al., 2016).

Strong evidence in the research suggests that holistic or complementary and integrative health practices are beneficial in decreasing symptoms related to posttraumatic stress, anger, depression, anxiety, substance misuse behaviors, as well as military suicidality. These practices are critical to the mission of Operation Military Counseling (OMC), which informs new strategies for clinical counselors to work with the military culture. Integrative approaches such as meditation work just as well as the evidence-based psychotherapy practices of cognitive behavioral therapy and prolonged exposure therapy endorsed by the U.S. Department of Veterans Affairs (VA) health care system (Steenkamp et al., 2020). Newer studies suggest that first-line psychotherapy treatment does not effectively treat complex PTSD because traditional approaches are effective in only 30%–50% of clients. In fact, newer studies suggest that first-line psychotherapeutic interventions to treat military PTSD have limited value because single and combined approaches, such as cognitive behavioral therapy and psychopharmacological approaches, are not effective treatment modalities for all military clients (Bauer et al., 2018; Benish et al., 2007; Herman et al., 2017; Steenkamp et al., 2020; Ysasi et al., 2016). Complementary and integrative health treatment approaches have shown significant potential for treating PTSD and co-occurring mental health conditions considering several different variables (e.g., stigma of interventions, return to treatment, motivation levels).

Multiple holistic approaches can be facilitated by competent practitioners within the therapeutic environment while connecting service members and veterans to other healing resources outside the session. In this chapter, I explore the use of complementary and integrative health approaches, as well as resiliency strategies, that are commonly utilized for self-care among service members, veterans, and their families. Resources and guidelines are offered to practitioners for the integration of mind, body, and spiritual practices to build resiliency.

WHAT IS INTEGRATIVE HEALTH IN THE MILITARY?

Most holistic researchers and practitioners use the terms *complementary* and *integrative health* because individuals rarely use only "alternative" physical or mental health approaches for serious conditions such as severe PTSD, TBI, cardiovascular diseases, musculoskeletal injuries, or chronic pain. The National Center for Complementary and Integrative Health (2018) has emphasized holistic patient-centered approaches to increase opportunities for health and wellness. The strategies and approaches used for self-care are included in the mental, emotional, functional, spiritual, social, and community domains with the intention of treating the whole person. The benefits of using various self-care modalities—such as yoga, expressive arts, mindfulness meditation, and acupuncture—are considerable and are supported by quantitative and qualitative research.

Many patients in the healing process have become frustrated with the traditional medical and mental health models of treatment. They have discovered how to optimize their body's natural ability to maintain health and wellness by integrating mind, body, and spiritual practices (Kabat-Zinn, 1990; Schlitz & Amorok, 2005; Tick, 2014; Weil, 1995). Historically, medical and mental health treatment providers have focused on strategies in one body system for healing illness, disease, or disability. For example, the *mind* is treated by psychologists and mental health counselors; the *body* is treated by medical providers; and the *spirit* is treated by chaplains, clergy, pastors, and other spiritual and religious leaders.

In traditional medical and mental health care, diagnosis and treatment of the patient are well defined. The provider has an ethical responsibility to provide evidence-based practices associated with their specialty area of medicine and mental health. The provider is typically seen as holding all the power. This arrangement provides the illusion that treatment within the medical and mental health model is the sole pathway to healing illness, disease, or disability. Considerations for the use of healing modalities outside clinical research and evidence-based practices of Western medicine are rarely recommended by medical and mental health practitioners (Stebnicki, 2016). Consequently, the prime focus on the medical and mental health model of treatment does not empower patients with responsibilities for coping and resiliency skills. It also does not allow individuals to explore the power and wisdom of self-care activities that invigorate their mind, body, and spirit for optimal health and well-being.

The military community now has a strong interest in using complementary and integrative health approaches. For instance, many veterans have successfully learned how to replace maladaptive behaviors with adaptive coping strategies using a three-pronged wellness approach of peer support, wellness strategies, and spirituality in combination with their medical and mental health treatment providers (http://mhaw.org/dwyer/programs-services/). The stigma of service members seeking traditional mental health treatment as well as their dissatisfaction with psychotherapy have been a disincentive to engage in such practices. However, the use of complementary and integrative health strategies—such as meditation, mindfulness-based stress reduction (MBSR), and yoga—is particularly beneficial in reducing the service member's or veteran's levels of stress, anxiety, depression, and substance misuse (Ysasi et al., 2016). It also teaches accountability for thriving optimally in mind, body, and spirit.

Within the last 5 years, some of the most common complementary and integrative health approaches utilized by civilian adults have been the use of nonpharmaceutical natural products, deep breathing and mindfulness meditation, yoga, tai chi, and chiropractic or osteopathic body manipulation (National Center for Complementary and Integrative Health, 2018). Evidence-based research has documented the benefits of using the natural healing treatments of prayer, breathing, meditation, visualization, body energy work, and intuitive or shamanic medicine (Stebnicki, 2016). They are frequently integrated into the daily routines of individuals with chronic illnesses and disabilities. Interestingly, complementary and integrative health approaches have existed for thousands of years. Most of these approaches were developed by indigenous cultures and are not recent innovations of modern Western medicine, psychology, or counseling.

HOW EFFECTIVE IS COMPLEMENTARY AND INTEGRATIVE HEALTH?

Many of the holistic treatment approaches previously identified as complementary or alternative are no longer considered on the fringe of traditional Western medicine and mental health. Rather, they have been validated throughout the military and civilian medical, psychological, and mental health counseling literature (Brintz et al., 2020; Evans et al., 2018; Gantt & Orina, 2020; Miller et al., 2017; Moodley & West, 2005; Stebnicki, 2016; Tick, 2014; Weil, 1995; Ysasi et al., 2016). Researchers have documented the effectiveness of complementary and integrative health approaches with several adverse physical and psychological conditions that were acquired during military service. The beneficial use of holistic treatment approaches is well documented, particularly for reducing the symptoms of posttraumatic stress, anger, depression, and substance abuse behaviors. The key elements associated with the integrative health movement have shown a positive outcome in improving the overall health and well-being of service members and veterans throughout the life span.

In a research study, Ysasi et al. (2016) found that the majority (80%) of service members and veterans were receptive and participated in the use of at least one complementary and integrative health approach, such as yoga, herbal supplements, massage, and acupuncture. Female service members, veterans, and those with a preexisting mental health diagnosis have reported that they are more likely to integrate holistic self-care approaches within their daily lives for both prevention and treatment (Evans et al., 2018; Ysasi et al., 2016). Other studies have shown that veterans who have participated in yoga on a regular basis have reported an 80% reduction in musculoskeletal pain, depression, and anxiety as well as increased energy levels (Miller et al., 2017).

One of the most widely studied Eastern mind-body-spirit traditions is the MBSR program (Kabat-Zinn, 1990). MBSR approaches center on mind-body techniques used for self-regulation, focusing on the present moment using one's emotions, thoughts, and experiences to release negative energy held within the mind, body, and spirit. MBSR techniques have been effective in improving physical and mental health conditions among active-duty service members and veterans (Brintz et al., 2020). Another Eastern tradition is the Japanese body energy work of Reiki, which has been provided for patients with chronic pain in military health care treatment facilities. The Reiki practitioner uses a hands-on or hands-above method opening the various body chakras. The intention is to release unwanted or blocked energy held in one's mind, body, and spirit. Much like acupuncture, which uses the various energy vortexes or meridians of the physical body, these toxins can be released by altering their energy path. In one study, 80% of veterans who participated in Reiki indicated that they would consider scheduling other appointments, whereas 70% indicated a desire for at least four Reiki sessions per month (Gantt & Orina, 2020).

The research in complementary and integrative health approaches, in nonmilitary populations, has grown substantially over the last 30 years. Thus, the U.S. Armed Forces have an abundance of studies to draw on for integrating these self-care approaches into a sustainable practice. Much of its acceptance into general military medical and mental health practice depends on a complicated system of evidence-based approaches mandated by the U.S. Department of Defense, the VA health care system, and TRICARE insurance coverage. It is beyond the scope of this chapter to fully discuss and evaluate the clinical effectiveness of specific complementary and integrative treatment approaches as well as other issues that hinder their use in military life. The interested reader is encouraged to review material in the reference section for further insight and discussion. Accordingly, the sections that follow describe the core foundations of holistic treatment approaches for use within the military culture.

MILITARY RESILIENCY

A new science has emerged within the last 20 years that uses a biopsychosocial approach of discovering one's own resiliency and coping characteristics after trauma exposure. The literature is robust, and researchers have suggested that persons who are more stress resistant have a higher capacity for expressing empathy and possess better overall health and wellness. These individuals enjoy what Siebert (2005) has referred to as the *resiliency advantage*, which comprises the following eight factors:

- Making a conscious choice in life,
- Power of positive thinking,
- Taking responsibility,
- Internal locus of control,
- Self-motivation,

- Not fearing trying out new and different things in life,
- Taking control of one's life, and
- Practicing positive approaches to life.

Military resiliency programs appear to integrate some of these essential elements. In fact, positive psychology and complementary and integrative health strategies significantly influence and strengthen the dynamics of resiliency programs in the military.

The acceleration of resiliency programs in the U.S. Armed Forces has occurred because of the obvious physical and mental health conditions that result from military life. Resiliency programs overall have the potential to empower the service member with effecting positive change within the family system and providing a practice of self-care. The early contributions of clinical researchers in resiliency psychology better identify why some service members and veterans are more stress hardy than others. Excellent resiliency models are available to choose from that provide guidance for integrating resiliency strategies into evidence-based practices for service members, veterans, and civilians struggling with conditions of stress and trauma. For example, research in posttraumatic growth (Updegraff & Taylor, 2000), resiliency (Siebert, 2005; Tedeschi & Calhoun, 2003, 2004), and positive psychology (Nakamura & Csikszentmihalyi, 2002) advocates for the person's ability to emerge from extraordinary stressful and traumatic experiences into a new depth of understanding. New understanding and awareness spring forth a renewed purpose for one's life. This attitudinal and perceptual shift transforms a sense of peaceful resolve that can assist in mending the mind, body, and spirit.

Military family members also benefit from resiliency programs, especially throughout the deployment cycle. Studies have shown that deployment is associated with poorer mental health functioning in military families as well as a higher risk for suicidality, maladaptive behaviors, problems with children and dependents, and divorce (Meadows et al., 2016; Robson, 2014). These issues have been corroborated by the Deployment Life Study—a large-sample longitudinal study (N = 2,700) of military families across all branches that evaluated the quality of marital and parental relationships along with the overall psychological, behavioral, and physical well-being of the family (Meadows et al., 2016). The key findings of this study include the following: (a) family relationships and other outcomes generally return to previous levels after the service member returns home; (b) preparation for deployment and communication during deployments are critical factors in the family's health; and (c) across a wide range of variables, little difference was found between families who deployed and those who did not. Readers are encouraged to review this study, as well as the other research presented in this chapter, for a comprehensive understanding of its application.

A RAND Corporation study specific to the U.S. Air Force—referred to as Total Force Fitness (Robson, 2014)—is another example of the U.S. military's interest in resiliency and wellness programs directed at improving the quality of life in the military. The key constructs of psychological fitness—including self-regulation, positive affect, perceived control, self-efficacy, self-esteem, and optimism—were integrated into this program. Total Force Fitness measured outcomes in the following domains: medical, nutritional, environmental, physical, social, spiritual, behavioral, and psychological. The intention, much like other studies, is to inform the U.S. Department of Defense leaders—in this case the U.S. Air Force command structure—of the salient features of living well in the military, with a focus on prevention and identification of a holistic set of conditions that are determinable factors for achieving optimal mind, body, and spiritual functioning.

Clearly, both civilian and military researchers support a wellness agenda for living optimally in mind, body, and spirit throughout one's career and beyond. The wellness paradigm is counter to the medical model of pathology in which illness, disease, and disability are conditions to be diagnosed and treated. Wellness models shift the focus from an illness orientation to an optimal functioning approach in which individuals make conscious choices to engage in healthy thoughts, emotions, experiences, and behaviors (Myers, 1992; Myers & Sweeney, 2005; Myers et al., 2000; Shannonhouse et al., 2016). Wellness can be applied regardless of physical or mental health functioning and status.

Wellness interventions are facilitated as both prevention and treatment because they have the advantage of viewing the *whole person* in terms of optimal physical, mental, cognitive, spiritual, occupational, social, emotional, and environmental health. Wellness approaches also have the benefit of being supported by the military culture, which has a natural support system of resources that potentially could increase group and unit cohesiveness, accountability, and shared responsibilities for maintaining optimal wellness.

INTEGRATION OF RESILIENCY, WELLNESS, AND HEALTH

Many in the resiliency, wellness, and complementary and integrative health community have suggested that specific personality traits, behaviors, and preexisting coping and resiliency skills are unique to each person and can predict their response or reaction to a critical event. The characteristics of each person depend on multiple variables that predispose or predict whether they will thrive or just survive. Most researchers and practitioners agree that one does not have to be born with resiliency traits. Rather, these skills can be self-taught and learned through mental health professionals, life and wellness coaches, and religious or spiritual mentors. One aspect of building resiliency and positive coping skills is that the individual can make a conscious choice to take responsibility for their mind, body, and spiritual well-being regardless of what challenges they must deal with in life. When military leaders want to cultivate resiliency among active-duty personnel to decrease combat operational stress, they build programs around the following intentions:

- Prepare service members for the physical and mental toughness required for combat operations with real-world training situations.
- Develop plans, options, and strategies during combat operations so that the service member can predict and prepare for both expected and unexpected critical events.
- Train for optimal mental and physical toughness in a mission-forward environment to create higher level warfighters or front-line personnel who can respond decisively without hesitation or questioning the combat mission and operation.
- Draw on experienced combat service members' past deployments to mentor and lead less experienced personnel.
- Provide constant reminders to personnel for developing faith in God, their branch of service, unit leaders and commanders, and each other to help get through the mission safely.
- Rely on natural support systems such as family members, unit buddies, chaplains, and the home-base environment from which they came.
- Advise service members to push away self-defeating thoughts, feelings, emotions, and experiences, with a conscious awareness of and focus on the mission.
- Seek short-term solutions to problems as they arise and develop coping strategies to assist service personnel through the combat mission, keeping them focused and safe.
- Reinforce coping and resiliency skills that serve to decrease combat operational stress.

At the intersection of Resiliency and Wellness Streets is a café that provides a menu of resources for military service members, veterans, veterans with disabilities, and their families. This metaphoric café can be self-serve, or it could come with your beloved barista to provide your favorite drink. The intention is not to provide an all-encompassing list of strategies, approaches, and resources. Rather, suggestions are offered for clients and providers to enhance or expand prevention and treatment resources commonly utilized in the military community. It is recommended that you use your preferred web browser to locate resources available in your regional and local communities. Military health providers may assist you in your search of the following items, which are listed in alphabetical order:

- *Acupuncture:* This body-energy, small-needle approach is based on ancient Chinese medicine used for the effective treatment of PTSD, depression, musculoskeletal conditions, and chronic pain.
- *Animal-assisted therapy:* Animals have been used for companionship, therapy, and service since ancient times. The K-9 Corps utilized canines beginning in World War II. Animals can be used in multiple ways, including search and rescue missions, to increase independence and safety for persons with physical disabilities, and—in particular—to assist veterans with mental health issues.
- *Biofeedback:* Biofeedback (or neurofeedback) assists persons to control heart rate variability, respirations, muscle tension, and other physiological functions, with the goal of being able to manipulate the body's systems at will. Commercially produced units are sold for many uses, including reduction of stress, chronic pain, depression, and PTSD.
- *Equine therapy and equine-facilitated psychotherapy:* These therapeutic approaches use horses as therapy. The approaches differ from recreational and competitive riding in that the focus is to use horses as therapeutic partners to connect with them emotionally and physically. Traditional psychotherapy makes use of intensive talk therapy approaches, whereas equine-facilitated psychotherapy relies on nonverbal approaches and animal attachment. The riders are challenged to communicate verbally and nonverbally with their horse, making unique mind-body connections to achieve optimal mental and physical well-being.
- *Expressive arts:* This form of therapy utilizes creative forms of art expression to communicate one's feelings, thoughts, and experiences both visually and sensorially. Expressive arts are a nontechnical, free-form type of healing therapy typically guided by a certified art therapist. Expressive arts take on many different forms, such as expressive writing, mandalas and other types of drawing, sketching, painting, use of clay or metals, dance expression, and other forms that connect with the individual.
- *Eye-movement desensitization and reprocessing therapy:* This therapy has been endorsed as an evidence-based practice utilized in the clinical setting to treat severe forms of PTSD. There is less reliance on lengthy verbalizations and disclosure of trauma experiences. Rather, the individual processes the trauma experience cognitively, which provides opportunities to regulate their stress and anxiety experiences and to exert more internal control.
- *Mindfulness training:* Dr. Jon Kabat-Zinn developed the MBSR program at the University of Massachusetts Medical Center in 1979. It was one of the first professional training programs to combine medicine and psychology with indigenous-cultivated mindfulness approaches. The approaches vary but fundamentally

integrate meditation, breathing, progressive relaxation, visualization, and other approaches that use the wisdom of one's mind, body, and spirit to assist with the reduction of pain, stress, illness, disease, and disability.

- *Operation REBOOT:* This national, peer-support, faith-based group is available to all military and veterans. The objectives are to enhance peer support for military persons interested in developing social connections, participating in recreational activities, and sharing life-affirming and faith-based experiences. The educational learning component of training provides veterans with prevention and treatment resources and illustrates how to maintain living well spiritually.
- *Outward Bound camps for veterans:* These outdoor-based therapeutic camps, led primarily by a recreational therapist, focus on nature attunement, developing individual trust in a team-building environment, and challenging the individual's physical and mental capacity at levels at which they are most comfortable.

OMC: STRATEGIES FOR A NEW CLINICAL COUNSELING PROFESSION

The mission I refer to as OMC began in 2015 when I developed one of the first graduate certificates in military counseling within a Council for Accreditation of Counseling and Related Educational Programs–accredited counselor education program. The mission and core values of OMC are reflected throughout this book, and key constructs of the role and function of a new clinical counseling profession are described more fully in the following sections. The voices of service members, veterans, veterans with disabilities, and military families are being heard. Instead of reacting to the needs of the military culture, counselor educators, researchers, and practitioners are progressively responding to the diversity of physical and mental health needs within the military community.

Clinical Military Counseling offers extensive research and qualitative data collected from focus groups of active-duty personnel, veterans, veterans with disabilities, and military families. Best clinical practices are offered for consideration in the assessment, diagnosis, and mental health treatment of military clients. Thus, this work advances the role and function of clinical military counselors as a dynamic and evolving specialty area, accentuating the needs for OMC training.

A PARADIGM SHIFT IN MILITARY COUNSELING

The changing military community for the 21st century has innovative programs and services offered to service personnel and veterans that were not utilized previously in military treatment facilities and the VA health care system. The combination of interventions listed earlier strongly suggests that many service members and veterans have abandoned sole reliance on traditional models of medical and mental health care. Some therapists have taken a somewhat different path and have integrated newer complementary mental health practices, as demonstrated by the following outcomes:

- Reduction of prescribed opioids along with stricter guidelines and protocols for military medical providers to follow;
- Congressional oversight committees aimed at improving veteran health care through (a) the coordination of military and civilian providers to deliver high-quality services, (b) easier access to care, and (c) better comprehensive inpatient and outpatient treatment within the VA health care system;
- Establishment of specialty clinics and inpatient facilities treating the signature wounds of today's service members and veterans (e.g., TBI, spinal cord injury, substance use and psychiatric disorders);
- Newer studies suggesting that first-line psychotherapy treatment does not effectively treat complex PTSD and is only effective in 30%–50% of clients;
- Newer studies suggesting that interventions that do not focus on the military trauma itself, such as traditional psychotherapy, open the door for complementary and integrative health approaches that have less stigma than receiving treatment for a mental health "disorder";
- Newer studies indicating that 85% of service members and veterans who have participated in nontraditional psychotherapy approaches (e.g., yoga, acupuncture, MBSR, animal-assisted therapy, expressive arts) continue to utilize these resources;
- Recognition that there is not just "one military"—rather, programs and services are offered that enhance and enforce the social justice and civil protections of women and other minority groups in the military;
- Appreciation that military families are an essential part of the service member's and veteran's physical and mental health care by offering enhanced family services that extend beyond the role and function of the Family Readiness Officer;
- Increased research and grants awarded to assist veterans who are at risk (e.g., homeless and rural veterans), who possess health disparities, or who have the signature wounds of today's military (e.g., complex PTSD, TBI, or blast injuries); and
- Improved body armor, emergency battlefield medicine, and advanced medical treatments and technology that have extended the lives of individuals who have served in the military.

The foundations of OMC consider the theories, knowledge, and skills in all specialty areas of psychology, counseling, and psychosocial rehabilitation. Building on the breadth of this research, OMC proposes a new specialty area within the counseling profession. Clinical military counseling within OMC has a strong foundation of facilitating military values within a multicultural context. Accordingly, competent and ethical clinical military counselors provide assessment, diagnosis, and treatment strategies that are facilitated within the cultural lens of the military. Overall, clinical military counselors are intentional with their military cultural awareness, knowledge, and skills; they work optimally with the medical, psychosocial, vocational, career transition, mental health, and family needs of active-duty service members, veterans, veterans with disabilities, and military families.

FOUNDATIONS OF OMC

OMC advocates working holistically with the mind, body, and spiritual needs of the military culture. Medical and mental health treatment models that diagnose and treat psychological "disorders" limit military clients' ability to utilize other coping resources and resiliency skills. Competent and ethical clinical military counselors open doors of unused opportunities and develop capacities for a transformational healing journey. Earning the circle of trust increases the prospects of a strong therapeutic working alliance. Guiding military client opportunities is enhanced by forming healing partnerships and coordinating care outside the traditional clinical setting.

Clinical Military Counseling delineates the framework of OMC through comprehensive research, practice, and training. The principles described within OMC propose a specialty area within the counseling profession given the unique and diverse cultural attributes of the military culture. The foundation of OMC supports, values, and advocates for military-focused mental health practices that demonstrate the following considerations:

- A service member or veteran is a unique individual but is part of the larger military culture and is affiliated with their branch of service.
- Military families are an integral resource for healing the mind, body, and spirit of the service member or veteran.
- Military families have also served and are an integral coping and emotional support system. The military family extends beyond spouses and dependents to the service member's or veteran's parents, brothers, sisters, grandparents, and all others they consider as family.
- Earning the circle of trust for clinical military counselors is essential in achieving a strong working alliance with clients. This alliance enhances the integration of therapeutic effectiveness for optimal military client wellness, accountability, and responsibility by partnering with family members and other healing resources.

CLINICAL MILITARY COUNSELING AS A NEW SPECIALTY WITHIN THE COUNSELING PROFESSION

There is a cultural identity of within-group differences in each branch of the U.S. Armed Forces (i.e., Army, Navy, Marine Corps, Air Force, Coast Guard, Space Force, as well as reservists and National Guard soldiers). When the United States is at war with foreign enemy combatants or a pandemic, some may perceive that there is just "one military." Yet, each branch has a separate mission and distinct military values. These differences are communicated through language, jargon, rank, and military occupational specialty. Today's military is composed of a diverse group of individuals who represent different cultural, ethnic, and racial backgrounds and who have different gender identities. Accordingly, the defining characteristics of becoming a culturally competent clinical military counselor involve the following principles.

Build the circle of trust first, then facilitate individualized approaches and strategies that maximize your client's coping resources, resiliency skills, and overall well-being. Common concerns reported by military clients are that previous therapists "did not understand the military culture." This lack of understanding was demonstrated by therapists who appeared uncomfortable with military clients when they discussed stressful and traumatic events experienced during military life. Many uninformed therapists shifted the conversation to another topic. Other therapists required military clients to repeat combat-related stories that would be retraumatizing for some. Newer research suggests that most evidence-based practices for complex PTSD have limited advantages because they typically provide a "one size fits all" approach to military clients. Overall, there is not one counseling theory or treatment strategy that works with all military clients. Thus, earning the circle of trust and building rapport remains a core value in the therapeutic relationship before implementing strategies and interventions.

Considerations for the assessment, diagnosis, and treatment of complex PTSD and co-occurring disorders are both the same and different in military versus civilian mental health. Compelling new research in military neuroscience is at the forefront of understanding the physiological, psychological, emotional, and neurocognitive intricacies of trauma survivors in military life. Indeed, the military brain is mapped differently. Multiple mediating variables within the brain's complex neuropathways record, transpose, replicate, and reproduce a wide range of psychological responses that underlie optimal brain health, functioning, and performance. The psychological response to military trauma cannot be simulated in civilian life. The physical, emotional, and psychological demands are different because the military brain is trained to "aggress not stress." Consequently, different psychological tools measure combat exposure, reaction time, blast injuries, and multiple other variables that do not exist in community or civilian clinical mental health settings. Interpreting psychological testing and choosing treatment strategies are much different than in civilian practices because of the timing of trauma exposure, the deployment cycle, and other critical aspects of military life. Thus, clinical military counselors are skilled in assessing, diagnosing, and treating military clients.

Finding meaning and purpose in one's military experiences, such as trauma or moral injury, involves an attitudinal shift of leaving the darkness and coming into the light. Finding meaning in one's physical and mental health and well-being—or in the loss, grief, and trauma experienced during military life—requires some level of attitudinal healing. For some, this healing begins as an existential or spiritual pursuit. Clinical military counselors can assist military clients in this deeper journey by helping with areas that affect optimal mental health and well-being, such as jobs and careers, social connections, intimate relationships, therapeutic recreational activities, and other aspects of life that bring some level of satisfaction or joy to the individual. Transforming one's attitude and perception toward self and others requires some level of hope, acceptance, letting go, reflection, and finding meaning and purpose in life's simplest tasks (e.g., driving, going grocery shopping, making new social or intimate connections).

Recognize your military client as a survivor. Individuals who view themselves as a "victim" of a negative critical event during military life devalue their coping and resiliency skills. The victim response is typically viewed as helplessness, hopelessness, dependency, and defenseless. Survivors are empowered to make both small and significant changes in their life circumstances. Clinical military counselors can facilitate strategies and interventions that empower their military clients to transform their perception and attitude as a survivor, not a victim.

Optimizing the healing system requires an understanding of health from a mind, body, and spiritual perspective. Dr. Andrew Weil (1995) has reminded us—on the basis of his comprehensive work as a medical researcher and practitioner—that the body can maintain and heal itself. He and many other mind-body medical practitioners challenge their patients to discover the body's natural ability to reproduce, transcribe, and replicate healthy tissue at the DNA or physiological level. The patient has some responsibility for optimal health through (a) maintaining basic lifestyle habits (e.g., good nutrition, elimination of toxic substances from the body), (b) performing regular movement or exercise (e.g., use of good body mechanics, mind-body activities such as tai chi and yoga), (c) achieving a deep-cleansing breath (e.g., deep breathing and mindfulness training for achieving balance in the sympathetic-parasympathetic nervous system), (d) increasing their immune response (e.g., combination of diet; exercise; and appropriate use of vitamins, minerals, and herbs), (e) increasing their positive thoughts and cognitions (e.g., being mindful of negative trigger events that begin the cascade of sympathetic-parasympathetic response), and (f) deepening their spiritual connections (e.g., seeking religious or spiritual helpers, connecting with spirit entities that are larger than oneself, believing in invisible forces that are helping spirits).

Holistic health approaches that integrate physical, mental, spiritual, psychosocial, and vocational needs are vital and essential in achieving optimal wellness. The defining characteristics of most chronic illnesses and disabilities involve one's perception and attitude toward the critical event itself and the meaning that they attribute to their overall well-being. Psychosocial adjustment to physical and mental health and well-being is different for service members and veterans than for civilians. This difference results from the exposure to extraordinary stressful and traumatic events, the nature of the loss and grief experienced, and other critical adaptations required in military life. Thus, military clients clearly benefit from holistic and integrated treatment approaches in which the military culture is at the center of their healing experiences.

Maintain good self-care as a professional to avoid empathy fatigue. Clinical military counselors spend a significant amount of time, energy, and compassion serving clients who have experienced extraordinary stressful and traumatic experiences and whose personal lives and careers may have been lost to chronic illness and disability resulting from physical and mental health conditions. Empathy fatigue (Stebnicki, 2008, 2017) results in a state of psychological, emotional, physical, spiritual, and occupational exhaustion that occurs as the counselor's own wounds are continually revisited by their clients' life stories of illness, disability, trauma, grief, and loss. Thus, it is of paramount importance that counselor educators, clinical supervisors, and clinicians themselves recognize this negative shift within their mind, body, and spirit that may impair their ability to serve the needs of their military clients.

CONCLUDING REMARKS

Complementary and integrative health as well as resiliency and wellness programs have been in existence for more than 30 years in the civilian counseling and psychology profession. The military as an occupation requires a shift in focus from medical and mental health pathology and illness to living well in mind, body, and spirit. Interestingly, many interventions that were once considered "complementary and alternative" are now supported by evidence-based practices and are utilized regularly by military treatment programs (e.g., MBSR, Reiki, wellness programs). Military researchers have reported that many service members and veterans who are offered complementary and integrative treatment approaches that promote wellness and resiliency continue to utilize these resources. These wellness strategies enhance unit cohesiveness, accountability, and responsibility and are a natural support system that can be carried throughout the life span.

REFERENCES

Bauer, A., Newbury-Birch, D., Robalino, S., Ferguson, J., & Wigham, S. (2018). Is prevention better than cure? A systematic review of the effectiveness of well-being interventions for military personnel adjusting to civilian life. *PLoS One, 13*(5), Article e0190144. https://doi.org/10.1371/journal.pone.0190144

Benish, S. G., Imel, Z. E., & Wamplod, B. E. (2007). The relative efficacy of bona fide psychotherapies for treating post-traumatic stress disorder: A meta-analysis of direct comparisons. *Clinical Psychology Review, 28*(5), 746–758. https://doi.org/10.1016/j.cpr.2007.10.005

Brintz, C. E., Miller, S., Olmstead, K. R., Bartoszek, M., Cartwright, J., Kizakevich, P. N., Butler, M., Asefnia, N., Buben, A., & Gaylord, S. A. (2020). Adapting mindfulness training for military service members with chronic pain. *Military Medicine, 185*(3–4), 385–393. https://doi.org/10.1093/milmed/usz312

Evans, E. A., Herman, P. M., Washington, D. L., Lorenz, K. A., Yuan, A., Upchurch, D. M., Marshall, N., Hamilton, A. B., & Taylor, S. L. (2018). Gender differences in use of complementary and integrative health by U.S. military veterans with chronic musculoskeletal pain. *Women's Health Issues, 28*(5), 379–386. https://doi.org/10.1016/j.whi.2018.07.003

France, D. (2018). *Combat vet don't mean crazy: Veteran mental health in post-military life.* NCO Historical Society.

Gantt, M., & Orina, J. A. T. (2020). Educate, try, and share: A feasibility study to assess the acceptance and use of Reiki as an adjunct therapy for chronic pain the military health care facilities. *Military Medicine, 185*(3–4), 394–400. https://doi.org/10.1093/milmed/usz271

Herman, P. M., Sorbero, M. E., & Sims-Columbia, A. C. (2017). Complementary and alternative medicine services in the military health system. *Journal of Complementary and Alternative Medicine, 23*(11), 837–843. https://doi.org/10.1089/acm.2017.0236

Kabat-Zinn, J. (1990). *Full catastrophe living: Using the wisdom of your body and mind to face stress, pain, and illness.* Dell Books.

Meadows, S. O., Tanielian, T., & Karney, B. (2016). *How military families respond before, during, and after deployment: Findings from the RAND Deployment Life Study.* RAND Corporation. https://www.rand.org/pubs/research_briefs/RB9906.html

Miller, S., Gaylord, S., Buben, A., Brintz, C., Olmstead, K. R., Asefnia, N., & Bartoszek, M. (2017). Literature review of research on chronic pain and yoga in military populations. *Medicines, 4*(3), Article 64. https://doi.org/10.3390/medicines4030064

Moodley, R., & West, W. (2005). *Integrating traditional healing practices in counseling and psychotherapy.* Sage.

Myers, J. E. (1992). Wellness, prevention, development: The cornerstones of the profession. *Journal of Counseling & Development, 71*(2), 136–139. https://doi.org/10.1002/j.1556-6676.1992.tb02188.x

Myers, J. E., & Sweeney, T. J. (Eds.). (2005). *Counseling for wellness: Theory, research, and practice.* American Counseling Association.

Myers, J. E., Sweeney, T. J., & Witmer, J. M. (2000). The Wheel of Wellness counseling for wellness: A holistic model for treatment planning. *Journal of Counseling & Development, 78*(3), 251–266. https://doi.org/10.1002/j.1556-6676.2000.tb01906.x

Nakamura, J., & Csikszentmihalyi, M. (2002). The concept of flow. In C. R. Snyder & S. J. Lopez (Eds.), *Handbook of positive psychology* (pp. 89–105). Oxford University Press.

National Center for Complementary and Integrative Health. (2018, July). *Complementary, alternative, or integrative health: What's in a name?* https://nccih.nih.gov/health/integrative-health

Robson, S. (2014). *Psychological fitness and resilience: A review of relevant constructs, measures, and links to well-being.* RAND Corporation. https://www.rand.org/pubs/research_reports/RR102.html

Schlitz, M., & Amorok, T. (2005). *Consciousness and healing: Integral approaches to mind-body medicine.* Elsevier.

Shannonhouse, L. R., Myers, J. E., & Sweeney, T. J. (2016). Counseling for wellness. In I. Marini & M. A. Stebnicki (Eds.), *The professional counselor's desk reference* (2nd ed., pp. 617–623). Springer.

Siebert, A. (2005). *The resiliency advantage: Master change, thrive under pressure, and bounce back from setbacks.* Berrett-Koehler.

Stebnicki, M. A. (2008). *Empathy fatigue: Healing the mind, body, and spirit of professional counselors.* Springer.

Stebnicki, M. A. (2016). Integrative approaches in counseling and psychotherapy: Foundations of mind, body, and spirit. In I. Marini & M. A. Stebnicki (Eds.), *The professional counselor's desk reference* (2nd ed., pp. 593–604). Springer.

Stebnicki, M. A. (2017). *Disaster mental health counseling: Responding to trauma in a multicultural context.* Springer.

Steenkamp, M. M., Litz, B. T., & Marmar, C. R. (2020). First-line psychotherapies for military-related PTSD. *Journal of the American Medical Association, 323*(7), 656–657. https://doi.org/10.1001/jama.2019.20825

Tedeschi, R. G., & Calhoun, L. G. (2003). Routes to posttraumatic growth through cognitive processing. In D. Patton, J. M. Violanti, & L. M. Smith (Eds.), *Promoting capabilities to manage posttraumatic tress: Perspectives on resilience* (pp. 12–26). Charles C Thomas.

Tedeschi, R. G., & Calhoun, L. G. (2004). Posttraumatic growth: Conceptual foundations and empirical evidence. *Psychological Inquiry, 15*(1), 1–18. https://www.jstor.org/stable/20447194

Tick, E. (2014). *Warrior's return: Restoring the soul after war.* Sounds True.

Updegraff, J. A., & Taylor, S. E. (2000). From vulnerability to growth: Positive and negative effects of stressful life events. In T. H. Harvey & E. Miller (Eds.), *Loss and trauma: General and close relationship perspectives* (pp. 3–23). Brunner-Routledge.

Weil, A. (1995). *Spontaneous healing: How to discover and enhance your body's natural ability to maintain and heal itself.* Fawcett Columbine.

Ysasi, N. A., Graf, N., Brown, A. D., & Sharma, R. (2016). Receptiveness toward complementary and alternative medicine by veterans and military servicepersons: Implications for counseling professionals. *Military Behavioral Health, 4*(1), 32–46. https://doi.org/10.1080/21635781.2015.1093977

INDEX

A

ACA Code of Ethics, 29
Academic performance of military children and adolescents, 212–213
Acceptance and commitment therapy, 275
Access to health care treatment
  civilians, 10
  Hispanics and Latinos/Latinas, 45–46
  suicide prevention and, 102–104
  veterans, 112
Accreditation, 3–4
Acculturation
  of Asian Americans and Pacific Islanders, 48
  of Hispanics and Latinos/Latinas, 46–47
  into military culture, 8–9, 57
Acknowledgment stage of psychosocial adjustment, 127
Active-duty service members
  adjustment disorders and, 265
  chronic pain and, 142, 146–147. *See also* Chronic pain
  combat death of, 209–212
  combat vs. noncombat operations and, 20–22
  disability benefits and, 25–26
  drunk while on duty, 281
  families and. *See* Family system
  LGBT concerns, 53–56
  military sexual trauma and, 38, 40
  psychiatric disabilities and, 23–25
  reservists vs., 208–209
  suicide prevention programs and, 102
  suicide rates, 96
  "thank you for your service" and, 22–23
  transition to civilian life, 223–233. *See also* Transition to civilian life
Acupuncture, 156, 189, 300, 305
Acute pain, 144
Acute stress
  chronic pain and, 148–149
  functional degradation and, 75
  suicide prevention and, 103
  sympathetic-parasympathetic response to, 80–81, 274
Ader, R., 72
Adjustment, integration, and growth stage of psychosocial adjustment, 127
Adjustment disorders, 23, 103, 263, 265–267. *See also specific disorders*
Adler, A. B., 9, 214, 272
Advocacy. *See* Social justice
African Americans in the military, 37, 41–43
After-action reports, 11–12

Age
chronic illness and disability and, 121
as suicide risk factor, 96
Air Force, 5, 21
Alaska Natives. *See* Native American Indians
Alcohol, Smoking and Substance Involvement Screening Test, 282
Alcohol use, 280–282, 287
Alcohol Use Disorder Identification Test, 282
Alternative treatments. *See* Complementary and integrative health
American Counseling Association (ACA), 29, 187
ACA Code of Ethics, 29
American Indians. *See* Native American Indians
American Military Partner Association, 55
American Psychiatric Association, 95
American Psychological Association, 4
American Revolutionary War, 41
Amputation. *See* Traumatic amputation
Amygdala, 78, 82
Anderson, R. N., 46
Anger
acute stress and, 76
amygdala and, 78
CIH approaches, 298, 300
deployment and, 209
diversion of feelings, 130
in military children and adolescents, 213–214
moral injury and, 193–194
as psychosocial adjustment stage, 126
PTSD co-occurrence, 273
TBIs and, 175
transition to civilian life and, 226
in younger service members, 93
Animal-assisted therapy, 189, 275, 305
Antihistamines, 278
Antonak, R. F., 123, 125
Anxiety disorders
best practices and guidelines, 274–275
blast injuries and, 166, 168, 178
chronic pain and, 147, 155
chronic stress and, 81–82
CIH approaches, 299–300
definition of, 274
deployment and, 209
insomnia co-occurrence, 278
MBSR and, 103
military children and adolescents and, 213–214
mind-body connection and, 118
psychosocial adjustment stage, 126
PTSD co-occurrence, 19, 268, 271, 273–275
somatic symptom disorders and, 148
spinal cord injuries and, 152
as suicide risk factor, 95, 99
TBI and, 166, 169, 178
warfighters and, 262, 273–274
women and, 39
Anxiolytics, 275
Armed Forces
branches of service, 5–6, 309
pain management strategy, 155
resiliency programs, 302
substance use disorder prevention, 285
suicide incidence, 91
Army
adjustment disorder statistics, 265
branch of Armed Services, 5
elite warfighters, 21, 27
Health Professions Scholarship Program, 4
overrepresentation in military health statistics, 264
Sharp, Ready, and Resilient directorate, 191
Army Dismounted Complex Blast Injury Task Force, 165
Army Study to Assess Risk and Resilience in Service members (Army STARRS), 49
Army Surgeon General, 155
The Art of War (Sun Tzu), 17
Asian Americans in the military, 47–50
Association for Spiritual, Ethical, and Religious Values in Counseling (ASERVIC), 187
Associative learning, 77–78
Attucks, Crispus, 41
Automated Neuropsychological Assessment Metric, 172

B

Back injuries, 121–122
Basic emotions theory of the brain, 74
Battle fatigue, 262
Battlefield documentation of blast injuries, 165

Battlemind training program, 272
Behavioral addictions, 287–288
Behavioral health and lifestyle
  chronic pain treatment and, 150
  high-risk factors, 57
Benzodiazepines, 275, 278
Bereavement. *See* Grief and bereavement
Best practices and guidelines
  for adjustment disorders, 266–267
  for anxiety disorders, 274–275
  for bereavement disorders, 277
  for blast injuries, 168–169, 177–179
  for chronic illness and disability treatment, 118–119
  for chronic pain treatment, 149–150
  for counseling minorities in the military, 56–57
  for defensive clients, 249
  for depressive disorders, 277
  for earning circle of trust, 245–249
  for family coping and resiliency, 217–218
  for grief and bereavement, 105–107
  military culture and, 12–13, 29–30, 56–57
  for moral injury screening, 195
  myths, stereotypes, and stigma in military culture and, 29–30
  for psychosocial adjustment, 131–134
  for PTS and PTSD, 271–273
  purpose of, 11
  for rapport building, 245–249
  for reluctant clients, 245–246
  for resistant clients, 247–248
  for spiritual care, 197
  for substance use disorders, 286–288
  for suicide assessment, 95–96, 100–101
  for suicide prevention, 103–104
  for TBIs, 177–179
  for wake-sleep disorders, 278–279
Bioethics of military neuroscience, 71
Biofeedback, 80, 305
Biomedical model of treatment, 113, 118, 120
Biopsychosocial factors of suicidality, 99
Biopsychosocial model of disability, 113, 123
Bipolar disorder, 95, 99
Bisexual service members. *See* LGBT service members
Blast injuries
  as chronic condition, 116–117
  as complex trauma, 163, 262
  documentation of, 164–166, 168
  explosion physics, 166–167
  military suicide and, 163, 166
  occurrence of, 164–169
  PTSD co-occurrence, 268
  severity of, 163–164
  symptoms of, 166–167
  TBI and, 166
Blood quantum of Native American Indians, 52
Blue Gene computer system, 70
Blue Star Families, 210
Body energy. *See* Reiki
Body image
  as measure of adaptation to chronic illness and disability, 124
  psychosocial adjustment and, 120–121
  traumatic amputation and, 153–155
The Body Keeps the Score (Van Der Kolk), 69
Bradshaw, B. S., 46
Brain function and structure, 173–175
Brain imaging
  amygdala activation, 82
  pathophysiological events, 79
  techniques, 73
Brain injuries. *See* Blast injuries; Traumatic brain injuries
Brief Traumatic Brain Injury Screen, 172
Broca's aphasia, 174
Brown, S. M., 41
Buffalo Soldiers, 41–42
Butler, J. S., 43

C

CACREP (Council for Accreditation of Counseling and Related Educational Programs), 3–4
Campbell, R., 40
Camp Lejeune, 42–43
Camp Montford Point, 42–43
Card-Mina, M. E., 243
Career counseling, 225, 229–233

Career development. *See also* Promotions
African Americans and, 43
Asian Americans and, 49
Career Resiliency Portfolio tool, 228
chronic pain and, 146
Hispanics and, 44–45
Latinos/Latinas and, 44–45
LGBT service members and, 55
Pacific Islanders and, 49
self-disclosure and, 101
transition to civilian life and, 225
Career One Stop, 231
Career resiliency, 224, 228–229
Career Resiliency Portfolio (CRP), 228–231
Career transitions, 223–233. *See also* Transition to civilian life
Carter, Ash, 27
Cashwell, C. S., 187
Castro, C. A., 9, 214
Catch a Serial Offender Program, 39
Center for Reiki Research, 156
Centers for Disease Control and Prevention (CDC), National Violent Death Reporting System, 93, 97
Cherokee Nation of Oklahoma blood quantum, 52
Chinese Exclusion Act of 1882, 48
Chiropractic body manipulation, 300
Chronic illness and disability, 111–135
adjustment and adaptation to. *See* Psychosocial adjustment to chronic illness and disability
complementary and integrative health approaches, 300
depressive disorder co-occurrence, 276
health disparities among veterans, 114–116
insomnia co-occurrence, 278
monitoring veterans' health needs, 112–114
transition to civilian life and, 226
treatment stages, 117
veterans and, 116
Chronic multisymptom illness (CMI), 81–82, 115
Chronic pain, 141–157
assessment of, 144–145, 149
best practices and guidelines, 149–150
complex trauma and, 262
definition of, 144
depressive disorder co-occurrence, 276
etiology of conditions, 142–143
management of, 155–157
medical conditions associated with, 150–155
mood disorders and, 147
phantom limb pain, 154
prevalence in the military, 142–143
psychosocial aspects of, 146–150
self-report questions, 145
somatic symptom disorders, 148
spinal cord injuries and, 151–152
traumatic amputation and, 152–155
treatment of, 155–157
Chronic stress, 75, 148–149
Chronic traumatic encephalopathy (CTE), 116, 169, 175–176
CIH treatments. *See* Complementary and integrative health
Circle of trust
best practices and guidelines, 245–249
clinical military counseling and, 240–242
defensiveness and, 248–249
empathy and, 84, 242–243, 251
Hispanics and Latinos/Latinas and, 47
importance of earning, 12, 133
intake interview and, 254–257
MST and, 40
multicultural counseling and, 36, 56
myths, stereotypes, and stigma of military culture and, 20
open-ended questions and, 252–254
person-centered interview and, 249–252
rapport building, 114, 245–249, 251–254, 309
reluctance and, 245–246
resistance and, 246–248
spiritual care and, 196–197
Stebnicki on, 239
Civilian life
transition to. *See* Transition to civilian life
trauma exposure, 9–10, 131, 264, 270, 289, 309–311
Civil War, 47
Clinical assessments
blast injuries, 164–165, 168, 177–179
intake interviews. *See* Intake interviews
military suicide, 98–101
moral injury, 194–195
MST evaluation, 40

TBIs, 171–173, 177–179
work readiness, 228
Clinical military counseling
art of, 240–242
best practices and guidelines. *See* Best practices and guidelines
brain injuries and, 163–179. *See also* Blast injuries; Traumatic brain injuries
career transitions and, 223–233. *See also* Transition to civilian life
chronic illness and disability and, 111–135. *See also* Chronic illness and disability
chronic pain conditions and, 141–157. *See also* Chronic pain
circle of trust and, 239–258. *See also* Circle of trust
cultural competency, 3–13, 56, 240, 309–311. *See also* Military culture
empathy fatigue, 311
family system and, 205–218. *See also* Family system
integrative treatment strategies, 297–312. *See also* Complementary and integrative health
military culture and, 3–57. *See also* Military culture
military health and, 69–179. *See also* Military health
military neuroscience and, 69–85. *See also* Military neuroscience
military suicide, 91–107. *See also* Military suicide
minority issues, 35–57. *See also* Minorities in the military; *specific minority groups*
myths, stereotypes, and stigma of military culture, 17–30. *See also* Myths, stereotypes, and stigma of military culture
OMC and, 306, 308–311
paradigm shift in, 306–308
person-centered counseling, 12
PTSD and co-occurring mental health conditions, 261–289. *See also* Complex PTSD
resiliency, 297–312. *See also* Resiliency
shortage of counselors, 6
as specialty profession, 306, 309–311
spiritual care, 185–198. *See also* Spiritual care
transition to civilian life, 223–233. *See also* Transition to civilian life
women's issues. *See* Women in the military
Clinical Military Counseling Certificate program, 3
Closed head brain injuries, 169
Coast Guard, 5
Code of Federal Regulations, Title 45, 40–41
Code talkers, 51
Coercive control, 40, 56
Cognitive behavioral therapy (CBT)
anxiety disorders and, 275
integrative approaches vs., 298
wake-sleep disorders and, 278
Cognitive functioning scales, 168
Cohen, M., 143
Combat Exposure Scale, 257
Combat operational stress and trauma exposure. *See also* Extraordinary stressful and traumatic events
amygdala changes and, 78
combat vs. noncombat situations, 20–22, 30
experience of, 270–273
military neuroscience and, 69–85. *See also* Military neuroscience
moral injury and, 192, 195
neuroscience of, 69–85
physical manifestations of, 118
sexual trauma. *See* Military sexual trauma
sympathetic-parasympathetic response to, 80
Combat Operational Stress Control program, 102
Combat vs. noncombat service members and veterans
myth regarding, 20–22
suicide and, 94, 96
trauma exposure in, 30
Coming out by LGBT service members, 54–57
Communications to employers, 232–233
Community-based counseling, 102, 112–113, 241
Compassion, 242
Complementary and integrative health (CIH), 297–312
chronic illness and disability, 118–119
chronic pain and, 149–150, 155–157
deployment impact on families and, 218

(Continued)

Complementary and integrative health (*continued*)
depressive disorders and, 277
description of, 298–300
effectiveness, 300–301
Operation Military Counseling and, 308–311
optimization of healing, 310–311
paradigm shift in military counseling, 306–308
remapping the military brain, 83
resiliency building, 303–304
resources, 304–306
spiritual care and, 188–189
stigma of, 299, 307
suicide prevention and, 103
therapeutic approaches, 305–306
utilization by service members and veterans, 157, 194
Complex PTSD, 261–289
anxiety disorder co-occurrence, 273–275
best practices and guidelines, 271–273
blast injuries and, 168, 268
depressive disorder co-occurrence, 275–277
diagnostic criteria, 267–268
eye movement desensitization and reprocessing therapy, 305
first-line treatment effectiveness, 307
intense stress as risk factor, 82, 297
military sexual trauma and, 28, 37, 39, 97
military vs. civilian, 270, 309–310
preferred terminology for, 268–269
remapping the military brain, 83–85
resiliency programs, 272–273
Stebnicki on, 261
stigma of, 268–269
substance use co-occurrence, 268, 271, 279–289
TBI blended with, 77–79, 117, 166, 169, 178, 268
traumatic experience as risk factor, 270–271
treatments, 298
veterans myth, 23–25, 30
wake-sleep disorder co-occurrence, 277–279
warfighters and, 261–262
Complex regional pain syndromes, 144
Comprehensive Airman Fitness program, 102
Comprehensive clinical assessments. *See* Clinical assessments
Comprehensive Soldier and Family Fitness program, 102, 191, 272
Comprehensive Soldier Fitness Program, 272
Conceptual act theory of emotions, 74
Concussions. *See* Traumatic brain injuries
Confidentiality. *See* Disclosure of information
Confucius, 17
Continuing education
on blast injuries, 177
on multicultural counseling, 56, 251
on spiritual care, 197
on TBIs, 177
Co-occurring mental health conditions
chronic pain and, 150–155
IPV and MST, 40
PTSD and. *See* Complex PTSD
TBIs and, 169
women and, 28
Coordination of care, 95, 187, 286
Coping strategies
compensation, 129–130
denial, 128
deployment impact on families, 217–218
diversion of feelings, 130
military suicide prevention, 101, 103
posttrauma recovery and, 133
psychosocial adjustment and, 120, 123
PTSS and, 78
rationalization, 130
regression, 129
resiliency advantage and, 301–302
skill building, 303–304, 309
Core competencies and skills
circle of trust and, 239–258. *See also* Circle of trust
military cultural competency, 3–13, 56, 250, 309–311
person-centered counseling, 12
spiritual care, 187
Coreil, J., 46
Corey, J., 258
Corey, M. S., 258
Coronavirus (COVID-19), 111, 115–116

Council for Accreditation of Counseling and Related Educational Programs (CACREP), 3–4
Cover letters, 232–233
COVID-19 pandemic, 111, 115–116
Critical life events
  coping and, 127
  as suicide risk factor, 95
Critical life events as suicide risk factor, 99, 103
CRP (Career Resiliency Portfolio), 228–231
CTE. *See* Chronic traumatic encephalopathy
Cultural competency, 3–13, 56, 240, 309–311. *See also* Military culture
Cultural expression of emotions, 83
Curanderismo, 47
Curthoys, K., 146
Cut-Down, Annoyed, Guilty, Eye-Opener test, 282

D

Data collection
  on mental health conditions, 264
  on military suicides, 93
Davis, Benjamin O., Sr., 42
Davis, Benjamin O., Jr., 42
DD-214 form, 227
Deaf culture, 131–132
Deep breathing, 299–300, 310
Defense Advanced Research Projects Agency, 71
Defense and Veterans Brain Injury Center (DVBIC), 172
Defense and Veterans Pain Rating Scale, 145
Defense Department (DoD)
  complex PTSD prevention, 268
  COVID-19 pandemic response, 115–116
  Exceptional Family Member Program, 212
  Joint VA Executive Committee strategic plan for 2019-2021, 112–113
  LGBT policies, 54–55
  mental health condition data collection, 264
  military suicide data collection, 93
  neuroscience research, 70–71
  suicide prevention programs, 102
  wellness program development, 191
Defense Enrollment Eligibility Reporting System, 206
Defense Health Agency, 113
Defense mechanisms, 78
Defensiveness, 248–249
Deliberate plans and acts of self-harm, 96, 98, 99, 194
Dementias, 116, 169, 176, 276
Demographics of service members
  Asian Americans, 48
  generally, 5
  Hispanics and Latinos/Latinas, 44
  military families, 206
  Native American Indians, 53
  Pacific Islanders, 48
  women, 27, 37
Denial
  as coping strategy, 128
  as psychosocial adjustment stage, 126
Department of ___. *See name of department*
Deployment
  academic performance of children and, 212–213
  combat operations myth, 20–22
  coping resiliency of families and, 217–218
  cycle models, 214–217
  as family stressor, 208–211
  intake interview questions on, 257
  military children and adolescents and, 211–212
  missions, 5
  of reservists, 208–209
Deployment Life Study, 217
Depression stage of psychosocial adjustment, 126
Depressive disorders
  blast injuries and, 166, 168, 178
  chronic pain and, 147, 155
  CIH approaches, 299–300
  deployment and, 209
  insomnia co-occurrence, 278
  military leadership and, 244
  PTSD co-occurrence, 19, 268, 271, 275–277
  reservists and, 208
  spinal cord injuries and, 152
  spiritual care and, 186, 192
  as suicide risk factor, 95, 99
  TBI co-occurrence, 166, 169, 178, 276
  transition to civilian life and, 226

(Continued)

Depressive disorders *(continued)*
traumatic amputation and, 153
warfighters and, 262
women and, 39
Developmental psychology perspective
of chronic illness and disability, 119–120
of spirituality, 190
Diagnostic and Statistical Manual of Mental Disorders (*DSM-IV*), 273
Disabilities. *See also* Chronic illness and disability; *specific disabilities and conditions*
adjustment and adaptation to. *See* Psychosocial adjustment to chronic illness and disability
blast injuries as, 165
chronic pain as, 141–157. *See also* Chronic pain
deaf culture and, 131–132
psychiatric, 23–25
Disability rating system, 25–26, 117, 227, 269
Disability rights, 114
Disclosure of information
intake interviews and, 254–256
LGBT service members and, 55
MST and HIPAA standards, 40–41
operational security and, 11–12, 255
self-disclosure impact on career development, 101
Discrimination in the military
against African Americans, 42
against LGBT service members, 54–55
Diversion of feelings as coping strategy, 130
Diversity in the military
African Americans, 43
Asian Americans, 48
Hispanics and Latinos/Latinas, 44
historic, 35
human resource issues and, 36–37
Pacific Islanders, 48
within-group differences and, 309
women, 37
DoD Medical Mortality Registry, 93
DoD Suicide Event Report, 93, 97
Don't Ask, Don't Tell, 54–55
Drug Abuse Screening Test, 282
Drug testing, 282
DVBIC 3 Question TBI Screen, 172

E

Earning the circle of trust. *See* Circle of trust
E-cigarettes, 288
Elite warfighters, 21, 27, 243
Emergency medical procedures for traumatic amputation, 153
EMIS-M (Expressions of Moral Injury Scale–Military Version), 194
Emotional brain
acute stress response, 80–81
biophysiological markers of PTSD, 78
chronic activation of, 83
empathy and, 85
Emotional freedom techniques, 275
Emotions
amygdala and, 82–83
cultural expression of, 83
healing potential of, 84
neurobiology of, 74
neuroscience of, 72
Empathy
circle of trust and, 12
counselor fatigue, 311
as leadership tool, 243–244
person-centered counseling and, 84–85, 251
Stebnicki on, 242
therapeutic relationship and, 240–243
Encephalopathy. *See* Chronic traumatic encephalopathy
Epidemiological characteristics
of Hispanics and Latinos/Latinas, 46
of military suicide, 92–94
of Native American Indians, 53
Equine therapy and equine-facilitated psychotherapy, 305
Estrada, A. X., 281
Ethics of military neuroscience, 71
Ethnic minorities in the military. *See* Minorities in the military
Evolutionary theories of neurobiology, 73–74
Exclusion Acts of 1875, 1917, and 1924, 48
Exclusionary policies and practices
Asian Americans and, 48
LGBT community and, 54–55
Executive Order 9981, establishing the Fair Employment Practices Commission, 42

Explosions, 152–153, 166–167. *See also* Blast injuries
Expressions of Moral Injury Scale–Military Version (EMIS-M), 194
Expressive arts, 83, 189, 275, 298, 305
Expressive writing, 230–231
Extraordinary stressful and traumatic events. *See also* Combat operational stress and trauma exposure
as chronic health condition risk factor, 116
denial as coping strategy, 128
individual pace of healing, 134
legitimacy of, 132
military vs. civilian exposure, 9–10, 131, 264, 270, 289, 309–311
moral injury and, 133, 186, 192
neurological mapping of, 74
perceptions of, 271
psychosocial adjustment and adaptation to, 124
resiliency and, 133
spiritual care and, 196–198
spiritual well-being and, 185, 189–190
stress inoculation effects, 75–76
as triggering events, 133
veteran's identity and, 226
Extremist activities in the military, 35
Eye movement desensitization and reprocessing therapy, 305

F

Factitious disorders, 148
Fair Employment Practices Commission, 42
Falvo, D. R., 128
Family system, 205–218
CIH approaches and, 307
clinician influence on, 20
combat death impact on, 209–212
coping resiliency and, 217–218
cultural values and, 57
deployment as stressor, 208–211, 302
deployment cycle and, 214–217
Hispanic paradox and, 47
intake interview questions on, 256
as measure of adaptation to chronic illness and disability, 124
military children and adolescents, 98, 211–214
military culture and, 12
military spouses, 98, 207–211
military suicide and, 91–92, 98, 105–107
models, 206–207
of National Guard members, 208
permanent change of duty station and, 209
psychosocial adjustment and, 120, 226
psychosocial stressors and, 206–211
of reservists, 208
resiliency programs and, 302
suicide rates for spouses and dependents, 98
"thank you for your service" and, 23
within-group differences, 207
Farley, J., 232
Fear, 274
Fibromyalgia, 148
Fight-or-flight response, 80, 274
Firearms
military suicide and, 100
ownership by service members and veterans, 28–29
veteran suicide and, 95
1st Special Forces Operational Detachment-Delta, 21
Fitness for duty
anxiety and, 274
clinician influence on, 20
disclosure standards, 41
LGBT service members and, 55
self-disclosure and, 101
traumatic experiences and, 270
Foran, H. M., 272
Frankl, Victor E., 80, 134
Freedom of Information Act requests, 43

G

GAO (Government Accountability Office), 113
Gay service members. *See* LGBT service members
Gender
Latinx, 44
military suicide and, 93
Gender dysphoria, 54–55
Generalized pain, 144

Genetics of neurobiology, 70, 73–74
Ghahramanlou-Holloway, M., 269
Glasgow Coma Scale (GCS), 168
Glucocorticoids, 82
Gold Star families, 210
Government Accountability Office (GAO), 113
Graduate programs in military cultural competence, 4
Grief and bereavement
    blast injuries and, 169
    delayed, 271
    depressive disorders and, 276–277
    spiritual care and, 186
    Stebnicki on, 205
    suicide and, 92, 105–107
    TBIs and, 178
Grossman, D., 273
Gulf War
    disability benefits, 26
    GWI/CMI, 81–82, 115
Gulf War illness (GWI), 81–82, 115, 148

H

Harlem Hellfighters, 42
Harm to Mission disclosure requirements, 41
Health Insurance Portability and Accountability Act of 1996 (HIPAA), 40–41
Health Professions Scholarship Program, 4
Hispanic paradox, 46–47
Hispanics in the military, 43–47
Holistic health practices. *See* Complementary and integrative health
Hollywood portrayal of military culture, 20
Homan, P., 78
Homelessness, 114–115, 226
Hostility, 126, 130, 213
Huang, J. Y., 70
Humana Military, 4
Human Brain Project, 70
Human rights losses of Asian Americans and Pacific Islanders, 48
Hyperarousal, 81–82
Hyperperfusion, 79
Hypervigilance, 10, 228, 261, 268
Hypoperfusion, 79

I

Identity
    Hispanics and Latinos/Latinas, 44
    within military culture, 6–9, 19, 29, 36
    spinal cord injuries and, 152
    spirituality and, 196
Immune system, 72, 81, 82
Immunologic memory, 81
Indian wars, 41
Indigenous cultural groups. *See also* Native American Indians
    distrust of American military, 19
    healing modalities, 83
Indoctrination process, 6–7, 19
Inpatient treatment
    of chronic health conditions, 117
    of signature wounds, 307
Insomnia, 277–279
Intake interviews
    family-related questions, 256
    general questions, 256
    information gathering, 254–256
    MST evaluation, 40, 255–256
    spirituality evaluation, 197–198
    substance use disorder screening, 283–284
Integrative treatment strategies, 297–312. *See also* Complementary and integrative health
International Association for the Study of Pain, 143
Intimate partner violence (IPV), 39–41, 56
Intimate relationships. *See* Sexual and intimate relationships

J

Japanese American relocation, 48
Jargon, 7–8, 11, 12–13
Job applications, 232–233
Job interviews, 232–233
Johnson, B. D., 190
Joint Executive Committee strategic plan for 2019-2021 (VA & DoD, 2019), 112–113
Judge Advocate General's Corps, 7

K

K-9 Corps, 305
Kabat-Zinn, Jon, 305

Kail, E., 243
Kaku, M., 70
Kardiner, Abram, 262
Kosal, M. E., 70

L

Labor Department, Career One Stop, 231
Latinos/Latinas in the military, 43–47
Latinx, 44
Leadership skills, 243–244
Leal, D. L., 43
LeDoux, J. E., 82
Left brain, 173–175
LGBT service members
  families of, 206, 207
  health outcomes, 112
  military culture and, 53–57
  suicide risk in, 97–98, 100, 103
Lieberman, H. R., 75
Lifestyle
  chronic pain treatment and, 150
  high-risk factors, 57
Livneh, H., 123, 125
Locus of control, 80, 150
Lozano, A., 44

M

MACE-2 (Military Acute Concussion Evaluation–2), 172
Major depressive disorder. *See* Depressive disorders
Mapping the military brain, 69–85. *See also* Military neuroscience
Marci, C., 84
Marine Corps
  branch of Armed Forces, 5
  career effects of seeking mental health care, 269
  elite warfighters, 21
  military culture of, 7
  segregation in, 42–43
Markham, Henry, 70
Markides, K. S., 46
Master Resilience Training Course, 191
MBSR. *See* Mindfulness-based stress reduction
McFarland, L. V., 155
Meals, ready-to-eat (MRE), 9
Measures of adaptation to chronic illness and disability, 123–124
Media portrayal of veteran mental health problems, 24–25
Medicalizing moral injury, 186
Medical records
  blast injury documentation, 164–166, 178
  chronic pain documentation, 142
  service-related disabilities, 269
  sexual orientation recorded in, 55
  treatment planning and, 121
Medical separation
  chronic health conditions and, 117
  chronic pain and, 146, 151
  family dynamics and, 120
  as retirement, 25–26, 265
  suicide risk and, 94
  traumatic amputation and, 154
  unhealthy denial and, 126, 128
  veteran mental health concerns, 267
Medicare, 4
Meditation. *See also* Mindfulness-based stress reduction
  as anxiety treatment, 275
  as CIH approach, 103, 194, 298–300, 306
  healing potential, 84
  as insomnia treatment, 278–279
  spiritual care and, 188
Mental Health First Aid program, 272
Mental health services-seeking behaviors. *See* Utilization of health services
Metacommunication, 20, 241
Mild TBIs, 163, 166, 169–170
Military Acute Concussion Evaluation–2 (MACE-2), 172
Military and Trauma Counseling certificate program, 3
Military children and adolescents, 209, 211–214
Military culture, 3–57
  acculturation into, 8–9
  best practices and guidelines, 12–13, 29–30, 56–57
  branches of service, 5–6, 309
  career and occupational focus, 224
  circle of trust and, 12
  client concerns, 6
  competency in, 3–13, 56, 240
  comprehensive clinical assessment and, 240
  demographics, 5, 27, 37
  history of OMC, 3–5
  identity and, 6–9
  indoctrination process, 6–7
  jargon, 7–8, 11, 12–13

(Continued)

Military culture *(continued)*
- military occupational specialty. *See* Military occupational specialty
- minority issues. *See* Minorities in the military; *specific minority groups*
- mission first objective, 214–215
- multicultural counseling and, 250
- myths surrounding, 17–30. *See also* Myths, stereotypes, and stigma of military culture
- person-centered interview and, 249–252
- punishment within, 7
- shortage of counselors, 6
- specialized training within, 8
- stereotypes surrounding, 17–30. *See also* Myths, stereotypes, and stigma of military culture
- stigmas surrounding, 17–30. *See also* Myths, stereotypes, and stigma of military culture
- training and, 5–6
- trauma exposure and, 9–10
- tribal aspects of, 193–194
- understanding of, 6–9
- war stories, 10–12
- within-group differences and, 309
- women's issues. *See* Women in the military

Military Entrance Processing Command, 282

Military families. *See* Family system

Military Family Appreciation Month, 218

Military Family Life Survey, 210

Military health, 69–179
- brain injuries, 163–179. *See also* Blast injuries; Traumatic brain injuries
- chronic illness and disability, 111–135. *See also* Chronic illness and disability
- chronic pain conditions, 141–157. *See also* Chronic pain
- military neuroscience and, 69–85. *See also* Military neuroscience
- military suicide, 91–107. *See also* Military suicide

Military justice
- demotion due to violation, 97
- disloyalty to Code, 193
- minorities and, 43
- MST and, 56
- SUDs and, 281
- system, 7

Military neuroscience, 69–85
- of anxiety, 274
- Complex PTSD and TBIs, 77–79
- early history of research, 71–72
- impact of combat operational stress, 75–76
- mental health and, 79–83
- modern technology and, 72–73
- neurobiological expression of stress and trauma, 73–75
- neuropathophysiology of the brain, 76–77
- remapping the military brain, 80, 83–85
- research agenda, 70–71
- trauma exposure and, 264

Military occupational specialty (MOS), 5, 21, 27, 37

Military PTSD. *See* Complex PTSD

Military Resources to Explore (MRE), 9, 14–16, 235–237

Military sexual trauma (MST)
- best practices and guidelines, 56
- as crime, 56
- pervasiveness, 38
- prevention programs, 39
- reporting, 39–40
- screening and assessment, 40, 255–256
- secondary victimization, 40
- suicide risk and, 96, 97
- women and, 27–28, 37–41

Military spouses. *See* Spouses

Military Stigma Scale, 18–19

Military suicide, 91–107
- Asian Americans and, 49
- assessment and diagnosis guidelines, 95–96
- blast injuries and, 163, 166
- chronic pain and, 155
- clinical assessment, 98–101
- combat vs. noncombat exposure, 94
- complex PTSD and, 268
- epidemiology and, 92–94
- firearms and, 28–29
- incidence vs. prevalence, 91
- insomnia co-occurrence, 278
- military family suicide, 98
- military leadership and, 244
- moral injury and, 194
- MST and, 97
- myths surrounding, 23
- Pacific Islanders and, 49
- prevention and treatment, 101–104

primary prevention strategy, 101–102
psychosocial aspects of, 91–92, 104–107
PTSD co-occurrence, 19
reservists and, 208–209
risk factors, 95–98, 103
secondary prevention strategy, 102
spinal cord injuries and, 152
spiritual care and, 186
TBI and, 163, 166, 169
tertiary prevention strategy, 102
transition to civilian life and, 226
veterans and, 94–95
Military Suicide Research Consortium, 93
Military Transition Assistance programs, 232
Miller, Doris "Dorrie," 42
Mind-body connection
anxiety and, 273–274
chronic pain and, 147–148
GWI/CMI, 81
optimization of healing system, 310
PTSS and, 263
Stebnicki on, 69
sympathetic-parasympathetic response, 80
treatment plans and, 118
Mindfulness-based stress reduction (MBSR)
as anxiety treatment, 275
as CIH approach, 103, 156, 189, 305–306, 310
effectiveness of, 300–301
as insomnia treatment, 279
remapping the military brain, 80
Minorities in the military, 35–57
African Americans, 37, 41–43
Alaska Natives, 50–53
American Indians, 50–53
Asian Americans, 47–50
best practices and guidelines, 56–57
CIH approaches and, 307
ethnicity categories, 37
health disparities among, 114
Hispanics, 43–47
identity and, 35–37
Latinos/Latinas, 43–47
LGBT service members. *See* LGBT service members
Pacific Islanders, 47–50
racial categories, 37
retention rates in psychotherapy treatment, 36
women. *See* Women in the military
Mission first concept, 214–215
Mission forward concept, 10
MISS-M (Moral Injury Symptom Scale–Military Version), 195
Mitchell, S. L., 153
Moderate TBIs, 169–171
Modern Military Association of America, 55
Moral injury
military suicide and, 96, 104, 194
PTSD vs., 30, 194
screening tools, 194–195
spiritual care and, 186, 192–196
spiritual well-being and, 189–190
Stebnicki on, 185
Moral Injury Symptom Scale–Military Version (MISS-M), 195
Moskos, C. C., 43
MREs
meals, ready-to-eat, 9
Military Resources to Explore, 9, 14–16, 235–237
MST. *See* Military sexual trauma
MTBIs. *See* Mild TBIs
Multicultural counseling
core competencies, 241, 250
expression of emotions and, 83
negative myths and stereotypes and, 30
rapport and, 35–37
Myers, J. E., 191
Myths, stereotypes, and stigma of military culture, 17–30
Asian stereotypes, 49
best practices and guidelines, 29–30
clinicians and, 20
combat operation service, 20–22
common myths, 20–29
disability benefits, 25–26
firearm ownership, 28–29
historical references and, 17
Hollywood portrayals, 20
impact of, 18–20
LGBT community and, 53–56
psychiatric disabilities, 23–25
reinforcement avoidance, 250
"thank you for your service," 22–23
women in the military, 27–28

N

National Center for Complementary and Integrative Health, 298
National Center for Complementary and Integrative Medicine (NIH), 143

National Defense Authorization Act for Fiscal Year 2010, 144–145
National Defense Authorization Act for Fiscal Year 2017, 113
National Guard families, 208–209
National Health Interview Survey, 280
National Institutes of Health (NIH), 70
  National Center for Complementary and Integrative Medicine, 143
  Patient-Reported Outcomes Measurement Information System, 145
National Veteran Suicide Prevention Annual Report (VA, 2019), 94–95
Native American Heritage Month, 50
Native American Indians
  military service of, 50–53
  soul loss and, 193
  sweat lodge ceremonies, 83, 194
  warrior ethos and, 154
Natural support systems
  benefits of, 133–134
  family as, 205, 218
  military family network as, 207, 209
  plan of care and, 119
  psychosocial adjustment and, 120
  resiliency and, 304
  wellness and, 303
  wellness strategies as, 312
Navajo code, 51
Navy, 5, 21, 27, 243
Negative myths and stereotypes of military culture. *See* Myths, stereotypes, and stigma of military culture
Neurocognitive Assessment Tool, 172
Neurocognitive deficits, 178
Neurofeedback, 80, 305
Neuroimaging and stimulation techniques, 73, 79, 82
Neuropathic pain, 142
Neuropathophysiology of the brain, 76–77
Neuropharmaceuticals, 71
Neurorehabilitation, 176–177
Neuroscience of military stress and trauma, 69–85. *See also* Military neuroscience
Newman, J. F., 46
Nociceptive pain, 142
Nontraditional psychotherapy approaches. *See* Complementary and integrative health

O

Office of Human Resources, 5
Open-ended questions, 252–254
Open head brain injuries, 169–170
Operational security, 11–12, 255
Operation Enduring Freedom (OEF)
  Asian American veteran health concerns, 49–50
  chronic pain, 143
  deployments, 205, 261
  disability benefits, 26
  health service utilization, 46
  mental health conditions, 262–263
  military suicide incidence and, 91
  Pacific Islander veteran health concerns, 49–50
  PTSD disability ratings, 19
  reservist component, 208
  SCI occurrence, 151
  traumatic amputation occurrence, 153
  women service members, 37
Operation Enduring Freedom (OEF) veterans
  TBI occurrence in, 116, 163, 169
  traumatic injury occurrence in, 119
Operation Inherent Resolve (OIR)
  deployments, 205
  PTSD disability ratings of veterans, 19
  traumatic injury occurrence in, 119
Operation Iraqi Freedom (OIF)
  Asian American veteran health concerns, 49–50
  chronic pain, 143
  deployments, 205, 261
  disability benefits, 26
  health service utilization, 46
  mental health conditions, 262–263
  military suicide incidence and, 91
  Pacific Islander veteran health concerns, 49–50
  PTSD disability ratings, 19
  reservist component, 208
  SCI occurrence, 151
  TBI occurrence, 116, 163, 169
  traumatic amputation occurrence, 153
  traumatic injury occurrence, 119
  women service members, 37
Operation Military Counseling (OMC)
  description of, 306
  foundations of, 308
  history of, 3–5
  training for, 5–6

Operation REBOOT, 306
Operation tempo
 definition of, 8
 leadership skills and, 243
 neuroscience and, 70–71, 80
 warfighter training and, 271
 in war on terror, 261
Operation Transition and Resiliency (OTR), 224–225
Opioids
 as pain treatment, 142, 146–147, 156–157
 prescription reduction, 307
 substance use disorders and, 143, 147, 285–286
Orthopedic injuries, 121–122
Osteopathic body manipulation, 300
OTR (Operation Transition and Resiliency), 224–225
Outcomes
 combat veterans and, 263
 deployment impact on families, 217
 Hispanics and, 46–47
 homelessness and, 114
 innovative mental health practices and, 307
 LGBT service members and, 55, 112
 reporting inaccuracies, 113
 stigma and, 18
 substance use disorder treatment, 287
 traumatic amputation, 153
 veteran women and, 39, 112
OutServe-SLDN, 55
Outward Bound camps for veterans, 306
Overcompensation as coping strategy, 130

P

Pacific Islanders in the military, 47–50
Pain
 acute, 144
 assessment of, 143–145
 chronic pain, 141–157. *See also* Chronic pain
 classification of, 143–144
 complex regional pain syndromes, 144
 health care costs of, 141–142
 perceptions of, 146
 psychosocial aspects of, 146–150
 rating scales, 144
 types of, 142
Pain Assessment Screening Tool and Outcomes Registry (PASTOR), 144–145
Pain Management Task Force, 155–156
Panetta, Leon, 37
Parity across counseling disciplines, 4–5
Parmar, B., 243
Patient Safety Plan (VA), 103
PCS (permanent change of duty station), 209
Peer support
 Operation REBOOT, 306
 suicide prevention and, 102–103
 wellness and, 299
Permanent change of duty station (PCS), 209
Personal care assistance, 121–122
Personal life story/testimonial, 230–231
Person-centered counseling
 core competencies and skills, 12
 elements of, 249–252
 intake interviews, 254–257
 open-ended questions, 252–254
 remapping the military brain, 84
 veterans and, 113–114
Pessoa, L., 74
Phantom sensation and limb pain, 154
Pharmaceuticals. *See also* Opioids
 antihistamines, 278
 benzodiazepines, 275, 278
 neuroscience research on, 71
Plans of care. *See* Treatment plans
Political rhetoric on military culture, 19
Postconcussive syndrome, 163
Post-Deployment Health Assessment, 272
Postdeployment stage
 description of, 216
 family dynamics during, 211
 medical screenings, 263
 mental health screenings, 268, 272
 TBI screen, 172
Posttraumatic stress (PTS), 268–270
Posttraumatic stress disorder (PTSD)
 biophysiological markers of, 78
 chronic pain co-occurrence, 143, 147, 155
 co-occurring mental health conditions and. *See* Complex PTSD
 as homelessness risk factor, 114–115
 military leadership and, 244
 military vs. civilian, 270
 moral injury vs., 30, 194

(Continued)

Posttraumatic stress disorder *(continued)*
neuropathophysiology of, 76–77
neuroscience research on, 71
pathophysiology of, 79
reservists and, 208
spinal cord injuries and, 152
spiritual care and, 192
as suicide risk factor, 95
transition to civilian life and, 226
traumatic amputation and, 153
VA disability rating, 19
warfighters and, 262
women and, 28
Posttraumatic stress symptoms (PTSS), 263
beta-blocker treatment of, 71
civilian trauma exposure and, 10
maladaptive associative learning and, 77–79
military trauma exposure and, 10
veterans and, 10
Predeployment stage
description of, 215–216
psychological screenings, 274
Preenlistment mental health conditions, 40
CIH and, 300
posttrauma recovery and, 132–133
substance use disorders, 282
women's issues and, 37–38
Primary strategy for suicide prevention, 101–102
Privacy. *See* Disclosure of information
Process addictions, 287
Promotions
chronic pain and, 146
clinician influence on, 20
military culture and, 8
minorities and, 36–37
racial discrimination against African Americans, 42
Prosthetic devices, 154
Psychiatric disability myth, 23–25
Psychogenic pain, 142
Psychoneuroimmunology, 72, 149
Psychosocial adjustment in transition to civilian life, 104, 131–134, 223, 226–227
Psychosocial adjustment to chronic illness and disability
acknowledgment stage, 127
adjustment, integration, and growth stage, 127
anger and hostility stage, 126
anxiety stage, 126
application to military culture, 134–135
best practices, 131–134
biopsychosocial model of disability, 113, 123
blast injuries and, 177–179
characteristics of, 120–121
chronic pain and, 150
coping strategies, 120, 123, 127–131
denial stage, 126
depression stage, 126
health symptoms and, 117–118
individual pace of healing, 134
integrative treatment plan, 118–119
losses and, 122, 178
measures of, 123–124
natural supports and, 133–134
preenlistment conditions and skills and, 132–133
rehabilitation process and, 119–124
shock and initial impact stage, 125–126
spinal cord injuries and, 151–152
stage models, 124–127
stigma and, 29
survivor vs. victim, 123, 131
TBIs and, 177–179
traumatic amputation, 153–155
treatment planning and, 121–122
Psychosocial impacts
of blast injuries, 176–179
of chronic illness and disability, 111–135. *See also* Chronic illness and disability
of combat operations myth, 21–22
of deployment, 208–211, 239
of disability benefits myth, 26
of firearm ownership myth, 28–29
of military suicide, 91–107. *See also* Military suicide
of negative military cultural myths, stereotypes, and stigma, 18–19
of psychiatric disabilities myth, 24–25
of TBIs, 176–179
of "thank you for your service" myth, 23
of women in the military myth, 27–28
Psychosocial stressors
on families, 206–211
on Native American Indian tribes, 52
psychosocial adjustment and, 121, 124
as suicide risk factor, 96

Psychospiritual issues in military counseling. *See* Spiritual care
PTSD. *See* Complex PTSD; Posttraumatic stress disorder
PTSS. *See* Posttraumatic stress symptoms
Punishment. *See* Military justice

Q

Quaternary and quinary blast injuries, 167

R

Racial minorities in the military. *See* Minorities in the military
Racism in the military, 35, 42
Raja, S., 40
Rancho Los Amigos Levels of Cognitive Functioning Scale, 168, 172
Rape. *See* Military sexual trauma
Rapport
  building process, 245–249, 251–254
  circle of trust and, 244–245
  multicultural counseling and, 35–37
Rationalization as coping strategy, 130
Rebooting the brain, 75, 78
Recognize, identify, interpret, and share (RIIS), 218
Regional perspective of the brain, 74–75
Regression, 129
Reiki, 83, 156, 300–301
Reimplantation of severed limb, 153
Reintegration and transition to civilian life, 223–233. *See also* Transition to civilian life
Reintegration stage of deployment, 216–217
Religiosity, 187–188, 192
Reluctance, 245–246
Remapping the military brain, 80, 83–85
Remembering therapeutic strategies, 106–107
Research in military neuroscience, 70–73
Reservist families, 208–209
Residual functional capacity, 117, 120, 173–175, 178
Resiliency, 297–312
  advantage, 301–302
  career resiliency, 224, 228–229
  CIH and, 297–301
  compensation and, 129–130
  complex PTSD and, 272–273
  deployment impact on families, 217–218
  emphasis on, 244
  Hispanic paradox and, 47
  military children and, 212
  military programs, 302–303
  military suicide prevention, 101, 103
  permanent change of duty station and, 209
  posttrauma recovery and, 133
  psychosocial adjustment and, 120, 123
  skill building, 303–304, 309
  spinal cord injuries and, 152
  spiritual well-being and, 185
  wellness programs and, 301–303
Resistance, 246–248
Resumes, 232–233
Retention rates in psychotherapy treatment, 36
Retirement. *See* Transition to civilian life
Reversal learning, 79
Richardson, A., 212
Riggar, T. F., 223
Riggs, D. S., 207
Riggs, S. A., 206
Right brain, 173–174
RIIS (recognize, identify, interpret, and share), 218
Risk assessment of suicide, 93–94
Risk factors
  blast injuries and, 168
  firearm ownership, 28–29
  of military suicide, 95–98, 103
Rogers, Carl R., 242
Roosevelt, Franklin D., 48

S

Sailor Assistance and Intercept for Life program, 102
Salinas, C., Jr., 44
Sapolsky, R. M., 72, 80
SCIs (spinal cord injuries), 151–152, 276
Screening and assessment. *See* Clinical assessments
Secondary posttraumatic stress, 270, 271
Secondary strategy for suicide prevention, 102
Secondary victimization, 40

Segregation
of Japanese Americans, 48
in the military, 42–43
of Native American Indians, 51–52
Self-care, 299–301, 310–311
Self-esteem, 154
as measure of adaptation to chronic illness and disability, 124
negative military cultural myths, stereotypes and stigma and, 18, 113–114
Self-harm. *See* Deliberate plans and acts of self-harm
Self-reflection, 231–232
Sensory deprivation, 84
Servicemembers Legal Defense Network, 55
Severe TBIs, 169–171
Sexual and intimate relationships
attitudinal healing and, 310
chronic illness and disability and, 122
as measure of adaptation to chronic illness and disability, 124
psychosocial adjustment and, 127
student veterans and, 227
as suicide risk factor, 100
younger service members and, 207
Sexual assault. *See* Military sexual trauma
Sexual harassment. *See* Military sexual trauma
Sexual orientation. *See* LGBT service members
Shamanic medicine, 84, 193, 300
Shay, J., 192
Shell shock, 262
Shock and initial impact stage of psychosocial adjustment, 125–126
Shrapnel, 167
Single service members, 207
Skin integrity, 121–122, 154
Skopp, N. A., 18
Sleep apnea, 277
Sleep hygiene and resting habits
as measure of adaptation to chronic illness and disability, 124
as therapeutic goal, 179
Smith, D. P., 46
Smoking prevention and cessation programs, 45
Social justice
CIH approaches and, 307
disability rights, 114
LGBT advocacy, 54–55
Social Security Disability Income, 25
Somatic symptom disorders, 147–148
Soul wounding or loss. *See* Moral injury
Space Force, 5–6
Specially Adaptive Housing program, 155
Special needs children, 212
Spinal cord injuries (SCIs), 151–152, 276
Spiritual care, 185–198
chronic pain treatment and, 150
conceptualizing spirituality, 186–188
core competencies and skills, 187
cultural values and, 57
integration into therapeutic process, 186, 188–192, 196–198
moral injury, 192–196. *See also* Moral injury
in person-centered interview, 250
religiosity and, 187–188
remapping the military brain, 83–84
spirituality vs. religiosity, 187–188
spiritual well-being scales, 189–190
treatment plan development and, 119
warfighting and, 11
wellness theories and, 190–192, 310
Spiritual Well-Being Scale (SWBS), 189–190
Spouses
deployment as stressor, 208–211, 214
homecoming as stressor, 210–211
within-group differences, 207
Stage models of psychosocial adjustment to chronic illness and disability, 124–127
States of consciousness, 84
Stebnicki, Mark A.
on chronic illnesses and disabilities, 111
on complex PTSD, 261
on empathy, 242
on grief and loss, 205
on healing, 297
on LGBT service member and veteran outcomes, 55
on mind-body connection, 69
on moral injury, 185
on trust, 239

Stereotypes of military culture, 17–30. *See also* Myths, stereotypes, and stigma of military culture
Stigma
of CIH, 299, 307
LGBT community and, 54–55
of military culture, 17–30. *See also* Myths, stereotypes, and stigma of military culture
Military Stigma Scale, 18–19
of MST reporting, 39
of seeking mental health services, 10, 20, 101–102, 112–113, 242, 244–245, 268–269, 272, 274
Story telling, 10–12
Stress. *See also* Combat operational stress and trauma exposure; Extraordinary stressful and traumatic events
adjustment disorders and, 265
chronic pain and, 148–149
CIH approaches, 299–300
military children and adolescents and, 213–214
neuroscience of, 69–85. *See also* Military neuroscience
resiliency advantage, 301–302
substance use disorders and, 279
wellness programs and, 192
Stress inoculation, 75–76
Student veterans, 227
Subjective universal ratings of pain, 144
Substance use disorders (SUDs)
best practices and guidelines, 286–288
blast injuries and, 166, 178
chronic pain co-occurrence, 155
CIH approaches, 299–300
deployment and, 209
insomnia co-occurrence, 278–279
military justice and, 281
military vs. civilian, 281
moral injury and, 194
myths surrounding, 24
opioids and, 143, 285–286
prevention, 284–285
PTSD co-occurrence, 19, 268, 271, 279–289
reservists and, 208
spinal cord injuries and, 152
as suicide risk factor, 95, 99
TBI and, 166, 169, 178
transition to civilian life and, 226
veteran suicide while undergoing treatment for, 95
women and, 39
"Suck it up" mentality, 19, 141, 146, 242, 271
Suicide
assessment and diagnosis guidelines, 95–96
in general population, 95, 98
LGBT individuals and, 98
by service members and veterans. *See* Military suicide
Sun Tzu, 17
Survival, Evasion, Resistance, and Escape (SERE) training, 75–76
Survivors
blast injuries and, 178
chronic pain and, 150
pace of healing, 134
TBIs and, 178
victims vs., 123, 131, 310
Survivor's guilt, 21–22, 105
Sustainment stage of deployment, 216
SWBS (Spiritual Well-Being Scale), 189–190
Sympathetic-parasympathetic response, 80–81, 274
Sympathy, 242

T

Tai chi, 300
Taoism, 17
Tart, C. T., 84
TBIs. *See* Traumatic brain injuries
Technology
life-extending advancements, 153, 262, 307
neuroscience and, 72–73
Teigen, J. M., 43
Tennant Biomodulator, 156
TENS (transcutaneous electrical nerve stimulation) devices, 156
Terrorism
blast injuries resulting from, 166
military children and adolescents and, 213–214
war on. *See* War on terrorism
Tertiary blast injuries, 167
Tertiary strategy for suicide prevention, 102
"Thank you for your service," 19, 22–23
Therapeutic relationship
circle of trust and, 239–258. *See also* Circle of trust
empathy and, 84–85, 240–243
spiritual care and, 186, 188–192, 196–198

Third-party private insurance, 4
369th Infantry, 42
Tick, E., 104, 154, 193
Tobacco use disorders, 45, 288–289
Total Force Fitness, 303
Training in clinical military counseling
lack of resources, 240
military culture and, 5–6, 36
Training programs in the military
resiliency building, 304
sleep deprivation, 277
Survival, Evasion, Resistance, and Escape (SERE) training, 75–76
for warfighters, 271
worker skills and, 224
Transcutaneous electrical nerve stimulation (TENS) devices, 156
Transgender, transsexual, or queer service members, 54–55. *See also* LGBT service members
Transition to civilian life, 223–233
career development and counseling, 228–233
career resiliency and, 228–229
career self-assessment, 231–232
chronic illness and disability and, 120
communications to employers, 232–233
as cultural shift, 13
homelessness risk and, 114–115
medical retirement, 25–26, 265
mental health concerns, 267
military children and adolescents and, 212
negative military cultural myths, stereotypes, and stigma and, 18, 29
Operation Transition and Resiliency, 224–225
persistence of mental health consequences after, 10
psychosocial adjustments, 104, 131–134, 223, 226–227
traumatic amputation and, 154
veterans with disabilities, 227–228
Trauma exposure. *See also* Combat operational stress and trauma exposure; Extraordinary stressful and traumatic events
neuroscience of, 69–85. *See also* Military neuroscience
substance use disorders and, 279
Traumatic amputation, 121, 152–155, 262
Traumatic brain injuries (TBIs), 163–179
assessments, 171–173
categorization of, 169–171
as chronic condition, 116–117
as complex trauma, 163
complex trauma and, 262
critical care, 171
early neuroscience research of, 72
functional deficits, 175
as homelessness risk factor, 114–115
maximum medical improvement, 121
mild TBIs, 163, 166, 169–170
military suicide and, 163, 166
occurrence of, 169
pathophysiology of, 79
psychosocial adjustment to, 121
PTSD blended with, 77–79, 117, 166, 178, 268
screenings, 171–173
The Traumatic Neuroses of War (Kardiner), 262
Treatment Episode Data Set, 281
Treatment plans
for blast injuries, 168–169, 177–179
for chronic illness and disability, 118–119, 121, 131–132
medical records and, 121
for TBIs, 177–179
TRICARE, 4, 115, 206
Troxel, W. M., 278
Truman, Harry S., 42
Trump administration, 54–55
Trust, 239–258. *See also* Circle of trust
Tuskegee Airmen, 42

U

Uniform Code of Military Justice. *See* Military justice
Unwanted sexual advances. *See* Military sexual trauma
Urinalysis drug screening, 282
Utilization of health services
by Asian Americans and Pacific Islanders, 49–50
CIH approaches, 307
destigmatization, 104–105
by Hispanics and Latinos/Latinas, 46–47
stigma of, 10, 20, 101–102, 112–113, 242, 244–245, 268–269, 272, 274
by veterans, 112

V

VA. *See* Veterans Affairs Department
Van Der Kolk, B., 69, 80
Vaping, 288
VA Video Connect, 111
Veteran organizations, 19, 112, 114, 133. *See also specific organizations*
Veterans. *See also specific wars and operations*
alcohol abuse and, 281
chronic illness and disability, 111–135. *See also* Chronic illness and disability; Psychosocial adjustment to chronic illness and disability
chronic pain and, 142–143, 147. *See also* Chronic pain
chronic traumatic encephalopathy, 116, 169, 175–176
CIH approaches and, 307
CIH utilization, 299–300
combat vs. noncombat, 20–22
disability benefits and, 25–26
disclosure restrictions, 255
firearm ownership and, 28–29
health disparities among, 57, 114–116
Hispanic health issues, 45–46
mental health concerns, 267
military sexual trauma and, 38, 40
military suicide in, 94–95
monitoring health needs of, 112–114
Outward Bound camps, 306
psychiatric disabilities and, 23–25
PTSS reactions, 10
as students, 227
suicide and, 28–29
"thank you for your service" and, 22–23
transition to civilian life, 223–233. *See also* Transition to civilian life
Veterans Affairs Department (VA)
congressional oversight of, 307
COVID-19 pandemic response, 115–116
disability program, 25–26
health disparity improvement goals, 114
Joint DoD Executive Committee strategic plan for 2019-2021, 112–113
military suicide data collection, 93
MST screening, 40
neurorehabilitation network, 151, 176–177
Patient Safety Plan, 103
revised standards for counselors, 4–5
suicide and treatment in health care system, 95
telemedicine programs, 111
treatment facilities, 112
Vietnam veteran treatment and benefits, 11, 19
wellness program development, 191
Veterans Crisis Line, 103
Veterans Health Administration (VHA), 4, 112, 114
Veterans of Foreign Wars, 11
Veterans with disabilities. *See also specific types of disabilities*
career transitions, 225
medical retirement, 25–26
work readiness, 227–228
VHA. *See* Veterans Health Administration
Victims and victimization
civilian trauma exposure, 9–10
secondary victimization from MST reporting, 40
survivor vs., 123, 131, 310
Vietnam War
segregation in, 43
stories of, 11
VA treatment and benefits of veterans, 11, 19
Visualization, 300
Volunteerism, 22–23

W

Wake-sleep disorders
blast injuries and, 166, 168, 179
moral injury and, 194
PTSD co-occurrence, 268, 271, 277–279
TBIs and, 170, 175, 179
Warfighters and warfighting
anxiety disorders and, 273–274
complex trauma in, 262
locus of control, 80
moral injury and. *See* Moral injury
myths regarding, 20–22, 24–25
neurobiology of, 75–76

(Continued)

Warfighters and warfighting *(continued)*
neuroscience research and, 70–71
spiritual care and, 11, 185, 192–196
story telling, 10–12
stress and trauma exposure, 132
in war on terrorism, 261
War neuroses, 262
War of 1812, 47
War on terrorism. *See also specific operations*
deployments, 205, 261
psychiatric disabilities and, 23
substance use disorders and, 280
Warrior ethos, 19, 154–155, 193, 243, 271
Weil, Andrew, 310
Wellness programs
integrative nature of, 299, 304–306, 309, 311
resiliency and, 301–303
resources, 191–192
as self-care, 299
spiritual care and, 186
therapeutic approaches, 305–306
Wernicke's aphasia, 174
Wheel of wellness (WoW), 191
Witkiewitz, K., 281
Women in the military
CIH treatment utilization, 157, 300, 307
demographics, 37–38
health outcomes, 112
military sexual trauma and, 27–28, 38–41, 112, 255
military suicide and, 93
myths surrounding, 27–28
suicide and, 29
Work readiness, 227–228
World Health Organization, 116
World War I
African Americans in, 42
Native American Indians in, 50–51
traumatic neuroses in veterans, 262
women service members in, 37
World War II
African Americans in, 42
Native American Indians in, 50–51
women service members in, 27, 37

Y

Yoga, 103, 156, 188, 275, 298–300, 310
Young, J. S., 187
Ysasi, N. A., 300